RISKY MOVE

TAMPA SUNS HOCKEY

ROBYN M. RYAN

Cover Photos: ©iStockPhoto/annebaek

Cover design by Bruiser Designs, a Division of L. Woods, LLC

Editors: Cara Lockwood, Mary Callaghan

ISBN-13: 978-1-7329590-3-3
ISBN-paperback: 978-17329590-40

Risky Move *is dedicated to*
Mary, my cousin and partner
In concocting schemes that sometimes come true.
Thinking Beach and Side-by-Side forever!

1

"Mom, you know I have my passport! I'm not a child." Cassie Johnson rolled her eyes in frustration as she pulled her suitcases from the trunk. She dropped them on a cart and walked around the car to the driver's window. "I promise—everything's under control."

"Just double checking." Her mother, Amanda, kept her tone light. "You realize that's my responsibility as your mom."

Cassie nailed her with a glare. "To treat me like a baby? I'm an adult. I'm moving to Tampa for a great job opportunity. I swear, I've got things covered."

"And Lauren's picking you up at the airport?"

Cassie handed her phone to Amanda. "Call her. Perhaps you'll believe her?" She knew she sounded like a bitch, but excitement, anxiety, and the desire to flee her mother's overprotective nest combined to bring out her worst trait—impatience. *Maybe she'll believe her sister... then again, perhaps not. She'd rather I stay a kid forever than admit I'm a capable independent adult.*

Memories of the recent family upheaval flashed through her mind. She knew she'd caused most of the stress by taking a twenty-four-hour "respite"...her location unknown to anyone. *The only way to get atten-*

tion. Rational discussions about the pros and cons of this "gap year" didn't work. Dad understood, so Mom dug in her heels with a "Hell no, you won't go."

Her Aunt Lauren—the only person who *got* Cassie—had tried to advocate on her behalf. But that turned into an epic shitstorm—Amanda learned that Lauren had ignored her advice and turned down a job offer in Europe. It didn't matter that Lauren continued as a partner in a successful public relations consultancy. Nor that she wanted to explore a relationship with a *man*—long-time friend Dave Martin, who played for the Tampa Suns professional hockey team. More than enough to incur the disdain and condemnation of Lauren's older sister—Cassie's mother.

She shook off the inner dialog, knowing that her mother had asked another question. "I have it covered," she snapped.

Amanda pressed the phone back into Cassie's hand. "I know you've thought of everything. It's hard to think of you living so far away."

Cassie released a breath. "I know, Mom. You've tried to shelter me and keep life from biting me in the…eh…tush. But I'm an adult—I need to have the freedom to make my own decisions or mistakes and decide what my future holds. And you know Lauren's right there, and you've spoken with Caryn. I couldn't have wished for a more perfect job than helping her and Andrew with the twins."

"Yes, I know you'll leave Mary Poppins in your shadow. Just give me a few days to adjust to my only child leaving the nest."

Cassie rolled her eyes. "It's only a few hours on a plane." She glanced behind her, noticing the line of cars waiting. "You need to go before you get a ticket, Mom." She pecked a kiss on her mother's cheek. "I'll let you know I've arrived."

Amanda sighed. "Enjoy this opportunity, Cassie. Please remember to explore your plans after this gap year ends."

By the time Cassie found the gate, passengers were boarding. She tried to suppress a smile when the flight attendant showed her the first-class seat that Andrew and Caryn had booked. She had a little private pod and snapped a quick photo to text to her mom and dad. "On the plane."

Cassie organized the area—plugged her iPhone in the supplied charger, stowed her carryon in a special compartment, and nodded with a grin when offered a glass of champagne. She took a selfie holding the flute in a mock toast. She tagged the photo "#adulting" before forwarding it to Lauren.

Cassie turned off the phone and settled into the plush leather seat. She experimented with the various positions available, looking forward to using the full-recline for the nap she needed after a sleepless night. Cassie followed the flight attendant's instructions as the plane taxied toward the runway. She allowed a smile to play across her face as the jet lumbered down the runway, gaining speed by the second. When the wheels left the ground, Cassie gazed out the window, giving Vancouver and her childhood a brief wave goodbye. *Time to explore my future.*

2

After clearing customs, Cassie followed the stream of travelers that funneled toward baggage claim. Lauren said she'd meet her once she exited the restricted security zone, and Cassie scanned the crowd—*make that mob. How the heck do I spot Lauren in this freaking mess? Unless Dave's with her, I'll never see her.* Unlike her aunt, Cassie stood taller than average, so she pushed her way through the crowd, hoping Lauren would notice her. *I can get my luggage and sit by the curb. Or…you could call her on her phone, Johnson…duh!*

Cassie fumbled with the carry-on bag, trying to locate her phone as she continued to squeeze through the crowd. She stopped walking when she couldn't find it. *Did I leave it on the plane?* Ignoring people bumping into her or muttering rude comments, she looked into the backpack, shaking it to rearrange the contents. *Finally!* Grabbing the phone, she slung the bag's strap over her shoulder and began walking again, her eyes on the phone. She stumbled against more people as she tried to find Lauren's name, murmured apologies, then bounced against what felt like a wall. She staggered backward; the phone flew from her hand, and she braced herself for a hard fall. Someone grabbed her shoulders, steadying her, and Cassie raised her face to look up…then further up. *Not a wall—just a tall, muscular, and…holy cannoli…HOT man.*

Dark golden-brown eyes hinted at amusement. "Cassie Johnson?"

"Who's asking?" Cassie countered as she stooped to grab the phone and then accepted the extended hand.

"I'm a friend of Lauren's. She and Caryn got tied up in a meeting—I volunteered to pick you up. Did you receive a text from her?"

Cassie glanced at the phone and turned the shattered screen toward him. *Can today get any worse? Not even out of the airport and I need a new phone.* "I didn't turn it on after we landed."

The handsome stranger grasped her arm and led her out of the crowded route to the baggage claim area. He pulled his phone from a pocket and swiped, then tapped the screen. He handed the phone to Cassie.

"Here's the photo she sent me via text."

Cassie bit her lip when she saw the picture, she sent several hours earlier. "So…you're not a serial killer?"

"Nope. I'm Tom Chadwick." He eyed her with a teasing smile. "Would you like to call Lauren?"

"No need, I sent that selfie from the jet. I'm Cassie Johnson."

He took the hand she offered. "Happy to meet you."

"Andrew's brother?" When he nodded, she added, "I should have recognized you from Caryn's photo. You and Andrew look alike." Her heart skipped a beat when he smiled.

"Shall we retrieve your luggage? Or did you travel light?" Tom gestured to her backpack.

"I may have packed a few things. Just a 'couple' of suitcases." She met the cinnamon-brown eyes, noticing the sparks of gold that outlined the pupils. "Eh…there wouldn't be an Apple Store on the way back?"

"You're in luck. Yes, we'll pass an Apple Store. Maybe they can replace your screen while we grab lunch?"

"That sounds wonderful." Something about this man caused Cassie to feel like the sun had just burst through the clouds after a prolonged, incessant Vancouver rain. *Spending my gap year in Tampa? Possibly the best decision ever.*

Tom glanced at Cassie as she watched bag after bag emerge from the baggage carousel. *Did Lauren mention her age? Know for sure she didn't tell me her niece is drop-dead gorgeous. Or an adult. She's not a giddy teenager.* He could see a slight resemblance to Lauren, but that's because he already knew the relationship. Instead of auburn hair like Lauren, Cassie's light brown hair featured soft pink highlights near her face and darker rose where the thick hair fell past her shoulders. Hazel eyes hinted playfulness, and her taller-than-average athletic figure suggested an interest in a variety of sports. Runner? Tennis? Swimmer? The tight jeans and form-fitting cotton top captured not only his attention but also that of almost every man who passed.

Tom followed when Cassie moved closer to the conveyer belt and asked which suitcase to grab. *Make that suitcases.* He pulled three bags from the carrousel, then glanced at her. "Any more?"

"Nope," Cassie laughed. "Remember, I had to pack for a year."

"Hope Lauren mentioned that Tampa only has two seasons…warm and hot."

"Oh, I hope so! I hate cold and rainy weather. Though, I may have packed a few sweaters and a jacket, just in case."

Tom reached for the two larger suitcases and asked Cassie if she could handle the roll-along bag.

"I managed all three when I checked in," Cassie said with a smile as she grabbed the handle and pulled the bag behind her.

While Cassie completed the paperwork for her phone's screen replacement, Tom contacted Lauren and Caryn to let them know the reason for the delay. Cassie met him at the entrance to the Apple Store.

"They said it'll take about an hour. Is that a problem, Tom? I can ask Lauren to bring me to pick it up later."

She watched Tom glance at his watch. "No trouble. Just enough time to get lunch. Both Lauren and Caryn said for you to take your time and don't worry." His slow smile made Cassie's heart twitch a bit. "Ready to dine like a local?"

"Absolutely, if you explain the local delicacies." Tom pressed his palm against her lower back as he guided her through the busy mall.

Could my luck get any better? Met at the airport by a gorgeous man and now getting my first taste of Florida cuisine. Sweet! Welcome to Tampa, Cassie Johnson. Hope it's a sign of a great year to come.

Tom took her to a charming, small restaurant that he said had a typical Florida vibe. One glance around the diner-like setup and Cassie approved of the atmosphere.

"Counter or booth?" The hostess approached them, menus in hand.

Cassie saw Tom look to her for an answer. "Whichever you prefer. I'm sleep-deprived and shouldn't make important decisions." She heard Tom's quiet chuckle as he led her to an empty booth.

"Then, I hope where to sit is the most important decision you need to make today, Cassie." Tom's eyes reflected the teasing tone.

"Works for me." She smothered a laugh as the hostess handed them menus and took their drink orders.

"What do you recommend?" Cassie asked, scanning the menu. "I've never heard of some of these…hush puppies? Shrimp with grits? Dolphin burger? Tell me Floridians don't eat those amazing creatures I hope to swim among one day?"

"Definitely not," Tom assured her with a smile. "This is the dolphin fish—sometimes called Mahi Mahi. Different species from dolphins—the mammals—you see in movies and on TV." He met her eyes. "The fish chowder's my favorite—you could try that with hush puppies if you're okay with fish?"

"I'm feeling adventurous…sounds wonderful. You going to tell me about hush puppies?"

"That's a great surprise. I think you'll enjoy them with honey butter. Did you know several places offer swimming with dolphins in central Florida?"

"I hope I can experience that while I'm here." Cassie paused for a moment. "But not in one of those concrete pools. I can't stand the thought of them in captivity."

"We can investigate options in the Gulf. I'd enjoy an up close and personal encounter with dolphins." Tom's smile caused Cassie's heart to flip. She felt her face growing warm and picked up the menu again, hoping to screen her face.

3

Tom opened the front door for Cassie, and they followed the sound of fussy babies to an enormous open room. Picture windows overlooked a landscaped pool and deck, covered on all sides by what Lauren called a lanai. She recognized it from photos that Lauren shared from Dave's nearby house.

Cassie's face reflected her delight when she saw the twins—Daniel and Jenna—nestled in her aunt's and Caryn's arms.

"Welcome to Tampa," Caryn greeted her.

"So happy you're here, Cassie," Lauren said as she hugged her with her free arm. "I don't think I need to introduce you to Caryn."

"I feel like I know you," Cassie said. "Thank you for trusting me to help with your sweet babies…and for the airline seats. I felt so pampered."

"Good." Caryn's smile was warm. "Please try to remember that when one of these angels spits up on you, or when they won't stop crying no matter what you do." She looked down at Daniel, who was now sleeping in her arms. "Would you like to help me put these darlings down for their nap?"

Cassie's grin spread across her face. "Please, I'd love to!"

Lauren placed Jenna in Cassie's arms. "You have her?"

Cassie nodded, gathering the baby against her chest. "You're just beautiful, you know that, Miss Jenna?" She followed Caryn to the nursery.

"Which bedroom, Car?" Tom asked. "I'll fetch Cassie's luggage."

"Thank you for meeting her at the airport, Tom," Lauren said as she walked beside him to retrieve Cassie's bags.

"No problem. At least after I convinced her I wasn't a serial killer." Tom watched as Lauren stopped and stared at him.

"What? Didn't she read…"

"Her cell phone screen broke before she received your message. Once I showed her the photo you sent me, she took the risk." His lips hinted at a smile.

Lauren laughed. "I guess I'm glad she didn't just say, 'okay,' and leave with a stranger."

"A healthy dose of skepticism never hurts." Tom beeped the trunk open and removed the bags. "Though, I expected someone much younger."

Lauren tried to hide a smirk. "Define 'much younger,' Tom."

"Seventeen, eighteen?"

"Try twenty. Worried about robbing the cradle?"

Tom shrugged. "Just curious…So, have the guys gone on to the arena?" He changed the subject.

"Thank God, yes! Dave's so tense, I told him to go early and skate it off."

"Big game tonight. The entire city's holding its breath."

"I hope the Suns just grab this win so we can get on with the Conference Final." Lauren took the handle of the roller bag and followed Tom to the bedroom Caryn mentioned.

"Caryn thinking about going to the game tonight?"

Lauren shook her head. "Not on Cassie's first day. Maybe during the Final."

"If I didn't need to work, I'd volunteer to stay here." Tom glanced at his watch. "Speaking of, I need to head out. Please tell Caryn and Cassie I'll catch up with them later."

Cassie looked up when Lauren joined them in the nursery. Enamored by the twins, Cassie leaned to kiss Jenna's forehead as she rocked back and forth. She saw her aunt's expression soften as she gazed at the babies.

"Ready to put them in their cribs for a nap?" Caryn asked.

Cassie shook her head. "I could rock them forever." She heard soft chuckles from both Caryn and Lauren.

"I'll show you how to settle them in bed," Caryn said as she stood, sleeping Daniel cradled in her arms. Cassie watched, then tried to duplicate Caryn's actions with Jenna. She covered her with a light blanket, and Caryn stepped beside her. "She loves this little teddy bear," Caryn whispered as she picked up the stuffed animal and placed it beside Jenna. She flipped the switch on the monitor and motioned for them to follow her from the nursery.

"Warning, they do not always go to sleep so easily," Caryn said as she led the way to Cassie's bedroom.

Cassie's excitement grew when she entered her room. French doors opened to the pool deck. The decor—beach blue and white drew her in. Besides the oversized bedroom, there was an ensuite bath. Caryn also opened the door to a walk-in closet, then showed her the dresser and nightstands.

"Think of this as your oasis—you definitely will need one after spending the day with the twins. The bathroom connects to another bedroom, the same as this one. You can choose the other if you prefer."

"I love this decor—very summery, my favorite season. It's more than perfect." *It's the size of two of the bedrooms combined at home. Lauren didn't prepare me for this. I may never leave.*

"Can I get you something to drink or a snack while you get settled?" Caryn asked.

Cassie waved her hand. "Thanks—we just had a wonderful lunch. I experienced my first hush puppies—yummy!"

"My weakness…always with honey butter." Caryn sighed, then looked at Lauren. "Did Tom leave for work?"

"He said he'll see you later."

Cassie felt a pang of disappointment. "I didn't get the chance to thank him." *Or get to know him better.*

"You'll have plenty of opportunities, Cass," Lauren said with a smile. Cassie ignored the mischief in her aunt's green eyes.

"Tom lives in the apartment at the back of the house." Caryn nodded toward the far end of the pool. "His schedule is crazy."

"Where does he work?"

"He's completing his residency in neurology at the Tampa hospital."

Doctor? Neurologist? Whoa…out of your league, Johnson. "So, does he work like a gazillion hours straight, then get a day or two off?"

Caryn laughed. "Something like that—unless he's on call or there's an emergency, then schedules go out the window."

"I had no idea…he doesn't look like any doctor I've seen."

"Because he's young and hot?" Lauren asked with a knowing smile.

"Maybe. I've never seen a young doctor except on TV." Cassie flipped her hair over her shoulder and pretended to focus on the pool. *Lauren's smiling like she can read my mind…Tom must be older than I thought. But maybe not too old? Enjoyed stopping for lunch, going to the Apple Store…But, you're not here to chase after sexy doctors, Cass. Remember that…Look, but do not touch. As if I'd have any chance.*

Days flew by in a blur as Cassie learned the routines and schedules Caryn tried to follow in caring for Jenna and Daniel. She told Cassie that she didn't expect them to eat or sleep on pre-determined schedules. When they were newborn preemies, she and Andrew had to feed them every two hours since they could swallow only two ounces of formula. But now that they'd reached seven months, Jenna and Daniel had exceeded the norm for height and weight on the pediatrician's growth charts.

Caryn said she waited for them to ask for a bottle, rather than force them into some arbitrary schedule for her convenience. Naps followed soon after meals, and with the recent addition of baby cereal, they slept through the night.

"How did you handle two babies with the every-two-hours schedule?" Cassie marveled at Caryn's ability to handle every challenge with patience and a sense of humor.

"Lots of help. Before Drew started playing again, he took on a lot of the work at night, so I could get uninterrupted sleep." Caryn looked at Cassie with a smile. "Once he began to play, he wanted me to hire someone to help full time. I resisted because I 'knew' I could handle it. I did, but I became a walking zombie. Total sleep deprivation. Tom and his 'friend,'" Caryn hooked her fingers in air quotes, "Katie helped as much as their schedules allow, and Lauren and our friends Kelly and Terri made sure I had plenty of breaks."

"I don't know how you did—and do—all this. I hope I can make things easier for you." Cassie lifted Jenna into her arms and kissed her forehead. She tried to hide her disappointment that Tom had a female "friend." *No huge surprise, Johnson. Friend? Sounds more like "girlfriend." Great-looking doctor, he has his choice of women.*

"You already have made things easier, Cassie. I'm so relieved we didn't have to hire a stranger to live in our home…When Lauren mentioned your gap year, I wondered if you'd be interested. I thought you'd rather travel around Europe or somewhere exotic."

Cassie laughed. "That's always a fun dream. But when you called, I couldn't think of anywhere I'd rather spend this year. And helping you with these beautiful children is so far beyond any expectations. Maybe the universe wanted our paths to cross?"

"Definitely," Caryn replied. "I don't know how I managed without you. You've spoiled me, and Jenna and Daniel love you, too. You're part of our family, Cassie."

Cassie's heart swelled, and she took a deep breath to prevent tears from slipping from her eyes. These lucky babies would grow up surrounded by love. Like she had during her youngest years—before her parent's bitter divorce and before she felt like a ping pong ball bouncing from house to house, parent to parent. Andrew and Caryn's love for each other radiated each time they were together—the same love they showered on the "peanuts," as Andrew called the twins. Cassie couldn't imagine either of them putting the twins in the crossfire of a divorce. She couldn't even imagine Caryn and Andrew arguing, much less divorced.

Cassie had stopped feeling she *belonged* to a family long ago, since they divided her days between two homes. When she lived with her mother, Amanda's bitterness toward her dad, Trevor, seeped into conversations. Even after Amanda convinced her own mother, Allyson—a virtual stranger to Cassie—to live with them last spring, she didn't feel any sense of family. If anything, tension had increased in the home.

When she visited her father, Trevor, and his wife, Tanya, Cassie felt guilty because she preferred their home. Her dad always spoke about Amanda with respect, and Tanya made a point of including Cassie in their celebrations, especially with her toddler sibling, Taylor. Even though Amanda insisted on referring to the baby as Cassie's "half-brother," Cassie loved Taylor as her brother in every sense of the word.

She spent as much time as possible playing with him or babysitting. Getting to see him as often as she wanted depended on her mother's mood. Whatever good vibes she absorbed while spending time with her dad faded when she returned home. Amanda clung to her bitterness like a shield. *Lays a good guilt trip on me just because I want to see my dad, Tanya, and Taylor.*

"These sweet angels are so blessed to have you and Andrew as their parents." Cassie didn't realize she had spoken the thought until she felt Caryn's hug.

"And we are all blessed to have you, Cassie."

4

When the Suns needed one win to progress to the Stanley Cup Final, Cassie encouraged Caryn to attend the game. Jenna and Daniel ran out of energy by dinner, and Cassie knew that the evening routine—dinner, bath, PJs, and the rocking chair—helped lull them into a deep slumber. She sensed Caryn wanted to watch the games in person rather than on TV and tried to assure her she could handle both babies.

"You want to go to the game, Caryn—I know you do," Cassie coaxed as she sat with Daniel in the rocking chair. "I promise to care for the twins as if they're my children. I won't let anything happen to them."

"Oh, Cassie, I know that. I just feel guilty leaving you with no backup. Lauren, Kelly, and Terri will be at the game. Tom's working... What if you need help?"

"What do *you* do when the munchkins get grumpy and you have no backup?"

"Cope." Caryn shook her head, suppressing a laugh as she sat beside Cassie. "I try to get both settled down, but sometimes one of these angels just has to wait—and cry—while I take care of the other."

Cassie recognized the hesitation in her eyes. "If—and that's a huge *if*—both give me a hard time, I'll stay calm and do what you would."

"You've heard the set of lungs they have when they're out of sorts."

"My little brother sometimes got so worked up he couldn't settle himself down. I swaddled him, held him, played soft music, sang to him—anything until he fell asleep. His cries sounded more like screams—I was sure the neighbors would call the police!" Cassie pressed her lips against Daniel's soft baby hair. "And I called my dad or Tanya. That only happened once."

"You'll call me if you get overwhelmed?"

"Promise."

Cassie's confidence faded when the twins realized their mother wasn't the person giving their baths. They looked for Caryn, then made their displeasure known, communicating the only way they could—with angry wails. Cassie spoke gently to them, completing Jenna's bath and dressing her for bed. After securing Jenna in the swing, she selected soft music and a slow, soothing pace.

Daniel started kicking the moment she lifted him from the second swing. He resisted sitting in the bath chair, arching his back, and screaming in Cassie's ears. Rather than force him into the bath chair, she dipped his toes in the warm water, hoping that soothed him. Daniel enjoyed bath time, but he wanted nothing to do with the water, the bath, or Cassie. His shrieks grew in volume, and Cassie watched his little face grow red with the effort.

After securing him on the changing table, she used a dampened washcloth to clean him as best as she could. "It's okay, Danny," she soothed. She reached across him to grasp a towel to dry him, and when Daniel chose that moment to pee, Cassie saw the laughter in his eyes as the warm water soaked her shirt.

"You are such a trickster!" Cassie kept her voice soft and humorous. "Let's get you cleaned and in a diaper, okay?" She covered her shirt with a towel and enjoyed a few minutes of calm while she dressed Daniel and then strapped him in his swing. She patted her shirt with the towel, wanting to change but unwilling to leave the twins alone.

Caryn called the swings a sanity-saver, and Cassie understood why as she kneeled between them, singing along with the music. Their eyes grew heavy, the lids at half-mast, and Cassie hoped to tuck them into their cribs before they fell asleep.

She grabbed a clean towel to cover her wet shirt. “Hey, cute girl,” she whispered as she gently drew Jenna from the swing and cradled her against her chest. Jenna’s eyes popped open, and she startled when she didn’t recognize her mom. Her face turned red, and after she drew in a breath, Jenna unleashed a high-pitched wail worthy of an opera soprano. Daniel soon joined in the protest with angry screams that also reached the upper decibels.

“Can you use a hand?”

Cassie turned in surprise when she heard Tom’s voice. “I thought you were working tonight?”

“Slow night. Put on call and sent home.” Tom lifted Daniel, and the infant’s tears and wails ceased when he recognized his uncle. “Are you giving Aunt Cassie a hard time?”

“In the middle of her bath, Jenna realized that I’m not her mom. She voiced her displeasure, and then Mr. Daniel protested.” Cassie grinned as she showed her soaked shirt. “They ne*arly* fell asleep in their swings…but as you heard, they’re not happy campers.”

She caught the twinkle in Tom’s eyes. “Daniel got you, eh? Join the club. Why don’t you let me rock both of them while you change?”

“Thank you—I smell like a soaked diaper.” She handed Jenna to him after he had settled in the rocker with Daniel. She watched them before she left the room. *Does he have any idea how extremely hot he looks holding the twins?* Her heart melted watching him settle the babies, each tucked into an arm. *Such a big guy with those babies—they looked so tiny in his arms.* Tom glanced at her, and Cassie’s cheeks reddened. He’d caught her gawking. “Eh…I’ll change and be back in a minute.”

“Take your time. Now that they’ve settled down, I hesitate to move them to their cribs.” His eyes held hers for a long moment, and

Cassie realized he'd enjoyed catching her staring. She broke eye contact and hurried from the nursery before she made an inane comment.

Tom and Cassie placed the exhausted babies in their cribs when sleep overcame their whimpers. She turned on the monitor and grabbed the receiver before following Tom to the great room.

"Can I get you something to drink?" Cassie asked as Tom picked up the TV remote and navigated to the Suns game in progress.

"Something cold with caffeine."

"Sure you don't want a beer?"

Tom turned to look at Cassie's eyebrows raised in question and a teasing expression across her face. *Does she know how adorable she looks?* "As good as that sounds, I can't take a chance when I'm on call. But don't let me stop you—you earned one tonight."

Cassie pulled two Cokes from the refrigerator. "Not when I'm caring for the twins. Besides, one beer puts me to sleep." She grabbed a bag of pretzels and settled on the couch.

"Thanks," Tom said and then pointed to the pretzels. "Dinner?"

Cassie laughed as she opened the bag and held it toward him. "Maybe."

Tom sat on the couch, careful to leave a space between them. "Your first time solo with Jen and Danny?"

"For dinner, bath, and bedtime. I didn't expect them to protest so vocally when they realized Caryn wasn't here." Tom watched Cassie shake her head with a wry smile. "But I'm so glad she went to the game. I promised her I could handle everything."

"You did, and you kept your cool even when Danny sprayed you, and both tested the sound barrier."

Cassie popped a pretzel in her mouth and chewed it before sipping her Coke. "With a timely assist from you."

"Nah, you had everything under control. Did you babysit much in Vancouver?" Tom turned to face her.

"Sure, but my brother, Taylor, is the only infant I've cared for before now." Cassie glanced away before eating another pretzel. "My dad's son with his new wife."

Something in her tone caused Tom to hesitate to ask another question. Cassie had turned her attention to the TV as the teams skated out to begin the second period. "Is Taylor as much of a prankster as Danny?"

Cassie giggled. "Well, today's not the first time a sweet little baby boy aimed his pistol at me." Her shoulders relaxed and Cassie leaned back against the soft leather. "As far as volume goes, I'd say all three have great lungs."

"No wonder you stayed calm." Tom stood and retrieved a large bowl from a cabinet. He emptied the bag of pretzels into it. "Can I get you a sandwich?"

"Not now, thanks. Don't miss the game." She met his eyes. "I'm a huge Suns fan—ever since Lauren introduced me to Dave, and he got traded here. Before, it was Blues all the way. I tend toward vocal while watching the games, so please stop me if I get too loud. Don't want to disturb my munchkins."

A week later, Cassie awoke before dawn and glanced at the clock. *Only two a.m.? Crap, I might not fall back asleep.* Cassie had occasional bouts with insomnia, but not since she'd moved to Tampa. She knew if she allowed herself to play "what if," she could give up on sleep. She thought of the sleep medicine her doctor had prescribed in Vancouver. *If I take it now, I might not wake up at five. At least not in a coherent state. Time to go with Plan B—warm decaf tea or milk.*

Cassie crept from her room and held her breath as she tip-toed past Caryn and Andrew's bedroom, and then the nursery. She didn't turn on a light for fear she'd wake someone, and the new moon added no extra illumination. Cassie navigated the great room from memory, guided by the kitchen's night light. With only several feet to reach the kitchen, she blinked her eyes—the semi-darkness caused her vision to blur. She shut her eyes and moved toward the kitchen, reaching to touch the counter.

Cassie didn't expect to collide with someone else in the dark. She bit back her urge to scream—*intruder?*—when hands gripped her shoulders, preventing her from tripping.

"Cassie?"

"Tom?" Cassie croaked as she clutched the hard body that had just smashed into hers. "I thought someone had broken in." She caught her breath and stepped closer, and Tom's arms closed around her.

"No burglar." His voice carried a hint of amusement.

Cassie exhaled a sigh of relief and took a deep breath. "What are you doing here?"

"I just came home. You?"

"Trying to defeat my dear friend insomnia." She realized her body still pressed against him. Her camisole and sleep shorts were not suitable for mixed company—*Gah! If he turns the light on, he'll see everything.*

Tom tightened his arms around her. "You okay?"

"As soon as my heart stops banging against my chest." She tried to ignore the goosebumps and hoped he didn't notice the sparks that coursed through her wherever her body touched his.

She didn't know how it happened and would wonder later if she had initiated contact. Suddenly his lips found hers, and she ignored the warning siren blasting her ears. His kiss was unlike any Cassie had ever received and caught in a rush of sensations, time stood still.

She moaned a protest when Tom pulled back. They spoke simultaneously.

"I'm sorry, I shouldn't have…"

"I didn't mean to…"

"…I'll just go back to my room," Cassie said.

"No, I'll go to the apartment."

They realized at the same instant that neither had broken contact. Cassie pulled her arms away from his solid chest and shivered when Tom dropped his hands and stepped back. Her eyes had adjusted to the dark, and she saw him gazing at her body.

"Cassie, I was out of line. Are you okay?"

Cassie self-consciously crossed her arms over her chest. "I'm fine, don't worry about it. Sometimes things just happen."

She caught the smile hinting at the corners of his mouth. "Yeah… that was…" He shrugged as he gently brushed his hand against her cheek. "I apologize, Cassie. That was inexcusable on so many levels."

Cassie blurted her reply without thinking. "Do you hear me complaining?"

Tom pressed his lips against her forehead as he chuckled. "This can't happen again."

He turned to leave. Cassie touched her lips as memories of the kiss flooded through her. *No one's ever kissed me like that…Guess I've never kissed a "real" man.*

She knew that nothing would ease her insomnia. Cassie turned and hurried to her room. *If she couldn't sleep, she'd just relive that kiss repeatedly.*

Tom splashed cold water on his face. *What were you thinking? Or not thinking? That should never have happened. It's like she cast a spell over me, and I acted by instinct. So wrong, but holding her felt just right.*

No excuse. I know better…she's the twins' nanny Lauren's niece… I can't even think about her that way. What if Andrew or Caryn had come to the kitchen? I wasn't aware of anything except how good she feels in my arms. Potential disaster…but that kiss? Very much worth the risk.

He headed to his bathroom, knowing he'd need a long, icy shower before he'd get any sleep.

Even though neither ever mentioned "the kiss," its memory hung in the air between them. Cassie held no expectation that Tom would ever think about her as more than Lauren's niece. Still, her imagination trumped reality whenever they found themselves together. In her alternate universe, Cassie and Tom crossed the line between friends and romance. *Tom gets me…in the short time we've spent together, he understands me…doesn't treat me like a kid. He brightens my day just by entering a room, and when he looks at me with that sexy smirk, he doesn't even realize that my heart does this little flip. I can see why Lauren thinks of him as her big brother. I would, too, if I didn't feel these tingly sensations whenever his hand brushes against mine or need to catch my breath every time I see him.* Conveniently, his "friend" Katie didn't exist in that universe.

5

The following weeks sped by with a frenzy of celebrations for the Suns' Stanley Cup Championship. Cassie's heart swelled with pride when Caryn and Andrew trusted her with the twins as they took part in the many city and state festivities. She sat in the VIP section for the massive parade in Tampa when Andrew and Caryn took the twins with them in the convertible. She didn't know any of the other VIPs, but felt a kinship with them when she saw family and new friends pass before them.

Both Dave and Andrew gave her championship T-shirts and hats, and Cassie started her own collection of Stanley Cup pins. Dave gave her the puck from one goal he scored, and Lauren supplied the case inscribed with the date.

"Do you know when Dave gets his day with the Cup?" Cassie asked Lauren, referring to the tradition that allowed each member of the team to take the Cup anywhere he wished for twenty-four hours.

"Not yet. Everything's too crazy right now with the 'Stand Up To Bullies' kick-off event next week. And after that, our Greek Islands cruise." Lauren's green eyes took on a dreamy look as she thought about the upcoming vacation with Dave.

"Color me envious," Cassie teased. "Is there anything I can do to help you with that?" The Tampa Suns' Cyber Bullying Awareness initiative had planned a public kick-off. Lauren agreed to address the consequences of rumors and nastiness, drawing upon her own recent experiences.

Cassie's mind replayed the devastation Lauren experienced only a few months ago. Her aunt's privacy and questionable decisions as a teen had become the target of a viral harassment campaign. Tears pricked Cassie's eyes as she thought of all the hateful posts and hashtags attacking Lauren…most lies from anonymous cowards who enjoyed spreading vicious rumors just because she and Dave were a couple.

Lauren's known him for years, but just because Dave's a man and a pro-athlete, Mom blamed him and questioned his motives…Even when Lauren came to Vancouver to deal with the fallout from the bullying, Cassie's mother treated Lauren like a child, not a successful twenty-something career woman. Thinking about their family dynamics threatened to produce a migraine.

"Hold my hand when I panic?" Lauren asked. "Remind me why I signed on for this? Pull my hair back when I lose whatever meal I just ate?"

Cassie hugged her aunt. "I'll do anything for you, Lauren. I'm so proud of you for speaking up on behalf of others in similar situations. Just remind yourself how much attention you'll direct to the problem of bullying. Perfect timing with the Suns just winning the Stanley Cup."

"I realize that up here." Lauren tapped her head. "The Suns' sponsorship should guarantee the program's success. But my heart and stomach keep forgetting that detail."

"You told Mom and Grandmother what you'd gone through during secondary school," Cassie reminded her. "After that, *nothing* should phase you."

Lauren nodded. "True. The hardest thing I've ever done—and I survived. You're right, speaking to a ballroom full of people—piece of cake."

"You can talk to me. I promise I'll sit in the front row, and I *know* Dave will stand right beside you. You've got this."

Cassie scanned the crowded ballroom, hoping to get a glimpse of Lauren. She didn't expect the large crowd. Andrew had mentioned that the entire team planned to attend, but hundreds of others had gathered. *I'd freeze if I had to speak in front of this audience. Geesh, over five people make me nervous. Maybe someday I'll have Lauren's courage.* She saw the Stanley Cup up on the stage near the podium and couldn't estimate the number of people waiting to take selfies with it.

She looked at Caryn, who stood beside her. "Thanks for making it possible for me to come with you today."

"You need to be here. And you know by now that Tom never turns down an opportunity to have the twins to himself."

"True." *Wonder if the famous Katie's helping him with the twins?* "Do you mind if I see if I can grab a front-row seat? So many people are here already."

"No, go ahead. I'll wait for Drew. He may have had to park quite a distance away."

"Save you guys seats?"

"Don't worry about us, Cassie. We'll find you afterward."

Cassie gave a little wave as she wove through the crowd toward the stage. *I promised Lauren I'd sit front and center. Today can't be easy for her. Before everything blew up, I never suspected she had such a rotten childhood...same as Mom. But Lauren was just a baby when Mom moved out, so Lauren had no one who cared about her.* How could anyone neglect a child? The only positive outcome? Lauren's childhood had helped shape her aunt into a self-confident and strong woman.

She rose on her tiptoes to scan the front row. She spotted an empty seat and then hustled to claim it. "Is this seat saved?"

The woman on one side said, "Not mine."

"It's yours," a male voice added. Cassie flopped onto the chair before she turned to thank both.

"Thanks so much! I wanted to sit up front. My aunt's a speaker…I guess one of the main speakers."

"Lauren Gentry?"

"Yes, she's my aunt..." Cassie's voice faded as she came face-to-face with a golden Greek god. *OMG! He's so hot, my face is burning! Messy blond hair, silver eyes...*She swallowed before she continued. "How do you know Lauren?"

"We're friends. We met last summer before training camp, and now she handles my social media. She's trying to tone down my indiscretions." He flashed a smile, causing Cassie to giggle.

"Shall I ask the type of indiscretions?"

"Ah...no. I'm Cliff Camden. Just about everyone calls me Cam."

"Cassie Johnson, from Vancouver." She saw him checking her out and ran her hands across her hair. *Another hockey hunk? He's spectacular...Hope he can't hear my heart thumping.*

"Here for vacation?"

She couldn't hold his gaze. "I'm helping Caryn Chadwick with..."

"...the twins," he finished for her. "I bet they're a handful. Do you live in their home?"

"Yes." *Why am I tongue-tied?*

He nodded with a megawatt smile. "Been there several times. A real hardship having to live in that house."

"Do you live in the same neighborhood?"

His rueful smile didn't hide the teasing spark in his silver eyes. "I wish. Entry-level contracts don't make a down payment on a condo in that neighborhood." He leaned against her shoulder to speak in a soft voice. "I stayed with John and Kelly Peterson for the second half of this season."

"But not any longer?"

"Got my own place. I found something near the Bay. I'm ready to have some privacy...you understand?"

Cassie's stomach did a little somersault when he winked. She replied as the curtain opened. "Perhaps we can chat later?"

Cassie let her mind wander while her aunt spoke about her experiences with cyber bullying. She knew what Lauren had faced, and it was too painful to hear the story again. *Luckily, she has Dave standing beside her...everything a girl could want in a guy...yet; it took them four years to admit their feelings for each other. At least Lauren. I'd have snatched him as fast as I could. Like I'd have a chance—I'm still a kid in his eyes...Lauren's "little sister."* The small age difference between them caused Lauren to treat her more like a younger sister. Growing up in the same home had forged a strong bond between them that went far beyond the typical aunt-niece relationship. *Lauren's my best friend.*

She snuck a glance at the guy beside her, as Cam listened to everything Lauren and Dave said. *Bet he has women chasing after him.*

As if feeling her eyes on him, Cam glanced her way and flashed a smile. He raised an eyebrow, and Cassie dropped her eyes, feeling her cheeks grow warm. She focused on the stage, realizing that Lauren and Dave wrapped up their talk. She jumped to her feet as the crowd rose and applauded them, then watched in stunned silence as Dave surprised Lauren by dropping to one knee to propose. *Say yes, Lauren. Don't keep him hanging!* She saw Lauren struggle to speak, then just nod furiously as she pulled him to his feet.

"So romantic." Cassie's vision blurred from tears of joy.

"Did you know?" Cam Camden's voice pulled her eyes away from the stage.

"About the proposal? Not a word. I don't think Lauren expected it either. I'm so excited for them!" *Maybe she'll ask me to be a bridesmaid?* Cassie dismissed the thought and looked at the man beside her. "You're *not* surprised?"

"Figured it was a matter of time. I got the message, and Mr. Martin realized we're only friends."

A giggle escaped her mouth. "What, did he tell you to back off?"

"One way to put it." Camden shook his head. "Took him a while to accept our friendship." He nodded toward the area in front of the stage where friends had gathered. "I'm heading over there. I can get you through the crowd."

"Thanks, I'll wait here for Caryn and Andrew."

"You want to get something to eat later?" His grey eyes captured hers.

Cassie hesitated. She hoped to visit with her favorite doctor or perhaps meet the famed Katie. "I'm not sure about tonight…Long day for everyone…" With a wink, Cam handed his phone to her.

"Maybe before I head home for the summer, then. Call yourself; I'll have your number—and you won't block me as an unknown caller."

"I'll think about it." She noticed that his eyes darkened at her teasing comment. "When do you leave for…?"

"Québéc, in a couple days. I'll call you. Do I need Lauren's blessing to ask you out?" His cocky grin caused Cassie to laugh.

"Nope. Only one permission slip required—my own."

"Look forward to it." A quick hug, along with another devilish grin, caused Cassie's legs to wobble like Jell-O. She sat down and watched him strut toward the crowd.

Have dinner with him...a date? Her eyes lingered on his broad shoulders before appreciating the way his tailored jeans hugged his lower body. He slid through the crowd, and Cassie sighed as he disappeared. *That's one smoking hot guy…who knows it.*

She heard Caryn and Andrew talking and stood to greet them. "Did you have any idea?"

"That's what I wanted to ask *you!"* Caryn said. "From her reaction, Lauren didn't expect it at all." She glanced at Andrew.

"Don't look at me. Not something guys discuss." Andrew's smirk reminded Cassie of Tom. *Maybe I can tell him the happy news…*

"Looks like Kelly and Terri plan to kidnap Lauren from that crowd." Caryn pulled her phone from her purse and tapped a text.

Andrew leaned to kiss Caryn's cheek. "I'll give Dave my congratulations. Just tell me when you're ready to leave."

"I'm checking in with Tom. We won't monopolize Lauren too long, will we, Cassie?"

"As if we could."

6

Cassie bit back a smile as she watched Caryn and Andrew transition to parent-mode the instant they entered the house. Both Jenna and Daniel's faces transformed from eyes at half-mast to excited delight when they spied their mom and dad.

Caryn plucked Daniel from Tom's arms, and Andrew unfastened Jenna from her bouncy seat. "You see where I rate on the twins' affection scale," Tom said to Cassie.

"You're definitely one up on me." Cassie brushed the hair away from her eyes as the sexy doctor-turned-babysitter stopped by her side. "I wish you could have seen the presentation today—Lauren and Dave made a huge impact on the audience."

"I caught a few minutes of the stream from the Suns' website… until my nephew and niece demanded more attention." He glanced over at them with a smile, then turned his grin toward Cassie. "Surprised by Dave's proposal?"

"You saw that?"

"Couldn't hear a thing with these chatter bugs, but easy to guess."

Cassie grabbed his arm without a thought. "I had no idea, but I'm not surprised Dave proposed. But in front of all those people? Lauren looked shell-shocked."

"Good thing she said yes, then." His cinnamon eyes sparked little electric bursts throughout Cassie's body.

She chuckled. "She told me no wedding planning until after their Greek Islands cruise. Darn it! I can't wait to help with that."

"In the meantime, how about helping me with dinner? It's my day to cook when I'm not working."

Those eyes! As if she'd resist his invitation. "What's on the menu, doctor?"

"Fresh vegetables. We have a community garden at the hospital. I've got squash, green beans, tomatoes, romaine, corn on the cob…I was thinking maybe some grilled chicken, corn, and a huge salad."

"Yum…put me to work."

When Caryn and Andrew took the twins to their room for a nap, Tom connected his phone to a Bluetooth speaker and handed it to her. "Pick some music, Cassie." She looked at him after she scrolled through some playlists.

"How about your Extra Golden Oldies?"

"That's a great list. Songs we listened to growing up—our mother's favorites. Brings back some great memories."

Cassie pressed "Play" and set the phone on the counter. "My mom has a playlist like that—my grandmother's favorites…from the sixties. No surprise, I prefer the oldies."

His smile threatened to melt her into a puddle. After a beat, Tom nodded toward the basket of fresh vegetables. "You want to figure out what to do with that while I finish marinating the chicken?"

"Got it."

Cassie chanced a glance at Tom as he flipped the chicken and brushed marinade over it. *Physician, son, brother, uncle, friend, chef… Even though he has a girlfriend, he must have women beating down the door? Maybe he does—at the hospital? I'd grab a number to stand in that line. Green scrubs or blue? Doesn't matter—with those looks, that smile, not to mention his smoking body, he'd look good in a burlap sack.* Her body still tingled when she allowed herself to think about "the kiss," and wished every day that Tom didn't top her "Forbidden/Do Not Touch" list.

Cassie yelped as the knife nicked her finger instead of slicing the zucchini. "Stupid move, Johnson." She reached for a paper towel, but Tom gently grasped her hand. He turned on the water and held her finger under the light stream. "Distracted dicing," she joked as she looked away from the blood.

"You did a number on your finger." Tom wrapped a paper towel around the finger and showed her where to apply pressure. Cassie nodded, still averting her face. Tom pulled a chair behind her and helped her to sit. "Dizzy?"

"It's just seeing the blood. Makes me woozy."

"Hold on for one second." Tom pulled the first aid kit from the pantry and set what he needed on the table. He gently lifted her hand above her shoulders and unwrapped the paper towel. Although the towel was red, blood now trickled from the cut. "Just need to clean and bandage it," he told Cassie.

"No stitches?"

"Not today." He rested his hand against her neck. "Water?" Cassie shook her head. "Give me a few minutes, we'll have this bandaged and ready to go."

Cassie nodded. *Klutz, squeamish, and the sight of blood makes me faint.* She closed her eyes as Tom cleaned and dressed the wound. *Does he notice that not so little flutter in my heartbeat each time he touches me? Probably the only person who gets turned on by a doctor cleaning a cut. Hope he doesn't hear my heart pounding...at least the nausea's easing.*

"Safe to open your eyes." Tom's voice held a humorous tinge. "However, I must replace you as my sous-chef today."

Cassie forced a laugh as she looked at him. "Thanks, doctor." She tried to look around him to see the mess on the counter, but Tom blocked her view.

"Just sit here a few minutes. I'll take care of the counter." He handed her a bottle of water. "Why don't you watch the birds at the feeder while I clean up?"

Cassie heard the tiny gold and black birds chattering nonstop as the goldfinches jockeyed for spots at the feeder. She chuckled as the birds also congregated on the edge of the birdbath, ducking their heads under water and flapping their wings to splash water for a communal bath.

Her head cleared, and she concentrated on her breathing. *Much better.* "So, are the veggies inedible?"

"No vegetables ruined…other than one zucchini," Tom reported as he met her eyes with a smile. "All evidence destroyed. Still feeling light-headed?"

"Better. Didn't realize I have such a weak stomach."

Tom smiled. "Many people react the same when it's their own blood. You did just fine."

"Instead of helping you, I wasted your time and a zucchini."

"We can spare a zucchini." Tom nodded toward her bandaged finger. "Throbbing?"

"Just a little. I think I'll survive." She met his brown eyes with a smile. "Can I help with anything that doesn't involve knives?"

She watched as he glanced at the counter space, then nodded toward the romaine lettuce. "It's rinsed and ready to tear for the salad." Cassie moved to stand, but Tom's hand guided her back to her seat. He set the salad bowl on the table and transferred the lettuce within reach. "I'll chop, you toss the salad and tell me details about today's anti-bullying kick-off."

7

SIX WEEKS LATER...

"Spectacular!" Cassie's eyes widened as she entered the hotel ballroom, transformed into a starry moonlit night. She glanced at Caryn, who laughed as Jenna reached to touch imaginary stars. Daniel, in his father's arms, appeared entranced by the twinkling lights. Jenna reached for Cassie.

"I'll take her, Caryn. I know *Mrs. Martin* is probably looking for you."

"Let's get you settled first. Drew, could you check where Lauren would like her Godchildren?"

Andrew nodded as Cassie took Daniel from him. "Just don't wander off somewhere," he said with a wink.

"Come here, little man. I bet Aunt Lauren chose a very special place for us." Cassie loved watching Caryn and Andrew interact. *It's so obvious they love each other and their beautiful twins—they act like newlyweds, even after...four?...five?... years of marriage. So freaking romantic. And now, Lauren and Dave. Can't believe they got married during their trip to Greece! Was so looking forward to being a bridesmaid...and getting paired with one of Dave's hunky teammates as a groomsman...maybe even Tom. Talk about missed opportunities.*

Plenty of eye candy here. She glanced at Caryn with a smile. "So, can you point out the single guys?"

Caryn shook her head as she laughed. "Cassie, I don't recognize everyone. Could be friends from the Blues or from Vancouver."

She kissed the squirming Daniel on his forehead. "Hang in there, champ. We'll get settled soon, and then you can get down." She followed Caryn when Andrew approached.

He guided them through the crowded room, greeting several teammates, and then stopped beside a toddler play area. Lauren and Dave had arranged for a plastic ball pit, pint-sized climbing area, dozens of toys, and a deep-cushioned floor that promised soft landings.

"Wonderful!" Cassie stepped over the low sides into the play area. Jenna and Daniel scooted around, grabbing toys and sitting next to each other as they examined them. She waved Caryn and Andrew away. "I've got this—go enjoy the party."

The afternoon passed swiftly as a steady number of Lauren's and Caryn's friends stopped to see the twins or checked to see if Cassie needed anything. Daniel and Jenna threatened to steal the party from the newlyweds' celebration, but Cassie knew Lauren didn't care. *Never seen her so happy—she wears this dreamy smile ever since they returned from their cruise and announced they'd married. And then everything went fine when they flew to Vancouver to deliver the news to my mother and grandmother, and to Dave's family. And now, happiness just radiates around them.*

When Jenna's eyes began shifting to half-mast, Cassie placed her in the portable crib Andrew had set up. She covered her with a light blanket and laughed as Jenna's thumb found its way to her mouth. She was fast asleep within a minute. A short while later, Daniel fussed. Unlike Jenna, he resisted his nap and continued to play with toys while he babbled and whined. Cassie scooped him into her arms and softly hummed a little tune. Most of the time, music calmed him, but in this different environment, nothing made him happy. He let out a frustrated cry.

Cassie rocked him, pressing lightly on his head until it rested on her shoulder. She stepped to the other side of the area, hoping Daniel's unhappy cries would not wake Jenna. She glanced at the crowd. No one seemed to notice, and she didn't know whether to feel relieved or panicked. "It's okay, Danny. Just close your eyes," she whispered. *He's not hungry, doesn't need changing—just an unhappy little guy.*

"Can I give you a hand?" Cassie whirled around and exhaled in relief when she saw Tom stepping beside her. Cassie kissed Daniel's head before passing him to Tom.

"Dr. Tom to the rescue," she said. "Did you just get here?"

"I congratulated Lauren and Dave, mingled, then decided I'd find my nephew and niece—and my favorite honorary aunt." Tom's brown eyes sparkled as he held the unhappy Daniel before him. "What's the problem, little buddy? You miss your Uncle Tommy?"

Cassie enjoyed watching him interact with Daniel. Actually, she enjoyed watching Tom any chance she got. With his schedule at the hospital, she didn't see him often, but that didn't stop her from fantasizing about him…or "that kiss" a lot. *He and Andrew look so much alike, almost like twins, except Tom's hair is darker, and he has those golden brown—cinnamon—eyes, and Andrew's eyes are that deep shade of blue…Did Tom play hockey before med school?…He's just as well-built…and just as swoon-worthy as his brother. Always calm, soft-spoken, Tom must be the best doctor ever. I wouldn't complain if he treated me in the ER.* She knew he was completing his residency in neurology at the same hospital where Andrew had recovered from a traumatic brain injury over a year ago. Her stomach fluttered a little whenever Tom's eyes met hers.

He quieted Daniel in just a few minutes.

"Do you want to take a break, Cassie? I can watch them for a while."

She hesitated. She preferred to chat with him. "Maybe just a few minutes to freshen up and see if I can find the happy couple. I don't think they'll make it to this side of the room."

"Take your time. I'm not needed anywhere."

"Just what the doctor ordered," Cassie said with a smile. "I won't stay away too long."

Tom watched as Cassie gave him a little wave before being swallowed by the crowd around Dave and Lauren. Her light brown hair today sported a hint of lavender around her face. *Definitely a free spirit. The changing colors in her hair suit her.* Taller than average, she stood out in the throng of people. He could see her head bob in the crowd. *Like her aunt in some ways, but Cassie's definitely her own person.* When she looked at him with those hazel eyes peeking through her hair, Tom had to remind himself that she's off-limits for too many reasons. *Andrew and Caryn's nanny, Lauren's niece. Not to mention that we live in the same home. At least the age difference's "acceptable," but the risks outweigh the positives—at least for now.* But the memory of their unspoken kiss called to him like a siren of the sea. *Don't go there, Chadwick. Too much of a risk to even think that way.*

Cassie told Caryn and Andrew that Tom was with the twins. "Jenna's sleeping. Uncle Tommy's working his magic with Daniel. I just want to congratulate Mr. and Mrs. Martin again."

"Good luck." Andrew nodded toward the center of the room. "Need an escort?"

"Nah, I'll slip through. Do you guys know everyone?"

"Just about," Caryn said. "A couple new teammates, some new girlfriends. I think Dave and Lauren are the only newlyweds."

"Wish me luck—see you soon!" Cassie looked over the crowd as she moved toward the newlyweds. She tried to focus on Dave—she could spot him more easily than Lauren.

She hugged Lauren when she reached them. "Having fun?"

"The best! Never expected so many would come."

"Everyone needs an excuse to relax a little now that training camp's over," Dave said. "Also, a good opportunity for the new players to meet people." Lauren leaned back against him as she stifled a yawn.

Cassie kissed Lauren's cheek, then hugged Dave. "Just wanted to add my congratulations…again. I'll see you later—Caryn may want to get the twins home soon."

"We'll catch up soon, Cassie," Lauren promised.

Cassie checked out the guys who played hockey as she walked back to find Caryn or relieve Tom. Not one compares to Tom and his panty-melting smile and those eyes that threaten to discover her deepest thoughts. As close to perfect a man as she could imagine. *He never ignores me, he listens when I talk with him and treats me like an adult. Why waste my time looking for a hockey player? Because your doctor may already have his own soulmate?* Cassie yearned to know the true relationship between Tom and Katie—the sooner, the better. She knew better than to think about anything developing with Tom. Her employer's brother, the obvious age difference, living under the same roof, and already involved with a woman. *He's off-limits for too many reasons... Dream on, Johnson.*

8

By the time Cassie found Caryn, Andrew had left. "Drew's helping Tom get the twins ready—they've done well."

"Because they're such sweethearts. Hopefully, I'll be that lucky someday."

Caryn smiled. "No time soon, right?"

"I'm talking years…lots of years." She looked over Caryn's shoulder and saw Andrew and Tom approaching, each carrying a sleeping baby.

Andrew handed Daniel to Caryn. "I'll get the rest of our things."

"I'll take care of it," Cassie offered. "Meet you at the car?"

"We'll pull up out front. Take your time," Andrew said.

"Back in a few." Cassie maneuvered through the thinning crowd to the play area. She grabbed the diaper bag and started loading the toys, blankets, pacifiers, bottles, and jars of baby food. *Packed enough for a weekend. Caryn and Andrew must think I'm clueless—if they even noticed.* She looked around and saw Jenna's favorite stuffed bear peeking out of the ball pit. *Nap and bedtime crisis if I missed that….* She grabbed the toy and slipped it into a side pocket on the bag, and slung it over her shoulder. Heavier than expected, she stumbled a bit as she stepped out of the enclosure. A hand gripped her elbow to steady her.

"Careful."

She looked at Tom, even as her skin tingled with electricity where he touched her arm. "Obviously, I overpacked," she stammered.

"I'll carry it—no tripping on my watch." Even his soft laugh made her heart flip.

"I almost fell because I'm a klutz. I'm okay now. Thank you for not watching me do a face plant."

A slow smile crossed his face. "No emergency room in my plans tonight."

Cassie hesitated before breaking contact, hoping he didn't notice the goosebumps or hear her racing heart.

"Thanks for coming back to help me," she said as he lifted the bag over his shoulder.

"Maybe you need to get used to that." She saw the smirk and his attempt to hold back a laugh. "I'm not leaving you behind."

"Cassie? Wait up!"

She stopped as Tom pushed the door open and saw the guy from the Stand Up to Bullies event and a gorgeous blonde date approaching. *Yikes! His name was…*

"Shall I stay?" Tom asked.

"Do you know his name?"

"Yes—Cliff Camden. How does he know you?"

"I met him at the anti-bullying kick-off." Cassie noticed the frown that flashed across his expression.

"Word of warning—he has quite the reputation." Tom had leaned close to her ear to keep his voice low.

"Thanks. This won't take a minute."

Tom made eye contact with Cam, nodding before continuing through the door.

"I didn't see you—avoiding me?" Cam greeted when he and his date stopped beside her.

"Why would I avoid you? I was watching the twins in the play area Lauren set up. They keep me busy." She glanced at the girl beside him. "I'm Cassie Johnson—Lauren's niece if you met the newlyweds."

"This is Amelia—my twin sister," Cam introduced.

Amelia smiled. "I'm glad to meet you. But, please call me Amelie —or Amie. I prefer the French spelling. Cliff mentioned you, perhaps?" She looked at her brother with a teasing smile. Unlike Cam, her voice carried a lovely French accent.

"Our paths crossed at a Suns' event," Cassie said. "Happy to meet you, Amelie. Are you in Tampa for a while?"

"Amelia's helping to set up my new condo. I may have mentioned it when we met?"

Cassie shrugged. "Maybe. Your sister's very kind to help you."

"She has an ulterior reason, don't you, 'Amelie?'" He ignored the glare she lasered toward him. "She just finished her second year at the University of Paris and is taking a semester off. Something about declaring a major."

Amelie laughed and swatted her brother. "Too many choices, Cassie. My parents refuse to pay for living expenses in Paris if I don't take a full schedule."

"I hear you. I'm in the same situation…except, I don't even know if I want to go to college. But I enjoy working as a nanny. Are you staying in Tampa a while?"

"Until Cliff kicks me out. I hope I can find a job, so he won't call me a freeloader."

Cassie glanced outside and saw the Chadwick's SUV pull in front of the entrance. She slipped her phone from her purse and handed it to Amelie. "Call your cell phone, please. Then we'll have each other's number. Maybe we can get together—if one of us can borrow a car."

"Don't worry about that. My fabulous *younger* brother will let me drive his."

"Ten minutes, sis. You're ten minutes older. I don't know about driving my car. Better if I lease something you can use while you're here."

Cassie laughed as she watched Amelie try to grab the keys from his pocket. "Great meeting you, Amelie. I hope we can get together soon."

Amelie gave up on the keys, then smiled with a small wave. "See you opening night?"

Cassie paused with the door half-open. "Maybe. Depends on Caryn—she may not want to take the babies to the games. Play by ear?"

"Bien sûr. I'll look forward to it."

Cassie pushed her way through the doorway, feeling a hint of excitement that she may have a new friend closer to her age—and irritation that Cam acted like he knew her. *Just a short chat after the event, then he never contacted me. Wasn't holding my breath, anyway.*

Tom waited for her outside the door. He pretended to groan as he carried the bag to the back of the car. "What did you and Caryn pack—bricks?"

Cassie laughed as he set the bag in the back of the SUV, then opened the door to the back seat. "It's all me. Just supplies, toys, you know, Tom."

She saw his lips twitch as he fought against a smile. "That bag weighs more than your suitcases when you arrived."

Cassie laughed. "Lucky for me, you came back to help. See you later?"

"Just going to check on some patients before I head home."

Cassie climbed into the seat beside Daniel and Jenna, and Tom closed the door with a wink.

Caryn caught Cassie's eyes. "So, you met Mr. Camden's girl of the day?"

"His twin sister, Amelie. She's going to the University of Paris and is taking some time off before she declares a major. Sounds like she'll be in Tampa for a few months. She's helping him set up his new condo. She says it's better than staying home in Montréal."

"How nice for him—I didn't know he's a twin. You might enjoy having someone closer to your age in the area. You need to get out. We didn't hire you to be on call twenty-four-seven."

"Amelie seems nice. Maybe we'll chat or text."

"I didn't know Cam was Québécois. He has no accent." Caryn

turned to face Cassie in the seat behind her. "Have you thought about enrolling in classes here?"

"Not really. I don't know what I want to do. I like dance but that's not much of a career path." Cassie made a face. "Besides, too much ballet when I was younger."

Caryn laughed. "I can relate to that. Remind me to tell you about my ballet lessons when I was a kid. You're more interested in contemporary dance, anyway, aren't you?"

"Anything from 1920s-forward. Love those dances from the first half of the Twentieth Century—Tango, Charleston, Shimmy…I love watching those old movies on Netflix. You know, actors had to dance —very dreamy." Cassie shrugged. "I think I was a flapper in a previous life."

"I can definitely see you in that role. Think about it. We can work your schedule around classes."

Tom stood by the stove in the kitchen early the next morning, and Cassie stopped to watch him a moment. *My lucky day. I get to see the hunky hot doctor two days in a row.* "Good day, Dr. Chadwick."

He turned and shook his head with a laugh. "I hear enough of that at the hospital. Just call me Tom, okay?"

Cassie pushed her hair to the side as she shrugged. "That just sounds...disrespectful." She allowed a teasing smile to cross her face.

Tom turned to face her. "Disrespectful, how? You call Caryn and Andrew by their first names."

Cassie shrugged as she brushed past him to grab a box of cereal and a bowl. "You're a doctor." She pulled a spoon from the drawer and set everything on the table before moving to the fridge.

She heard Tom's chuckle. "When I'm home, I'm just Tom. None of that doctor stuff. You're making me feel old."

Cassie cocked her head. "My mom taught me to respect my elders." She giggled as she set the milk on the table.

"Just how old do you think I am?"

Cassie took her time before replying, enjoying the opportunity to look him over. *Too old to be interested in me, that's for sure.* "Eh, I don't know. How long does it take to become a neurologist?"

"Not as long as you assume. Andrew's my *older* brother. I'm sure 'respect your elders' does not include anyone in their twenties."

"So...you're like twenty-seven?"

"Not quite. Next birthday. Not that much older than you, Ms. Etiquette."

She couldn't suppress a chuckle. "Etiquette is not one of my strengths, *Tom*. You must have flown through your undergrad?"

His brown eyes pinned her with amusement. "Not entirely. Not taking summers off made a huge difference."

"Well, I'll be twenty-one next spring and do not know what I want to be when I grow up." She swallowed a laugh. "My mom thought she could homeschool me. I did okay while in the primary level, but after my parents divorced, she lost interest. To catch up, I had to go to summer school, and I still ended up two years behind my age-group."

"That must have been rough."

"It only bothered me when I reached my teens. My classmates wanted to play hopscotch, jump rope, and other kid games during recess. My hormones had kicked in, and I spent recess hanging around the edges of the secondary school playground. Forbidden fruit," Cassie said with a laugh.

"You never felt you belonged with either group?"

Cassie paused. *Tom understands how isolated I felt.* "Age wise, I wanted friends in my age group, but they didn't want to hang out with someone two grades below. Most people just assumed I needed to repeat two grades because I couldn't pass the first time."

"That's rough. I can understand why you felt out of place with either group. But didn't you graduate?"

She nodded. "Last May. The thought of more school makes me ill. Just a tad burned out. Thus, the gap year, much to my mother's er... let's call it disdain."

"Take your time—I'd feel burned out, too. You can explore options while saving Caryn's sanity."

"Caryn's amazing. I hope I'll be half the mom she is..." Cassie let her voice trail off and watched as Tom gathered what looked like the ingredients for an egg dish. *He cooks breakfast, too.*

"Can I make you an omelet?"

"I'm good. But, thanks. I don't know many guys who cook."

Tom glanced over his shoulder and winked. "I prefer to eat clean and steer clear of fast food. That's the only way to survive the long shifts."

"I still can't figure out your schedule. You're not here when I think you should be and vice versa."

She saw him glancing at the streaks she'd added to her light brown hair. "So, today it's pastel blue *and* green. Yesterday it was lavender. Any secret meaning to the colors?"

"Not really. Just trying things I couldn't do at home. My mom freaked when I tried subtle pink highlights."

Tom laughed. "The colors complement your eyes. I like it."

"I'll send Mom a selfie. You'll see how fast my phone rings." The sound of unhappy babies echoed from the nursery. "Well, there's my cue." She took her bowl to the sink, rinsed it, and opened the dishwasher. "See you later...*Tom.*"

9

Tom tossed his scrubs in the bin and showered, ready to get home and sleep after another long shift. *Home…if you can call freeloading at your brother's house "home."* He enjoyed the privacy of the apartment that was part of their home—but every time he brought up the subject of paying rent, both Andrew and Caryn protested and refused to discuss it. *Maybe now that I'm completing the residency, Andrew will accept rent payments.*

Money was not an issue. His brother signed a lucrative contract with the Suns over two years ago—but if he continued to live in the apartment, Tom wanted to contribute more than babysitting the twins or serving as the resident doctor on call. He'd hash it out with his brother.

He saw the Chief of Neurology in the hallway as he walked toward the exit. "Got a minute, Tom?" Dan Forster asked.

"Sure, Dan, what's up?"

The physician nodded toward his office. "Help yourself to coffee or soda."

"Caffeine sounds good." Tom grabbed a Coke from the small refrigerator in the office, then took the seat Forster indicated.

"We've an opportunity you may find interesting." Forster reached across his desk to grab a piece of paper before sitting beside Tom. "The Suns wish to hire a neurologist to help evaluate players—on either team—who may sustain a concussion during the game."

"A concussion spotter?"

"No, they wish to take it one step further. The league will continue to monitor games for signs that a player needs assessment for the concussion protocol. The Suns want to ensure no player steps back on the ice without a neurological assessment."

"Good for them. The league's rules leave room for misinterpretation—with the play-at-all-costs mentality among some players. I've seen guys playing who had no business on the ice."

"That's why I thought about you for the position. Your residency is winding down. I know you're exploring options. If this enhances your chances of staying here in Tampa, we'll work around the game schedule." Forster's smile bordered on a smirk. "You'd also get to see your brother play more frequently."

"I'm in," Tom replied without hesitation. "I want to stay in Tampa—just waiting for the hospital to offer a full-time position."

"You don't want to enter private practice? I know you have multiple offers." The surprise in his voice caused Tom to shake his head.

"Dan, I like what I'm doing now. No two days are alike. I enjoy rotating through the ER, ICU, step-down, and post-injury therapy. I knew that from watching Andrew progress through the program. You stayed involved until we cleared him to play."

"I'll have an offer put together in a few days. Consider each department—you may gravitate to a particular area. ER/ICU, for example. Or even a teaching supervisor for the new residents. Make your wishes known—this is the time to think about yourself," Dan advised.

He stood and Tom followed. "In the meantime, I'll get back to the Suns. You realize, Dr. Chadwick, that some of your decisions may cause some dissension among the players and coaches?"

Tom laughed. "They wouldn't play hockey without the mindset of playing through pain…blurred vision…unsteadiness…" He held his hand out to his mentor. "I'll check with Andrew, see if he has any objections. But I can handle the verbal abuse. My brother desensitized me before I reached my teens."

Tom entered the house and found Andrew attempting to calm two furious babies. "What have you done with my nephew and niece?" He grabbed Jenna and held her against his shoulder, looking at his brother with a snicker.

Andrew scowled as he stood with Daniel. "Caryn thinks it's a combination of the vaccine yesterday and teething today. They were fine until about thirty minutes ago."

Tom winced. "Did you give them some Tylenol?"

"Yes, Dr. Turner recommended something to rub on their gums, so she's gone to the pharmacy."

"Each by itself can make them upset, but combined, you have two very uncomfortable children."

"No kidding. Caryn would have postponed the shots if she had an inkling that teething would flare up." Andrew kissed Daniel's forehead. "You're exhausted, little buddy. How about a walk around the pool?"

Jenna had also calmed, so Tom followed his brother out to the pool deck. The sun had dipped low in the sky, casting a comfortable shade over the lanai. "Andrew, did you know the Suns want to hire a neurologist as their concussion specialist during home games?"

"No, but that's a good idea. The concussion spotters the league hires have limitations. Most are trainers, not doctors. How'd you learn that?" Andrew glanced at Tom.

"Dan said the Suns want to partner with the hospital's neurology department. Once he signed off on the idea, they discussed the staffing. He offered me the part-time gig. I said yes, unless you had objections."

"Why would I object, Tom? I know to take concussions seriously."

"Even if I decide Reese Ekstrom needs to come out of a game?" Tom referred to the team's all-star goaltender. "Or your top center or D-man? Will you get shit from your teammates when I sideline someone from playing?"

Andrew shrugged. "Probably. But, if you think there's cause for concern, then they'll just have to deal with it. I have no problem if that happens."

"So, the coach and training staff told Dan. But I know how intense you guys get during a game. You might get some resentment from your teammates. I'd do the same function for the visiting team."

Andrew glanced at him with a speculative expression. "So, we could bribe you to pull the starting goaltender before a game goes into overtime?"

"You could try, but I wouldn't. Think of me like Switzerland during the game."

Andrew sat on a chair and nodded at the one beside him. He set Daniel on his legs and bumped him up and down. "That's not a full-time job."

"No, but I will receive an offer from the hospital. Dan said to decide where I'd prefer to work, but I enjoy rotating through the departments. I like the variety."

"Congratulations, doctor. So, you'd moonlight as the concussion specialist?" Andrew nodded toward Daniel, whose tears had turned into giggles.

"Not moonlight." Tom checked to see if Jenna still slept, her little hand pressed against her mouth as she relaxed against his shoulder. "Dan said he'd work my schedule around games, just a little supplemental pay for forty to sixty games. And only for home games. I would like a regular schedule as much as possible."

"So, you'd get paid to watch us play. Tough job."

"Someone has to do it. So, you have no reservations? None?"

"Of all people, I will not question if you think someone needs to leave the ice. If anyone has a problem, I'll share my experience dealing with the mother of all concussions."

10

"Shall we try the pool today?" Cassie asked as she and Caryn ate lunch with the twins. "Perfect day. Not too hot...and no direct sunlight on the shallow end."

Caryn bit back a wry smile when she glanced at Cassie. "Might as well get over my pool phobia. We can surprise Drew when he gets back in town. With the exhibition schedule wrapping up, this is my chance to get over the anxiety I have about the pool—so I don't drive him crazy."

Cassie touched Caryn's arm. "Not that we'll need it, but just remember I passed those CPR and lifeguard courses at the hospital and the Y."

Caryn's laughed, sounding only a bit forced. "That's my insurance policy that we'll never need them." Her eyes fell on Jenna, then Daniel. "Why not? I think I can take it more slowly with you. Drew would probably want to take them underwater first thing."

"Have you thought about swimming lessons?"

"I have. I found a company that will send someone to your home for lessons, and they have a certified instructor for infant lessons. Guess I should get on the waiting list?"

"When you're comfortable," Cassie said. "We can just try getting their toes wet today."

"I think I can handle that." Caryn lifted Daniel from his seat. "I'll get the swim diapers while Miss Jenna finishes her lunch."

Afraid she might miss something, Jenna squawked when Caryn and Daniel disappeared around the corner. She shook her head and clamped her mouth shut, refusing more food.

"No peaches today, Jen?" Cassie teased her lips with the spoon. "I promise you won't miss out on anything." After trying several times, Cassie set the food aside and cleaned her face. "Okay, sweets, we'll go find your brother."

An hour later, Lauren, and their friends Kelly Peterson and Terri Rogers joined them at the pool, all wishing to document the twins' first swim with photos and videos.

"Does Andrew know you're taking the plunge today?" Kelly tried to ask with a straight face that soon dissolved into laughter.

"No way. Big surprise if we're successful. No need to know if we're not."

"Could I take Daniel?" Terri asked. "You're the official photographer, Cassie, aren't you?"

"Sure." She sat on the side of the pool and dipped her feet into the water. "Perfect temperature, Caryn."

"Remember, you're the lifeguard if anything goes wrong."

Lauren and Kelly sat beside Cassie. "Nothing's going wrong," Lauren teased Caryn. "This is one of those days you'll always remember." She nudged Cassie. "Where's your whistle and emergency float?"

Cassie laughed and then glanced behind her. "We need some emergency supplies. I'll look through the materials the Y gave me. I'm surprised Tom hasn't already covered this." She held her phone to record the milestone. As soon as her feet touched the water, Jenna jerked back. She wanted nothing to do with it. Daniel, however, squealed in delight—kicking his feet, then splashing with his hands as Terri walked a few steps away from the edge. Cassie bit back a grin as

Jenna turned to see why Daniel giggled, and suddenly she squirmed in Caryn's arms until she submerged her feet. She mimicked Daniel's kicking, as she learned to splash water.

Caryn visibly relaxed as the twins enjoyed the water. Terri dipped lower until Daniel's belly sank below the surface, and he expressed further delight in the sensation.

"I take it this one loves his baths?" Terri laughed.

"Not this much," Caryn replied as she brought Jenna to Daniel's side. Soon, Jenna shrieked and giggled when the water lapped against her tummy. Cassie stopped the video and caught Caryn's eyes.

"I think they're ready for swimming lessons."

"Now I wish I'd signed up for that waiting list," Caryn said. "But we have plenty of time."

"Want to take them underwater?" Terri asked.

"Eh, not just yet. I think we're doing great for the first time." Caryn kissed Jenna's forehead. "I don't want to take the chance on scaring them—or me!"

"I don't think Mr. Daniel scares easily." Cassie laughed.

"Mr. Camden's stopping by the day after tomorrow, Caryn," Lauren said.

"Uh-oh, is he misbehaving?" Kelly asked. "I've wondered how he's doing living in an apartment. Hope he's not over enjoying this 'freedom.'"

"His sister lives with him," Cassie spoke up. "I don't know if Amelie's a party girl like her brother."

"You want me to ask him to invite Amelie with him? You two could enjoy some girl time together."

Cassie nodded. "Sure, if she's available. I'd enjoy girl chat."

When Cam dropped his sister at the Chadwick's house two days later, Caryn suggested they get snacks and drinks and enjoy the fresh air on the pool deck or take a walk.

"I'll help you get the munchkins ready for their nap," Cassie offered, but Caryn declined.

"You're off the clock, Cassie. Relax, enjoy, go for a walk, swim. Have some fun."

The girls walked around the vast neighborhood to see if they could meet any others—preferably male—in their age group.

"How do you like Tampa?" Cassie asked as they headed toward the far back of the subdivision.

"It's nice. I get a bit of cabin fever when Cliff's gone, and I'm stuck without a car. But if I get a job, he can co-sign a loan for me." Amelie looked at Cassie with a smirk.

"Or buy you a car? I know how you feel. I haven't asked, and Lauren hasn't offered to let me drive her Mustang." Cassie slipped on her sunglasses as they rounded a curve, suddenly facing the sun. "And I don't want to ask Caryn if I can drive her car. The insurance and liability could get crazy. If I stay in Tampa, I could afford a car payment…nothing fancy." Cassie glanced at Amelie. "I honestly didn't realize when we met just how much you and your brother look alike. Your eyes, your expressions…much prettier on you."

Amelie laughed. "The joy of having a fraternal twin."

"So, where are you looking for a job?"

Amelie shrugged, then pointed at a tree in the distance, "A bald eagle."

"Let's see if we can get closer. I've never seen one." They walked in silence a while, their eyes trained on the tree.

"I've applied for a job at a boutique near Cliff's place," Amelie answered Cassie's earlier question. "The hours are flexible, so I can still get out and go to games and sometimes tag along for open practices. Surprised the ice doesn't melt with all that hotness on skates. Hard to know where to look first." She grabbed Cassie's arm. "Oh, I met this new guy from Québéc. I could barely stutter when he spoke to me. So gorgeous, with the French accent. *Oh la la!*"

"Older guy?" Cassie said. "I think I saw him at Lauren and Dave's celebration. Beyond tall, dark, long hair?"

"Oh, yes! The French guy, 'Chance' something. I'd *love* to get together with him."

"Friends with your brother?"

"Who knows? I met him…briefly…after practice before Cliff

pulled the protective brother crap." Amelie wrinkled her nose. "Says he's too old for me, reputation as a player, blah, blah, blah."

"So that didn't discourage you one bit?" Cassie guessed.

"You got it. If I get a 'chance'—*ha-ha*—with him, I'm going for it." She grabbed Cassie's arm. "I got his cell number. We've texted a few times—but please don't say anything."

"Asked you out yet?"

Amelie's grey eyes danced as she shook her head. "Just some text flirting and he's called a few times when they're away." She glanced at Cassie. "And that accent...He's very smooth with his words, but it's difficult to get him to answer questions."

"Mysterious? Hiding something? A wife or fiancée somewhere?"

"I hope not. Maybe just a private person? I can't ask Cliff about him."

Cassie thought a minute. "Maybe Caryn or Lauren works with him or his agent—you know, they do PR and social media stuff. Not sure they'd tell me anything. Probably confidential stuff. So, you've called dibs on him?"

"Hey, if you have the opportunity, go for it." Amelie nudged her. "Now, if I hook up with him, then..."

"I get it. The 'code' like the guys say. They don't know we have our own version." Her eyes drifted toward the tree where the large bird had perched. "We may not get an up-close view of our bird tonight. It appears the eagle has flown."

Cam waited at the Chadwick's until Cassie and Amelie returned. "Thought you two had gotten lost," he smirked. He sat at the kitchen counter, watching as Caryn and Andrew fed the twins.

"I can do that, Andrew," Cassie protested. "Time got away from us. I'm sorry, Caryn."

"For what? I told you to enjoy yourselves. Just try to get that spoon away from Drew."

Andrew looked at Cassie with a smile. "Bonding time with my peanuts. Not giving that up."

Cassie focused her gaze on Jenna, who eagerly awaited the next spoonful of peaches and then laughed as Jenna spit a mouthful of pureed peaches at her father.

"And you denied your children would ever do that," Caryn teased as she handed him a towel.

"I'll finish feeding Jenna," Cassie offered. "Caryn and I both know how it feels to have baby food in our hair."

Andrew wiped the towel over his face before he kissed his daughter and pushed back the chair. "Your children are incorrigible, Cary." He handed the spoon to Cassie. "Thanks."

As soon as she sat, Caryn whispered, "His children are perfect angels—*my* children are incorrigible."

"We're taking off," Cam said. "Thanks for letting me hang out while I waited for my time-challenged sister to return." He raised his hands in surrender as two sets of eyes nailed him. "No offense, ladies. Just saying."

"Amelie, you're welcome here any time," Caryn said.

"Thanks. A bientôt, Cassie."

11

Tom met with the Suns' management, coaches, training staff, team captain, and assistant captains to discuss his role as the concussion specialist during home games. Everyone stated they stood behind the process one hundred percent. Tom glanced around the table. "And when I say one of your top players needs to sit during a crucial moment in a game, no complaints?"

"At that moment, you may hear some choice words from me," Head Coach Harper predicted. "But no one will keep you from doing your job. I know the training staff will back you."

"Damn straight we will." Jim Pettit's reply more than confirmed his support. "You know these guys—they fight you every step of the way. Even when they can't see straight or walk without stumbling. Before his accident, Andrew was one of the hardest to take off the ice."

Tom chuckled. "No surprise there. So, the others don't take concussions more seriously after what Andrew went through?"

"Some do. Others think it can't happen to them." Pettit met Tom's gaze. "Welcome to the team, doc."

"I scheduled a team meeting tomorrow after morning skate." Harper glanced at John Peterson. "Expect any resistance?"

John shrugged. "Some—especially the older players and the rookies. I'll handle them. Those on the team two years ago shouldn't protest at all."

John walked with Tom to his car. "Thanks for taking this on. No one wants to hear they need to leave the game, but the more we've learned about concussions, the less easy it is to shrug it away. Now, the players on the other teams…I can't make any promises, but with Pettit briefing their training staff on the protocol before each series and the front office speaking with the GMs, no one should be surprised."

Tom shrugged. "When someone's health's at risk, there's zero tolerance for debate. You know that Andrew would have been back on the ice long before they cleared him." He laughed as he rested his arm against the top of his car. "If I could tolerate his frustration, I should be able to handle anyone else's complaints."

"You headed back to the hospital?"

"Off until after tomorrow night's game. I'll be transitioning to a more defined schedule. Fewer multi-day shifts."

"Maybe time for a life outside the hospital. Stop by later—I'll buy you a beer to celebrate." John slapped Tom's shoulder before heading to his car. "Thanks for what you've taken on, Chadwick."

Later, stepping out on the pool deck to swim laps, Cassie caught Tom's attention. He stopped a minute when his gaze fell on her bikini-clad body. Her body curved in just the right places, her legs stretched for miles, and Tom suddenly realized he was not looking at her like Jenna and Daniel's nanny. Cassie stirred something unexpected inside him—even before "the kiss"—definitely not an older brother instinct.

Tom forced his mind elsewhere as he walked over to the other side of the pool and dropped his towel on a chair. He slipped into the pool and hoped that swimming laps would draw his attention to a more appropriate subject than his friend's niece and brother's nanny.

Cassie opened her eyes, realizing she'd drifted off to sleep in the sun's warmth despite the music pounding in her ears. She stopped the playlist and glanced at her watch, relieved that she hadn't slept the afternoon away. Jenna and Daniel should still be napping. She sat up, reached for her water, and for the first time, realized she had company. It took her a minute to decide that Tom, not Andrew, was swimming laps, and a playful smile spread across her face as Cassie walked to the side of the pool. She waited until he was in range, and using both hands heaved a wave of water toward him, striking Tom in the face as he turned his head for a breath. *Crap, I didn't mean to do that.* Cassie slipped into the water, an apology on her lips as Tom stood and coughed until he caught his breath.

His brown eyes met Cassie's, and before she could apologize, he pounced, pushing her under the water. Cassie tried to retaliate by knocking him over, but she might as well have been trying to move a concrete wall. She pushed away and broke the surface, taking a quick breath before Tom dunked her again. This time, she swam away from him and cautiously emerged on the other side of the pool.

"I didn't mean to splash water on your face!"

His brown eyes narrowed but held a playful gleam. "Just where did you intend to hit me?"

"Um, maybe the other side of your head. Bad timing. I'm sorry. What are you doing here, anyway?"

"Day off, but don't change the subject. A couple of dunks aren't enough." He started toward her, but Cassie took off, swimming diagonally to the far corner of the pool. She hoped he wouldn't realize her direction, but she had only swum a few yards before Tom grabbed her leg and pulled her underwater. This time, when she squealed, she received a mouth full of water and quickly pushed to the surface, coughing and trying to catch her breath.

"Trying…to…drown…me?" She got one word in between each cough.

He was beside her in a moment, his arm wrapped around her waist until she caught her breath. "You all right now?"

Her hazel eyes looked at him warily. "Are we even?"

Tom laughed and fought the urge to hug her. Instead, he withdrew his arm from her waist. "More than even. I wasn't trying to drown you."

"That would make a great headline, wouldn't it, doctor?" Cassie moved to the edge of the pool and rested against it. She laughed, but it triggered more coughing.

"Hey, did you swallow water?"

She shook her head. "If I did, it was because I was laughing. I'm fine." She ducked underwater to smooth her hair away from her face. When she emerged, she teased him. "So, there is a fun side to our good doctor." She looked toward the house and saw Caryn en route to the nursery. "I'd better get inside to help Caryn. I think nap time just ended."

Tom pushed himself onto the side of the pool and offered a hand to help Cassie. She grasped his hand with a smile but didn't speak until she stood beside him on the tile. "You don't know how tempting it is to pull you in."

"Yeah, I thought about that. Truce?"

"Sure…until next time."

Cassie quickly entered the nursery, a coverup thrown over her swimsuit and her hair still soaked.

"I'm sorry, Caryn. I lost track of time. Do you want me to take Daniel?"

"You deserved the break. Go ahead, shower, and change. You'll get chilled with Drew's preferred setting on the AC. They can play for a while before dinner."

"Thanks, I won't be long."

"Take your time."

Cassie couldn't contain a smile when she thought about playing water tag with Tom. *Really haven't laughed that hard in a long time. How could I have dozed off and not heard him get into the pool? Glad I didn't sleep through his work out.*

She loved the impromptu battle in the pool. She hadn't had that much fun in…*forever? Never with a guy who made my heart skip a beat just by looking at me. I hope he doesn't think of me as some pesky little sister...no, surely not after "the kiss." But he's the forbidden one...the gorgeous doc who's off-limits for too many reasons—topping that list—his girlfriend, Katie.*

Revived by the warm shower, Cassie threw on some cut-offs and a T-shirt and ran a comb through her hair. She brushed it behind her ears and frowned when she saw all traces of her "accent color" washed away. *Not worth it if I'll swim. Though I didn't plan to get in the water. But sooo glad I did.* She tingled just thinking about Tom putting his arm around her waist. *Maybe I should have just continued to cough...*

When she returned to the family room, both Andrew and Tom were keeping the twins busy bouncing balls back and forth.

"What, no hockey sticks yet?" Cassie teased.

"Give them six months!" Caryn responded from the kitchen.

"Maybe basketball?" She watched as Jenna heaved the ball up into the air.

"That or maybe a quarterback." Tom caught her eye with a wink. "What if neither pursues athletics?" he taunted his brother.

Andrew didn't look at him as he rolled the ball back to Jenna. "In the unlikely event that occurs, I'll encourage them to find something they enjoy." He glanced at Caryn. "We know the pitfalls of trying to plan a child's future."

"Amen." Caryn looked at Andrew with a knowing smile.

Cassie walked into the kitchen. Watching Andrew and Caryn interact always made her long for her own someone to share that kind of love. *Caryn told me she wasn't much older than I am when she met Andrew. She didn't meet him at college—though they bumped into each other on the campus. Andrew just cut across her path on his daily run...So freaking romantic. And random.*

"What can I do to help, Caryn?"

"Since Jenna and Daniel are happy for now, would you mind cutting up the banana? Otherwise, you-know-who will just mash it around on his tray."

Cassie giggled. "My mom has a picture of me feeding myself SpaghettiOs...I was literally covered with them and had decorated the tray and the floor. They started putting a plastic tarp under the high-chair to protect the wood floor!"

"Maybe we'll skip the SpaghettiOs," Caryn said. "Though, I guess any pasta has the same potential."

"Spaghetti's easier to throw," Andrew warned.

Cassie exchanged a look with Caryn before they both laughed. She enjoyed working in the kitchen with Caryn. They chatted about all topics, especially when they were alone.

"Have you and Amelie talked recently?"

"She got the job she applied for at that boutique. It's close so she can walk."

"Maybe she gets a friend and family discount?"

"I'd enjoy that!" Cassie lowered her voice. "Her brother nearly had a stroke when she applied at The Center Ice Lounge. Isn't that the place where the team goes after games?"

Caryn nodded. "He probably didn't want her to cramp his style or hookup with someone on the team."

"But isn't there some kind of code like 'Don't date another player's sister?'"

Caryn laughed. "You'd have to ask Dave or Andrew…nieces and nannies may fall on that list, too."

Cassie chuckled. "No doubt." *At least she didn't mention brothers or doctors.*

12

Tom's introduction to the Suns as the arena's in-house concussion expert ended up a non-event. Those who had been on the team when his brother was injured spoke in a positive tone. He read the *"It'll never happen to me"* expression on the young players, and a hint of combativeness from the veterans new to the team.

"This some new bullshit from the commissioner?" Chance Gagné grumbled.

"That's a hard no," Captain John Peterson replied immediately. "This initiative originated in the Suns front office. The league concussion spotters don't have the expertise to properly recognize the more subtle signs of a concussion."

"I've gone back on the ice with my equilibrium questionable. You learn to fake it, right?" Steve Rogers said. "If you've read the stories about athletes diagnosed with CTE, it's not a joking matter. Remember the player who committed suicide because he couldn't tolerate the cumulative effect?"

"And those who retired after multiple concussions," Jason Hart added. "Many don't want to take the chance of permanent damage. This is serious shit." He addressed the younger players. "No more pressure to suck it up and push yourself when you know you're not *right.* The Suns front office has our backs. I, for one, am grateful."

"See if you feel the same when Ekstrom gets yanked during a game." Gagné didn't hide his skepticism. "You know you'll do everything you can to prove you're okay to get back on the ice."

"I would expect nothing less," Tom said. "Keep in mind I'll be working with the visiting team. We will evaluate everyone with the same criteria. Hopefully, not too often."

"Don't bother trying to bribe him," Andrew said. "I already got shot down."

Most of the team left the meeting in a positive mood, and many stopped to thank Tom for taking on the responsibility. Jim Pettit stood beside him, watching the last player leave. "We know the guys who'll fight us every step of the way. But if we can get through to the young kids, it's worth it. They feel the pressure to perform and worry their place on the team will evaporate if they're hurt. Maybe when they see a clear path outlined for clearance to play, it will ease that worry. Ready for introductions to the visiting training staff and coaches?"

Tom shrugged. "Why not? Better now than in the third period with the game on the line."

After the first few games passed with only minor questionable hits to the head, and no push-back or negative feedback from either team's players or coaching staff, Tom relaxed a bit. He had yet to prevent a player from returning to the ice after a head hit. Coach Harper offered him a place behind the bench, but Tom preferred to monitor the games from the trainer's office. Multiple feeds broadcast the entire ice, which enabled him to view the big picture of a game. Both teams' trainers served as first responders when a player's head hit the boards or the ice. Many went to the team's concussion protocol room, where Tom performed a quick, but thorough evaluation. Mostly, the players expressed gratitude for the second evaluation.

Just wait until I have to tell someone to sit for the rest of the period, the game, or transport to the hospital for further tests. Hopefully, never an injury that requires transport...Memories of his brother's long recovery from a Traumatic Brain Injury that resulted from unintentionally blocking a shot with his head stayed fresh in Tom's mind. Playing a role in Andrew's recovery led to an opportunity to complete his residency in neurology—at the same hospital where Tom had assisted with his brother's treatment and recovery plan. When the Chief of Neurology, Dan Forster, offered Tom a position, it felt more like a gift, not work.

Except for the games and during emergencies, Tom's schedule settled into a more structured format. For the first time since he'd begun medical school in Toronto, he had time for a social life. Andrew teased him about his hospital groupies, but after trying to maintain an exclusive relationship with Katie, he preferred not to get involved with anyone at the hospital. Different schedules and few opportunities to explore the mutual attraction left both unsatisfied. When Katie recently moved home to accept a job in Minnesota, they agreed to remain "friends." Without benefits.

He didn't plan to accept invitations to post-game celebrations—though his friends on the Suns assured him he'd be welcomed. *Don't want to cross that line between professionalism on the job by hanging out with them. The guys I'm already friends with—one thing. The new guys and the younger players could resent the intrusion into their private lives. Even Andrew understands that. Though he warned me about the puck bunnies who might trail me in the arena's parking lot.*

"You could meet your soulmate," Andrew said with a straight face.

"Until she discovers I'm not a hockey player."

"Doctors trump jocks every time, brother. Don't overlook an opportunity because you think someone's looking for an athlete."

Tom laughed and clapped a hand on Andrew's shoulder. "Thanks, but no. I've heard enough about puck bunnies to walk the other way."

"That leaves it up to the wives. Word gets out we have a single doctor on the payroll, you'll receive a shit ton of dinner invitations to meet sisters, friends, daughters. Just saying, Tom."

"Well, I'm not on the Suns' payroll, and I *know* you guys don't normally share information of that sort. I'm good. If my potential soulmate's in Tampa, our paths will cross at the right time—you know, just like you and Caryn."

13

Several knocks on the front door finally caught Lauren's attention as she completed a recommended appearance schedule for a new client. "Coming!" she called, even though she could guess who she'd find on the other side of the door.

As soon as she turned the lock, Cassie practically danced through the doorway. "I have the best news—just couldn't wait to tell you!"

Lauren barely restrained her smile as her niece bounded in. "Something to drink first?" She guided Cassie toward the kitchen counter.

"Maybe in a minute." Cassie practically bounced from excitement on the counter-height bar chair. "Guess what?"

"The twins took their first steps today?"

Cassie stopped a second, imagining that moment. "No, but that will be a huge milestone." She drank from the water bottle Lauren placed in front of her. "You know how Caryn keeps telling me I need to get out and take some time for myself?"

"I agree." Lauren leaned against the counter and faced her niece. "That's got you so excited?" A teasing smile played across her face.

"No, of course not. But I appreciate it. I talked to my dad last night."

"How are they doing?"

"Great, if you don't count Taylor's going through the Terrible Three's." Cassie laughed, then continued. "Anyway, I asked Dad if he would co-sign a car loan for me. I need to get something I can drive without worrying about denting it or parallel parking."

"And he agreed," Lauren prompted.

"He did some research and asked me to choose among four cars." Cassie's smile widened. "I picked this cute little Honda Civic because I knew I could afford the payments. He said he'd call me back today. He did and guess what? He bought the car! It's ready for me to pick up whenever. He's taken care of the insurance, all those complicated taxes, and he won't let me pay him back. Said it's a graduation present to me from his family. Can you believe that, Lauren?"

Her aunt laughed when Cassie took a breath. "You know you have your dad wrapped around your finger. Trevor doesn't surprise me at all. Congratulations, Cass! Tell me he's not sending you a gas card, also?"

"Gas and maintenance come from my pocket, and maybe the insurance next year. He said he wants to see where I am first. Mom was *less than thrilled* when I told her." Cassie made a face. "Hopefully, I'll make good decisions and don't mess anything up."

"When in doubt, ask. I know it's hard stuck in the middle of divorced parents. Just focus on *your* future—they'll be proud no matter which road you choose." Cassie saw a speculative look cross Lauren's face. "So…you need a ride to pick up your car? Where's the dealership?"

Cassie pulled her phone from her pocket and opened a window before handing it to Lauren. "Please tell me it's not on the other side of Tampa."

"Actually, it's not too far. We can pick it up, then grab some dinner if Caryn doesn't need you."

Cassie sat in the driveway, inspecting every feature of her new car. *Everything I could want—or need.* She loved the sunroof that allowed the sunshine to roll across her. The GPS, once she figured it out, would take her wherever she wanted—like visit Amelie or drive out to the beach. The safety features freaked her out—she nearly slammed on the brakes when the lane departure warning caused the steering wheel to vibrate. The automatic braking system made some sense, but that orange "BRAKE" warning light flashing on the control panel caused her to slow down. *But it's all mine, and I love this car. Dad knew I'd choose this bright red color—though Lauren says it's a radar magnet. Probably the reason Dad chose it.*

She leaned back against the headrest and inhaled the new car scent. She knew how lucky she was to have her father support her. *Mom's pissed that Dad bought me the car, though she can't say much. Just stay out of trouble and don't make the same mistakes Lauren did. Will she ever let that go? Lauren and Dave are perfect together. Mom needs to accept that not all marriages end like hers.* A light rapping on the window startled her. A smile crossed her face when she saw Tom, and she quickly opened the door to greet him.

"Nice wheels, Cassie."

"I still can't believe it's mine. If you hadn't knocked on the window, I probably would have fallen asleep out here."

"Just pick it up?"

"About an hour ago. Lauren took me, then I followed her here. Even with this GPS that I don't know how to set up." Cassie shook her head. "Then I drove around the neighborhood to get used to all the safety cameras, brake warning, lane departure warnings…you know, this can make a driver nervous!"

"Good thing you practiced. Tampa traffic can be rough…brutal. Avoid the busy times, and you'll do fine," Tom said. He leaned to glance at the interior of the car. "Leather seats—nice. Heated?"

"Think so."

"Let's hope you don't need it while you're in Tampa."

Cassie dug the key out of her pocket and offered it to him. "Want to drive it?"

"Maybe we can go for a ride later—after the munchkins go to bed. See if we can figure out your GPS."

"Sounds like fun." Cassie closed the car door before she walked away. She smiled when the beep sounded, automatically locking the doors.

"Fancy," Tom teased as he headed toward his private entrance. "See you later."

Cassie allowed her eyes to trail after him as she walked to the front door. Every time he smiled, her heart did a tiny somersault. If his hand brushed hers, her body felt an electrical surge. *Forbidden territory. Silly to hope he might think of me as someone other than his brother's nanny. Not anyone he'd take out on a date. Keep dreaming, Johnson. Besides, there's his relationship with Katie. When does he have time to see her outside the hospital? He hasn't brought her to the house. At least not when I'm there. Maybe he goes to her place?*

Amelie squealed in delight when Cassie told her about the car. "We can go to the beach now! And check out anything that's not within walking distance of this condo."

"I haven't even seen what's around you. We'll have plenty to do on my days off."

"Like tomorrow?"

"Free. I want to see your neighborhood and the beach. If you send me your address, I should find you okay. Then we can figure out how to get to the Gulf." Cassie put her bikini and a towel on the dresser and then added a T-shirt cover-up.

"We could check out this area, go to the beach, then have a late lunch when we get back. Would that work for you, Cassie?"

"Just tell me the time. I'm a very early riser…more than ever since I've helped with the twins."

"So am I. Shops open at nine o'clock. Call or text when you leave —I'll stand by the entrance gate, so you don't miss it."

Cassie organized her all-purpose tote with everything she thought she might need. *Sunscreen. Glad Caryn has almost a case of different types. She said the sun's much stronger than in Canada. Amelie's hoping to meet some guys tomorrow…well, maybe me too. Just a fun, stress-free day with a girlfriend. And possibly some flirting with a few beach guys…surfers? Are there even waves in the Gulf? Guess I'll see.*

She heard Tom's voice, and like a moth attracted to light, she followed the sound.

"You're just in time for some pizza," he said as he greeted her. "My dinner contribution for today."

Cassie took a moment to appreciate the way the blue polo shirt stretched across his broad chest and noted the casual shorts he wore. *Tom does casual, very well.* She reached for the plates Caryn had just pulled from the cabinets.

"I invited Lauren to join us," Caryn said. "Terri and Kelly are still shopping."

"They won't miss the game?" Cassie asked.

"No, I seriously doubt that. Shall we eat in the sunroom?"

Cassie nodded and added silverware and napkins before moving to the sunroom. She heard the door open and Lauren's greeting. She laughed when Tom set the pizza boxes in the middle of the table. "Outnumbered again, Dr. Tom."

"And I should mind that?"

"Well, you have Daniel to help even the odds," Cassie said.

"My boy, Danny. Though, you realize I'm usually outnumbered by my brother's and his friends' wives."

Cassie saw the smirk hinting at his mouth.

"Well, Jenna and I aren't married," she added.

"Jenna, I can handle. You? Not so sure about that."

Cassie leaned against the table, her eyes challenging him playfully. "You don't think you can handle me?"

His response was interrupted when Caryn and Lauren brought drinks to the table. Cassie hugged her aunt, though her eyes drifted back toward Tom, silently questioning him. He merely winked in response, but that was enough to cause goosebumps to erupt all over her skin. *Is he teasing me or maybe something more?*

"Cass, what are you drinking?" Lauren caught her attention. "A glass of wine?"

"You don't mind, Caryn?"

"Of course not. You're legal age at home and if Lauren doesn't care…"

"Not planning to take your new car for a spin?" Lauren teased her niece.

"Not if I have a drink."

"Good answer," Tom said as he helped her finish setting the table. Their fingers brushed against each other, and Cassie swallowed a gasp as sparks sent tingles up her arm. She glanced to see if he noticed, but Tom had already taken the napkins to set beside each plate. She felt her aunt's eyes on her but averted her glance. *The less anyone knows about my crush, the better.*

14

"Hey, Cassie. Look at this."

Cassie reluctantly flipped over and balanced on an elbow to see what Amelie wanted to show her. The sun's warmth and the gentle sound of waves lapping at the shore had lulled her into a dream-like state. She took the card Amelie held toward her and squinted at it in the bright afternoon sun.

"Why did you get a Florida driver's license? Do you need it for work?"

"Check my age."

Cassie did some quick calculations, then looked at Amelie. "This is a fake?"

"It's just to get into clubs. Cliff has one, so I badgered him until he took me to get one. Don't tell anyone."

"Who would I tell?" Cassie laughed. She handed the ID back to Amelie and resumed her position on the beach towel.

"This beach is obviously not the place to meet guys," Amelie moaned. "Great for parents and little kids, though."

"Yeah, I can see Daniel and Jenna running around in the sand in a year. It's a nice beach, anyway."

"But absolutely no action."

Cassie heard the hint of disappointment in Amelie's tone. "You only wanted to come to the beach to meet guys?"

"Well…yeah."

Cassie swallowed a giggle as she sat up. "We could drive down the coast further. Maybe Clearwater's not the place college kids gather."

"That's obvious."

Cassie watched as Amelie's eyes swept across the beach. "Did Cam tell you where the college kids hang out?"

"Haven't asked him. Guess I will now. This place is d-e-a-d."

A glance at her watch confirmed they'd only been at the beach for about an hour. "Why don't we just relax and enjoy the sun? This is my first time at a beach. The water's so beautiful."

"Oh, you should see the Mediterranean…unbelievably blue. Gorgeous." Amelie lay on her stomach and pushed up on her elbows as she continued to scan the people.

Her eyes closed, Cassie resumed her fantasizing about the sexy doctor who probably has no clue what he does to her. *He can't know that he makes my temperature rise just by entering a room? Or how much I want to touch his biceps or those abs? Geez, when he swims his laps, I can't take my eyes off him. Wish he could treat me if I was ever in the ER. Though, my luck, I'd wind up with some older doctor who's ready to retire.* She closed her mind when her thoughts drifted to Jenna and Daniel. She'd never wish anything that could take them to the Emergency Room. *Can't believe that even flashed through my mind. No, he needs to notice me at home. Like the night we kissed, the other day in the swimming pool…maybe he can catch me skinny dipping some night?* She laughed to herself. The only one who'd likely discover her was Caryn or Andrew. *Total non-starter.*

After an additional thirty minutes in the sun, Cassie reluctantly agreed to scout other beaches in the area to find people their age. The GPS guided them to several areas south of Tampa, but none of the beaches appealed to Amelie. Finally, Cassie suggested they just head back to Tampa.

"It's getting toward mid-afternoon. I don't want to get stuck in traffic."

Amelie asked Cassie to stop at the grocery store on the way back.

Conveniently, a liquor store shared space in the same strip mall. After putting her sack of groceries in the car, Amelie headed toward that store. Cassie watched for a bit, thoughts of her mother's and grandmother's tendency to drink excessively crowding her brain. She knew they went to AA periodically, but neither thought social drinking—a glass of wine with lunch or a martini before dinner—presented a problem. Now that Cassie lived elsewhere, she could look at the situation more objectively.

She knew Lauren had talked to Amanda and encouraged her to take AA seriously. But Lauren refused to discuss the subject with her own mother, Cassie's grandmother. Not that Cassie blamed her. *With Lauren's nightmare childhood, I can see how hard it is for her to spend time with her mother, Allyson—which may be the reason she and Dave eloped instead of planning a big wedding.*

Amelie interrupted her thoughts when she called back to her. "Are you coming?"

"I'll wait here. I need to check in with Caryn. It's getting late." Sometimes the thought of falling into the same pattern as her mother and grandmother caused Cassie to detest the sight of alcohol. Things had improved, though, since moving to Tampa. She couldn't ask for better role models than Lauren, Caryn, and their friends. *Can't imagine any of them acting irresponsibly with alcohol.* But it didn't take much to remind her of the path her mother had chosen.

Lauren and Caryn sat by the pool when Cassie walked in after fighting early rush hour traffic. She asked if Caryn needed her to help with anything. "I'm sorry it's late. I need to figure out the traffic patterns—like when rush hour begins."

"Come, sit and relax," Caryn invited, patting the side of the pool. "Dip your feet in the water—guaranteed antidote for crazy Tampa traffic."

Cassie saw Lauren's surprised expression as she lowered herself to the tile.

"I thought you drove to the beach. Was it cloudy by the Gulf?"

"Yes, we spent about an hour at the beach in Clearwater. Sunny and beautiful."

"That's a wonderful area," Caryn added.

"And a great place to take the twins, maybe next summer. Downside, we were the only young people there." She shrugged. "I didn't care—just enjoyed soaking up the sun and listening to beach sounds. Almost fell asleep."

"Too tame for Amelie?" Lauren guessed.

"No guys to check out or flirt with. We were only there an hour before Amelie suggested we look elsewhere for a beach with more action." Cassie's laugh sounded forced. "I got more sun driving with the sunroof open than sitting on a beach. Drove about thirty miles—found nothing she wanted to try."

"I'll go to the beach with you soon," Lauren promised. "A crowded beach is not my idea of relaxation. We need to go to the restaurant Dave found south of here. The beach and the sunset were unlike anything I'd ever seen. Just spectacular—plus, the menu's wonderful."

"I'm sure Dave would rather spend a romantic evening with only you," Cassie teased. "You're still newlyweds."

"Nah, the honeymoon's over. We've had our first fight."

"I don't believe that," Caryn said. "What caused the argument?"

Lauren laughed, shaking her head. "Sounds so stupid now, but for a while things got hot." She looked at Caryn. "Remember when Jim Wesley recently called to see if we were interested in taking on some of those seminars, they thought they'd handle in-house?"

Cassie saw the look of disgust cross Caryn's expression. "We declined that. What did Dave find objectionable about that?"

"I mentioned it in passing, but before I could tell him that we said, 'No way in hell,' he started telling me he didn't want me working for 'that man.'" Lauren made a face. "And you know how much I enjoy someone telling me what to do."

"Even such a gorgeous, hunky husband?" Cassie teased.

"Especially not my husband. I told him he was acting like a caveman…one comment led to another until the whole thing got ridiculous. When I said we declined the contract, he's like, 'Why didn't you say so?' So, I informed my 'gorgeous, hunky husband' that had he contained his inner cave-dweller, I could have told him." She giggled, along with Cassie and Caryn.

"So, how was the make-up sex?" Caryn teased.

"Unbelievable! If I'd known…"

"Just remember to pick a fight every so often," Caryn replied with a wink.

"You don't do that with Andrew?" Cassie demanded.

"My secret. Just something to store in the back of your mind for future reference."

15

Tom's first official action as the concussion specialist came during the Suns second homestead. Chance Gagné took a massive hit against the boards. His head crashed against the glass, then in the ensuing retaliation, he somehow got shoved to the ice where his head took another blow. The Suns' trainer, Jim Pettit, hurried across the ice, and Tom watched on the monitor as the veteran pushed aside any offers of help and climbed back up on his skates. Gagné definitely did not want to leave the ice—his body language spoke volumes. He turned to skate away while the officials sorted out penalties, but Pettit grabbed his arm as did John Peterson. As they skated him off the ice, arguing the entire time, Tom grabbed what he needed and stood outside the dimly lit evaluation room.

"Come on, I don't need to get checked out. I'm fine. At least I'll be once I get back on the ice," Gagné grumbled.

The buzzer sounded, marking the end of the period, and Tom noted the involuntary cringe cross the defenseman's face. He caught Pettit's eyes and nodded toward the darkened room.

"Let us do our job, and you could get back in time for the third period," Pettit said. "Hop up on the table."

"This is bullshit, and you know it."

"Humor us." Tom resisted helping Chance up on the table, wanting to prove a point.

"Freaking skates."

Both Pettit and Tom grabbed arms before he could pitch forward, guiding, then lifting him up on the table. Tom kept his focus on the evaluation, even as Gagné resisted complying with the assessment. He ignored the string of F-Bombs the player muttered.

"Look, you say you're okay," he said finally. "If you'd shut up and cooperate, maybe we'll complete this in time to get you back on the ice." *Or to the hospital.* He kept that thought to himself, although Pettit's body language showed he agreed with the unspoken comment.

Tom knew he'd order a scan if Gagné presented at the ER. His eyes met Pettit's, who nodded his agreement. "I'll step out for a minute. Why not lie back and relax, Chance?"

He walked across the hallway to find Coach Harper waiting for him in the training room.

"What's the verdict, doc?"

"I'd prefer to send him to the hospital for a scan. Precautionary, but with those two head hits in succession…"

"Do what you need," Harper. "Cooperating, or do I need to speak with him?"

"I think he got the message." Tom first alerted the ER, per the procedure he and Dan Forster had devised. Either a senior Neurology Resident or Forster would meet the ambulance. The paramedics employed by the Suns had already positioned a gurney in the hallway. Tom nodded to them, then re-entered the darkened room. The smell of vomit did not surprise him, and Chance's demeanor had changed.

"What's the verdict, doc?"

"I've ordered a scan at the hospital. You have a concussion—the scan will rule out any complications. We'll monitor you for several hours, probably overnight, then hopefully we'll release you with recovery instructions or discuss treatment options." He watched the man's expression darken. "Can we call anyone for you? Wife? Girlfriend? Anyone at the game?"

"No need to call anyone. Let's just get this over and done with."

"The paramedics are ready to transport you," Pettit said. "Blakely has your wallet and clothes." He referred to assistant trainer Lucas Blakely. "You want to get out of the skates and pads before you go?" When Gagné nodded, Pettit stepped to the end of the exam table and quickly removed the skates. "Let's get you into some sweats."

"I'll see you either later tonight or tomorrow morning," Tom said when they were ready to transport. "Hopefully, to sign off on your discharge."

"I'd better hear you say that." Chance scowled as the paramedics moved him to the gurney.

Tom touched his shoulder. "I hope that, too. Just remember, you'll have the best doctors over at the hospital."

"Gotcha." Gagné finally closed his eyes as the gurney left the room.

Amelie invited Cassie to join her for dinner at The Center Ice Lounge. Amelie flashed her fake ID the moment they sat in a booth near the dance floor. Cassie ordered sparkling water and a tapas appetizer. She'd have ordered dinner had she'd known she would spend the evening watching Amelie flirt and dance with a constant stream of different guys. While Amelie danced, Cassie monitored the drinks her friend continually left on the table. *Surely, she knows the danger, right? Or is that why Amelie wanted me to go out with her—free ride and someone to make sure no one slips anything into her drinks? She should know better. Rather be home with the twins…*

Cassie had many guys approach her—some to chat for a while, others looking for a hook-up. She declined all invitations, even to dance. She'd loved dancing but knew she wouldn't enjoy herself if she lost track of her friend. Especially with Amelie's third—*or fourth?*—drink sitting on the table. She kept an eye on the Suns home game broadcasted on several large screen TVs.

Jenna and Daniel had seemed especially fussy earlier, so Caryn opted to stay home with the twins and had encouraged Cassie to enjoy an evening off. Now she wished she'd gone to the game. *Tom's working for the Suns tonight. I could have seen him if I'd gone with Lauren.*

Cassie glanced at the TV as Chance Gagné took the big hit into the boards. She cringed when she watched his head hit the glass and shuddered when two members of the team assisted him off the ice. *Holy crap! Wonder if he needs to get checked for a concussion? Is this the first player Tom's had to evaluate?*

When Gagné did not return to the ice at the start of the next period, she sent a text to Lauren.

Cassie: Chance all right?
Lauren: Not sure. Going to hospital for eval. Conscious, complaining
Cassie: Can I do anything?
Lauren: Don't think so. Will check in with you after the game.

Cassie waited until Amelie stopped by the table to quench her thirst before she told her about Chance.

"OMG! We need to go to the hospital. He's all alone." She drained the contents of her glass and grabbed Cassie's arm. "Let's go."

She ignored the slightly slurred words. "I don't know where they took Chance. Lauren will call when she knows something."

Amelie stared at her. "How can you just sit there so calm?"

"He didn't leave the ice on a gurney, Amelie." Cassie reached for her purse. "Have you settled your bill? By the time you get home, Cam should have an update."

"Soooo, no more dancing for you?" Amelie's worried expression morphed into a pout.

Cassie chose not to mention that she'd never left the table. "I'm tired. I think I should go home and relieve Caryn with the twins."

"Go ahead. I'll call Uber when I'm ready to leave."

"Seriously, Amelie? You don't want to get into an Uber alone. Come on, I'll drop you off."

Amelie rolled her eyes. "Yes, mother."

Cassie's cheeks burned as she led Amelie from the sports bar. *Wow, she's as self-absorbed as her twin. Acts like I'm the Fun Police.*

They drove in silence to Cam's condo, and Amelie exited the car with a muttered, "See you later, Cass."

After the game, Tom stopped by the hospital to check on Gagné. Once assured that no complications appeared on the scan, he looked for Lucas Blakely in the designated waiting area. John and Kelly Peterson arrived as Tom spotted Lucas. He updated the trio and tried again to obtain information on Gagné's family.

"There's nothing in his medical file," Lucas said.

"Never talks about himself either," John added.

"Who'd he list as emergency contacts?"

"Micky and Minnie Mouse."

Tom shook his head. "That needs to change. I know the guys don't take this seriously or think they could get hurt. I hate that we have no family contact information."

"I'll see if Pettit can touch base with his former team," Lucas said as he pulled his phone from his jacket pocket.

"They're running his name through the medical information database. Something may pop up," Tom added.

Blakely returned to the group. "Pettit's already on it. I'll hang around here for a while just in case Chance wants company."

Peterson laughed quietly. "Not likely, but we can stay, too."

Tom shook his head. "No need. He's out for the night. Any changes, I'll get the call."

"Thanks, Tom," John said. "We'll stay with Lucas until he hears from Pettit. Let us know if there's anything we need to do."

"You know the routine as well as I do." Tom referred to the days of uncertainty while Andrew fought to survive his TBI. The Petersons and Steve and Terri Rogers had encircled Caryn–and him—with support. His family owed a huge debt of gratitude for the many ways they'd supported Andrew on the long recovery. He said a silent prayer of thanks that Gagné's injury did not appear serious.

Cassie set the GPS for the Chadwick's and struggled to concentrate on driving while her mind wanted to scream in frustration. *So much for my new friend—if I wanted to chauffeur people, I'd work for Lyft or Uber. I will not screw up this opportunity. Why not just go out and enjoy dinner and dancing—forget about the drinking? Thought we'd do that tonight. Different agendas?*

The warning sound and vibrating steering wheel jerked Cassie's thoughts to the road. She hadn't even realized she'd drifted toward the adjacent lane. *Concentrate, Cassie. You can think about Amelie later.*

She arrived home before Andrew had returned from the game. Caryn dozed on the sofa and sat up reluctantly when Cassie walked in.

"Not a good evening for Jenna and Daniel?"

Caryn shook her head with a wan smile. "Teething again, I think. Just got them asleep."

"I'm sorry—I should have stayed home and helped you."

Caryn brushed the hair away from her face. "No, you need to get out. Have a good time with Amelie?"

Cassie shrugged. "It was okay, different." She laughed softly when she saw Caryn's perplexed expression. "She needs a designated driver and someone to make sure no one slips anything into her drinks…I think she's a lot like Cam, if I understand his reputation."

"Possibly. They *are* twins. You didn't drink?"

"Nothing but water. I promised myself I'll never drink, then drive. When I wouldn't let Amie stay and call Uber or Lyft for a ride later, Amelie got slightly peeved. She definitely had at least one too many drinks."

Caryn hugged her sympathetically. "I'm sorry. That's not exactly the type evening you had in mind."

"We'll see if she calls tomorrow—or even remembers tonight. Have you heard anything about Chance?"

"Drew said he's good. They're keeping him at the hospital tonight for observation." Caryn stifled a yawn. "Drew said he'll run by the hospital—no need to wait up for him."

"Why not get some sleep?" Cassie picked up the monitor. "I'll check on the munchkins and listen out. I'm kind of wired, so I won't be sleeping soon."

"I'm not arguing with you on this one. I'm exhausted." Caryn squeezed Cassie's hand. "Thank you. I'm proud that you played the responsible party tonight. I know that couldn't have been much fun."

"Honestly, I wish I'd stayed home or gone to the game. But, all's good, Caryn. Get some rest while you can."

About an hour later, Andrew and Tom entered the house together.

"My peanuts cranky this evening?" Andrew smiled when he saw Cassie.

"They fussed a bit…well, let's say they were cranky earlier. Caryn thinks they're teething again." Cassie bit back a smile. "She didn't argue when I suggested she get some sleep."

"Thanks, Cassie." Andrew opened the refrigerator and set two bottles of beer on the counter.

"How's Chance? That looked scary."

"He's okay," Tom said. "We're keeping him overnight as a precaution. Definitely has a concussion."

Cassie started to respond but glanced at her phone as a ringtone sounded. *Cam? What could he want? Maybe it's Amelie.*

"Excuse me," she said as she swiped to accept the call.

"Cassie. Do I need to pick up Amelie? Are you downtown? She's not answering her phone." Cam didn't wait for her to answer questions.

"Battery's dead," Cassie interrupted. "Have you checked her bedroom? I dropped her off a couple hours ago. She's probably deep in dreamland."

"Hang on." Cassie saw the question on both Tom's and Andrew's faces. She shrugged and waited for Cam to confirm that Amelie had fallen asleep. "When did you drop her off?" His question and tone surprised her.

"Not long after Chance left the game. She wanted to stop by the hospital, but Lauren said he was okay."

"Why the hell did she want to go there?"

"I don't know, Cam. Maybe they're friends? We were at a club, and I was ready to go. She wanted to stay and grab an Uber, but I asked her to leave with me." Cassie stopped to take a deep breath. "I dropped her off at your building's front door."

"Shit," he muttered. "Where were you tonight? Drinking?"

"Center Ice Lounge," Cassie said.

"How many drinks did she have?"

Cassie's patience ran its course. "I don't know. I wasn't counting."

"Drunk?"

"No, maybe buzzed, but definitely not drunk."

"Why the hell did you take her there, Cassie?"

She didn't like the implication in his tone. "I've never been there. She suggested it. I wanted to eat dinner, not drink it."

"You let her drink?"

"Hey, you got her the fake ID. I didn't know I was supposed to babysit. She had a few drinks and danced. With a lot of different guys. I assume you've taken her there. I'd never heard about it."

"Did she say she wanted to go anywhere else?"

"I. Don't. Know!" Cassie snapped. "The hospital? Back to the sports bar? Somewhere else? How would I know?"

She looked up when Andrew stepped beside her and held out his hand for the phone. Cassie didn't hesitate, giving him her phone and walking away, breathing deeply to calm her emotions. *How can he imply it's my fault?* She vaguely heard Andrew's sharp tone as he spoke with Cam, blinking back tears of frustration as she stared out the window toward the pool. She listened as Andrew suggested Cam contact Uber and Lyft or go back to the sports bar.

"I'll call Peterson at the hospital in case she's there or shows up later." Andrew listened a minute. "Don't panic. If she's using your Uber app, you can see where she's gone. Maybe check the clubs within walking distance of your place. If you need help, most of the guys were planning to go to Center Ice after the game. Call *me* back either way. And get your head out of your ass—you owe Cassie one huge apology."

16

She hadn't noticed that Tom stood beside her until Andrew returned the phone. He squeezed her shoulder. "Forget anything he said. You did nothing wrong."

"Thanks," she whispered. "Just so you both know, I don't drink, then drive."

"Thought never entered my mind," Andrew said. "Absolutely no reason to treat you rudely."

"That's not your fault, Andrew, but thanks for the backup. I might have said something I'd regret."

She heard Tom's quiet laugh. "There's more to this story?"

Cassie sank to the couch and swiped a finger under her eyes. "Maybe Cam's the same way…Amelie left her drinks on the table while she danced. Either she's clueless, naïve, or taking advantage of me. That's what I did tonight—chauffeur and make sure no one slipped anything into her drinks. Then stay alert in case I needed to stop her from leaving with someone."

Tom handed her a bottle of water as he sat beside her. "Not much different from babysitting the boy last season, right?" He looked at Andrew. "No common sense."

"Nice way to put it. So, Cassie, your evening out sounds more like hazardous duty," Andrew leaned against the back of the sofa.

"Did you at least get dinner?" Tom asked. "Center Ice has a great menu."

"Amelie wanted to have a drink before dinner, so I ordered some tapas. Amelie never stayed at the table long enough to eat."

"I missed dinner. Would you care to join me for an omelet?"

Cassie saw the smile that hinted at Tom's mouth. "You're cooking?"

"You bet." The wink caused Cassie's heart to flutter as Tom looked at his brother. "Give me your phone. I'll talk to Mr. Camden if he calls back. You may not get much sleep if the twins fuss again."

Andrew plugged the phone into a charger on the counter. "Get me if I'm needed. If Amelie's at Center Ice, one of the guys or wives should recognize her. In fact, Steve and Terri Rogers were heading there." He looked at Cassie and smiled. "Amelie's in for a rude surprise if Camden catches her flirting with any of the guys."

Tom refused Cassie's offer to help and suggested she relax while pushing the disastrous evening to the back of her mind. Content to watch him grate the cheese, then chop up green and yellow peppers, her gaze traveled from the doctor's broad shoulders to his perfect ass. The blue Suns' polo shirt only enhanced his athletic build...*definitely Dr. McHottie. None of my personal physicians back home ever came close...not even in the same universe.*

She shook her head and tried to stop staring. "So, you survived pulling a player from the ice?"

Tom glanced at her with a wry smile. "Not willingly, that's for sure. Unless they're unconscious or have a compound fracture, guys who play hockey never think they need to leave the ice."

"Did you play?"

She heard his quiet chuckle. "I played until major juniors. It was hard to accept that I didn't have the talent to go pro. Especially with my hot-shot brother. Coaches encouraged me to look elsewhere, go to college. So, I had no problem walking away when it came time to seriously concentrate on getting into med school." He cracked the eggs into a bowl and used a whisk to stir the mixture. "Following my super-talented brother left skates too big for me to fill."

"Andrew could say the same thing about you." Her phone interrupted the conversation.

"If that's Cam…"

"Lauren's ring tone." She picked up the phone. "You just get back from the game?"

"We went by the hospital first. Just checking that you're back home safely."

Cassie groaned. "Been home over an hour."

"Terri called to say a pretty buzzed Amelie came in Center Ice. We wanted to make sure you're okay."

"Did you call Cam?"

"Yes, on his way now." Cassie heard Lauren's laugh. "Getting a taste of his own actions and consequences. Anyway, Terri persuaded her to join the team's post-game meal. They were more concerned about you since Amelie told them she didn't know where you'd gone."

"She acted like I deserted her there? What an ungrateful…." Cassie bit her tongue.

"Terri said she made little sense. I just wanted to check in on my favorite niece. I know you wouldn't do anything irresponsible."

"I try not to do anything stupid." She looked up as Tom set a plate on the counter for her as she heard Lauren's soft laughter.

"You? Do something stupid? I know better than that."

Tom watched Cassie as she slowly savored her omelet. Her hair hid her eyes when she looked at the food, and he fought the urge to brush it aside.

"No highlights today?" Tom noticed the missing kaleidoscope of colors she used to highlight her hair. "Isn't this fuchsia day?"

She giggled as she swallowed. "Actually, I'd planned to use teal."

"Out of stock?"

"No, my new friend said it made me look…I don't know…juvenile. Translated—not classy." She met his eyes with a mischievous grin. "Maybe if I'd used three different colors, I'd have passed the sophistication test."

"Those colors are cute and…sexy."

Cassie rested her chin on her hand. "Are you color blind or something?"

Tom drank some water to keep from laughing. "Nope, I look forward to seeing what colors you choose each day. Suits your personality—and the highlights enhance your…" He paused, searching for the word he wanted. "Let's just say, you're gorgeous but edgy." He watched pink splotches forming on her neck and face. "I think your 'friend' doesn't want you to outshine her."

"Thank you, doctor, but don't worry about Amelie hurting my feelings. I just planned to have a fun evening with a new friend." She shrugged. "No big deal."

"Don't change for anyone, Cassie. No one who cares for you wants that." Tom watched her hazel eyes sparkle as she ate the last tiny bite of her omelet.

She slid off the stool and carried the dishes to the sink. "Bet you have a great bedside manner. You know just the right thing to say." She rinsed the plates and slipped them into the dishwasher. She took the silverware from him. "Tomorrow, I'll pick a color especially for you." She unsuccessfully contained the giggle that followed and turned her attention to the sink.

They heard a soft squawk on the baby monitor. Cassie quickly dried her hands. "I hope I can soothe them, so they don't wake Caryn." Tom followed as she quietly sprinted to the nursery. Once both had fresh diapers, Cassie caught Tom's eye and gestured toward the kitchen. "If they take a bottle now, maybe they'll sleep through the night," she whispered.

17

Cassie didn't hear from Amelie over the next few days—not that it bothered her…much. In her free time, she touched base with some friends from home. Most had scattered across Canada and some to the US, and she enjoyed chatting with them about campus experiences. *Parties, games, guys, fraternities, more parties, and oh yeah, studying, too.* Her inner voice questioned her decision to take a gap year…*maybe I should have gone to school in Toronto like Lauren? Perhaps I'd have more than one new friend. Or even a guy…*Tom flashed through her mind. She knew she had it bad for the doctor but didn't know how to interpret his playful teasing or flirtatious winks. *Interested in me?* But she knew he was off-limits for too many reasons. She had no one to confide in about her secret crush. *Definitely not Lauren. Last thing I need is for Tom to find out and avoid me.*

She gritted her teeth in frustration as she carefully applied a hint of rose gold to her hair. Using a slim brush, she added just enough to highlight her face. Then, because sunny days always lifted her spirits, she dipped the ends of her hair into a brighter rose hue.

Caryn had surprised her earlier in the day when she suggested Cassie attend the Suns game that night.

"Don't you want to go?"

Caryn shrugged. "More tired than usual. I'll enjoy a quiet evening with Jenna and Daniel, and no one will know if I fall asleep before the third period."

"If I help you, you could fall asleep before the game begins."

"Cassie, you're the most giving person I know. Enjoy an evening out. You can ride in with the girls. Go to Center Ice after the game and have fun! You know, I was about your age when I met Andrew." Caryn smiled mysteriously. "Who knows? You could meet your special guy."

Cassie felt her cheeks burning. "Unlikely, but I'd love to go to the game. As long as you really don't need me? I'll happily play with my cuddle bugs."

"Not tonight. You have fun—I insist."

Lauren had game credentials for Cassie, and she slipped the lanyard over her head. "Thanks, Lauren. Did Dave get these?"

"Picked them up at morning skate. Dave said to tell you he doesn't want to see you wearing another player's number."

"Like that will happen. If I get a jersey, I'll choose his. Family first, you know."

Terri looked over her shoulder from the front seat. "Don't count on that if you meet one of the cute young guys on the roster."

"Like that will happen." Cassie snorted.

"Maybe after the game, we can go to Center Ice—you can decide for yourself." Kelly showed her parking pass to the attendant and parked near the entry door reserved for players, family, and VIPs.

Cassie's eyes widened when she saw the suite reserved for family and friends. "You have this every game?" She asked Lauren, her voice barely above a whisper.

"Different menus, but yes, all you could ever want to eat or drink." Lauren took Cassie's arm. "I'll give you the tour. We'll get something to eat and drink before we go to our seats."

While waiting for her turn at the buffet, Cassie glimpsed Amelie across the room. *Will she acknowledge me? Or should I approach her?* She filled her plate with small samples of many foods and then followed Lauren down the stairs to the suite's front-row. She placed her drink in a cupholder, set her plate on the ledge, and took a few minutes to watch the team warm-up.

"I can recognize the guys I know without the helmets. I love Steve's hair, Terri. Just kinda flows with him. You know how…um… sexy he looks right now?"

"Definitely on my radar," Terri laughed. "I'll point out the available guys for you."

Since everyone seemed to have a preferred seat, Cassie indicated the one on the aisle. "This seat claimed?"

"It is now," Terri said. "We're not superstitious or anything, but we sit in the same place every game."

"Not superstitious?" Kelly added. "Just try to take that second spot."

Cassie giggled as she sat on the plush leather seat. "This is perfect. I love that Dave, Andrew, and John skate together."

"Especially when a certain defenseman joins in the rush," Lauren added.

"Speaking of…Jason Hart is single," Terri whispered. "Check him out, number twenty-six. Nice guy, too."

"Another hunk," Cassie sighed. "A girl can dream, can't she?"

"You never know what fate has in store for you. I grew up in the same neighborhood as Steve. My brother's best friend. I had such a crush on him—but all he saw was the tomboy sister and resident babysitter for my younger brothers."

"And how did you get him to break the bro-code? I know you had no problem getting his attention."

Terri laughed in memory. "Fate. He gave me a ride home from school when I was a senior. A storm was approaching, and my brother Bill said he'd pick up our younger brothers, so Steve volunteered to take me home. We stopped for the usual snow supplies, and when we left the store, the storm had already turned into a blizzard. We should have stayed at the store, but…" Terri shrugged. "We both thought we could get through it in Steve's four-wheel drive. Ten minutes later, the road disappeared, we couldn't see a thing and had to pull over."

"Yikes!" Cassie's eyes widened. "But maybe kinda romantic?"

Terri laughed. "No, not at all. I didn't panic until the snow started drifting over the hood of the car." She shuddered at the memory. "I'll never forget that. So cold, then dark when the snow buried the entire car."

"What did you do?"

"Steve called our parents to let them know we were okay, but stuck. They got his location from his phone's Find Friend app. We had to wait it out." Terri laughed softly. "Like an Eagle Scout, Steve had blankets, battery lanterns, emergency food, water…plus what we'd bought at the store."

"How long were you stranded?"

"Twenty-four hours."

"How'd you stay warm?" Cassie wondered.

"Body heat. We climbed in the back and wrapped ourselves in blankets. I'd have lost it if not for Steve's calm and the warmth…make that the *hot heat* that he generates. Eh, that's when things turned romantic."

"So, the end of Tomboy Terri in Steve's eyes?" Lauren guessed.

"Pretty much. When you're freezing cold, that bro-code flies right out the window."

"Details?"

"One of these days I'll tell you the story."

"Promise?" Cassie pictured an ultra-romantic scene. She turned when she felt a hand touch her shoulder. Her…*friend*…flashed a smile. "Amelie, nice to see you."

"Hey, Cassie. I hope you're not too angry with me. I don't remember much after you took me home, but I know I acted like a bitch." She sniffled and wiped her eyes. "I'm so sorry. I hope I didn't ruin our friendship?"

Sincere? Give her the benefit of the doubt? "Not ruined, but I'm not your designated driver the next time you want to go dancing and drinking." Her smile softened the words. "Anything new?"

"Working." Amelie looked around the box and waved at a group of women. "Your first time here?"

"Enjoying every minute, especially the view as the guys warm-up." She watched as Amelie's eyes turned toward the ice. "So,

Chance is cleared to play? That should cheer him up," Cassie commented.

Amelia grinned but didn't respond.

"You've seen Chance?"

"Just texting and chatting. Guess the concussion recovery took longer than he wanted."

Terri leaned forward to reply. "Post-concussion headaches are no joke. Glad he passed all the tests to clear him."

"If he weren't so stubborn, I could have brought him chicken soup or something." Amelie's expression morphed into a hint of a pout. "Said he needed nothing but dim lighting and quiet. So, I sent him a care package via Uber Eats."

"Thoughtful," Cassie said. "Does he live close to you and Cam?"

"A few blocks over." Amelie smiled coyly. "I'll surprise him one of these days."

"You may want to call first," Terri warned. "He's got a reputation. Be careful."

"Absolutely will." Amelie touched Cassie's arm. "Want to go to the beach or shopping this weekend? I'm tired of the stores within walking distance."

"Sounds like fun. I'll check with Caryn and let you know."

18

Like clockwork, Cassie's mother, Amanda, called each Saturday morning at ten a.m. Tampa-time. While she bristled a bit at the thought her mother felt she needed to check on her weekly, Cassie enjoyed hearing the news from Vancouver. Fall had given way to winter's chill early, and when Amanda mentioned the first snowfall, Cassie shuddered.

"I probably shouldn't tell you how beautiful and warm Tampa is right now?" Cassie said. "Or that we're going to the beach later today?"

"Only if you want to hear me cry!"

"Forget I said that. It's raining and miserable here."

Amanda laughed. "Have you started thinking about your next steps after this gap year ends? The year's quickly passing."

Cassie paused before answering, a sudden feeling of dread dropping over her like a shroud. "I'm looking at a lot of options. I'm torn between taking dance, teaching preschool, or maybe even communications like Lauren and Caryn."

"Cassandra, that's all over the map. Have you analyzed each option and identified where you'd study?"

"Working on it." Cassie tried to keep the prickly tone from her voice. "Trying to decide where I want to spend the next four years. I like Tampa, and there are opportunities here."

"And the universities that accepted you last year?"

"I need to see if any offer the programs I'm considering." Cassie absently played with her hair, wrapping some around her finger.

"Maybe try to narrow it down, Cassie," her mother suggested. "You can take dance classes anywhere. Maybe think about teaching versus communications. I'm sure many universities offer both programs, and Lauren can help you narrow your choices. That would be a place to start."

"Always the practical answers." *I can't tell her I'm considering not going to college. Not yet. Not everyone needs to go to the uni.*

"Don't wait too long," her mother advised. "I'm sure deadlines for applications aren't too far in the future. Have you made arrangements to visit us at Christmas?"

"I need to talk with Caryn. Andrew has a three-day break over Christmas, so if I come, I won't have much time. But I'd miss seeing you, Dad, and Taylor."

"Speak with your dad. Last I heard, he planned to book a Disney Christmas cruise. But your grandmother and I would love to have you visit. I don't suppose Lauren's mentioned their plans?"

"We haven't even thought about Christmas. With this weather, it's tough remembering what month it is." Cassie glanced at her watch, double-checking that October still had another week. "I'll start working on all the above. Maybe I'll have narrowed my choices in a few weeks."

Phone conversations with her mother left Cassie feeling anxious. She liked to live in the moment, not plan years into the future. She loved her job, loved living close to Lauren and Dave, and loved the twins more every day. *I need to find a way to do both—work for Caryn and Andrew and enroll in school to study...something? Can't keep putting it off. Maybe more research into the schools here?*

She opened her laptop and quickly checked the universities that had accepted her last year. All offered Early Childhood Education, but Communications programs proved not as easy to find. The university in Tampa offered a wide choice of communication majors. *Public Relations? Marketing? Something like Lauren and Caryn's company? Wonder if they'll eventually hire an assistant? Lauren could tell me what I'd need to choose as my major.*

Cassie logged off her computer and wandered to the living area. The twins had pulled every toy from the bin, or most of them, dragging them to all corners of their play area.

"They look so pleased with themselves," she told Caryn with a laugh.

"Very proud. I tried to contain the hazard to just part of the room." She showed the soft cushions that prevented Jenna and Daniel's access to the entire open area. "Once they figure out how to climb…we may have to consider a playpen."

"Somehow, I don't see them…" Cassie stopped mid-sentence when Andrew and Tom entered the house. Tom's face was flushed as if he'd just come from practice. "Is the team doc working out during practice?" She captured Tom's brown eyes as a teasing smile crossed her face. "Or trying out for a spot on the roster?"

"Hardly. Checked in on some patients, then hit the wellness center afterward." He nodded toward the toy-strewn play area. "It appears Jenna and Daniel had the same idea."

"You mean make more work for Cassie and me?" Caryn challenged. She turned to Andrew. "Remember, swimming lesson this afternoon."

"You bet—looking forward to finally getting in the pool with these peanuts. You ready to swim, Danny?" Both babies' faces lit up when they saw Andrew kneel beside the cushions. They crawled toward him, then fussed when they couldn't reach him. Jenna batted at a pillow, trying to move it.

"Drew, please don't let them discover how to climb over the barricade." Caryn quickly lifted Daniel before he focused on the cushions. Andrew laughed, then did the same with Jenna.

"How about I help you with lunch?"

"How about you maneuver your peanuts into their highchairs while

I prepare lunch?" Caryn countered with a saucy grin. "Maybe they can get a nap in before the swim lesson."

Caryn glanced over her shoulder to double-check that the door to the lanai was closed. Cassie knew Caryn's greatest fear—*obsession*— that one or both twins might accidentally slip into the pool. She'd already installed child-proof locks on every door and cabinet—even Cassie had difficulty bypassing them. *Hope the swimming lessons help with that anxiety...hers and mine.*

Cassie stepped over the cushions and began collecting toys to return to the toy bins. A moment later, Tom joined her.

"Looks like a disaster area," he said as he gathered several toys.

"They have fun tossing these around. Jenna has quite an arm." Cassie stole a glance at Tom and saw the teasing sparkle in his eyes,

"Baseball, you think?"

"Maybe. Or volleyball?" *Does Tom know how incredibly sexy and irresistible he looks right now? With those brown eyes...and that smirk. I'd like to wipe that away with a kiss. Or three.* She startled as a nerf ball bounced off her shoulder.

"Earth to Cassie—you were supposed to catch that."

Cassie bent to pick up the orange ball, then eyed Tom while biting back a smile. "So, you waited until I didn't see it coming?"

"Maybe." Tom gathered additional toys and tossed them into a basket. "You're an attractive target."

Cassie tossed the ball at his head when he reached for several toys that had landed outside the barrier. He glimpsed the ball just as it approached his face and caught it with one hand, and then immediately threw it back, striking Cassie squarely in her face.

She pretended to collapse against the cushions, covering her face with her hands. "I surrender!"

Tom collected the remaining toys, then grabbed the bin containing all the nerf toys and dumped it over the prone Cassie. She glared at him before the laughter bubbled up within her.

"You rat!" She grabbed toy after toy to fling back at him, jumping over the cushions to duck and avoid the next attack. Cassie laughed so hard she couldn't catch her breath, finally lifting both arms in surrender. Tom flopped on the cushions opposite her.

"Admitting defeat?" The corners of his mouth quirked, stopping just short of a smirk.

Cassie tucked her hair behind her ears while she attempted to control her giggles. Tom waved a nerf dinosaur in her face, and she swatted at his hand. "Enough!" she begged. Tom caught her hand, and a sudden surge of electricity pulsed through her body. From the expression that briefly flashed across Tom's face, Cassie thought he felt the spark, too. Their eyes met, and although she wanted to turn away, the intensity in his eyes held her captive. She saw him glance at her lips, and without thinking, Cassie leaned toward him. He dropped her hand and lightly ran his fingers across her lips. Cassie opened her mouth slightly, inviting the kiss. She closed her eyes in anticipation.

Tom cleared his throat, and Cassie looked up, noting that his gaze traveled behind her. She covered her face in embarrassment when she heard Caryn's voice.

"Drew, I think we just solved the mystery of where Jen and Danny learned to throw toys."

"Thought you guys were cleaning up? You've expanded the disaster area." Andrew didn't hide his amusement.

Tom pushed to his feet and offered his hand to Cassie. "Just an impromptu indoor snowball fight."

"Snowball fight, eh? With the twins' soft toys. Clever, brother."

Cassie didn't dare look at them. "We'll get everything picked up now." She knew her face and neck had splotched red. "We just got a little carried away."

"Looks like you had fun," Caryn teased them. "We'll see if these two settle down for a nap before swim lessons. Drew and I may sneak in a little nap of our own."

19

Over the following days, neither Tom nor Cassie mentioned the "snowball fight," and both acted as if nothing had changed between them. However, Tom's thoughts wandered to Cassie unexpectedly throughout the day. *What guy wouldn't be attracted to her?* He'd seen the hope and invitation in her eyes, and he would have kissed her if Caryn and Andrew hadn't interrupted. *Took that chance once before. Nothing's changed since then. Any misstep and Cassie could leave her job, Caryn would no longer have her nanny, and I'd need to look for a new place to live. Not to mention incurring Lauren's wrath. We played with fire once before and no one knows, but that luck could turn in an instant.*

The problem? *Cassie's not only drop-dead gorgeous, she's also a free spirit. Full of energy and positivity that never dims.* He enjoyed her optimistic personality, which only added to her enticing aura. She made Tom realize there's more to life than existing in the halls of the hospital. As long as he and Katie had dated each other casually, their infrequent free evenings inevitably found them discussing work. He wanted a life outside medicine and the hospital.

Cassie made him laugh, maybe feel his age again? With her, he could leave the hospital behind and just enjoy life as a twenty-something. The age difference didn't bother him—five or six years? *Not much different than Andrew and Caryn.*

His personal life had languished while he focused on his education. When Andrew suffered the brain injury, Tom moved to Tampa to support Andrew and Caryn through the fifteen-month rehabilitation program. During that period, he also entered the neurology residency program, which also had its own demanding schedule.

When Andrew first entered the NHL, Tom had enjoyed going out with him after games. He had his share of girls hitting on him, and he made the most of it for a while. When the pre-med studies demanded more and more of his time, Tom reluctantly excused himself from most team gatherings. Soon, he had no free time to even think about girls, much less begin a relationship.

He had to talk with Andrew and Caryn—and Lauren—before exploring any kind of non-platonic relationship with Cassie. She may have no desire to go out with him, could be thinking about the single guys on the Suns. *Harmless flirting? She might not even think about me that way. But did she also feel that electrical current when our hands touched?* Cassie could see him as honorary big-brother, the same relationship he enjoyed with Caryn and Lauren. But neither of his "little sisters" had ever produced that spark, and he definitely did not look at Cassie in that way.

Cassie invited Amelie to spend an afternoon at the Chadwick's after Caryn had mentioned that Amelie might feel lonely with the Suns on a four-game road trip. Tom offered to pick her up on his way home from the hospital, saving Cassie the trip, and suddenly the afternoon by the pool morphed into an impromptu get together.

"You're sure, Caryn? Feels like I'm slacking off on my job?" Cassie asked for the tenth time.

"How so?"

"I should help you feed Jenna and Daniel dinner and get them ready for bed instead of hanging out with a friend."

"Don't worry about me, Cassie." Caryn laugh was lighthearted. "I have plenty of back-up. Not sure what you and Amelie have planned, but Tom's grilling barbecue for Terri, Kelly, Lauren, and me. You're welcome to join us."

Cassie smiled as she flashed on the last meal he'd cooked for her. "Can't think of a better option than that!" *Plus, no barhopping with Amelie and perhaps extra time with Tom. Sweet.*

Within the hour, Cassie regretted extending the invitation. Amelie openly flirted with Tom and entertained the entire group with tales about student life in Paris. *If she bats those eyes one more time when she looks at him, I'll scream. So obvious.* She couldn't read Tom's expression, but he laughed with everyone else as Amelie spun her stories.

Lauren caught Cassie's expression and winked before she spoke. "I guess you're eager to get back to Paris. I loved visiting a few days after our cruise. I think I could spend months as a Parisienne."

"We all could," Kelly added. "You grew up in Québéc, so communicating in French is not a difficulty for you?"

"Maybe just a little. I had to lose my Québécois accent—no one understood me. Or chose to understand me. I did a quick immersion course the week before classes started."

"My grandparents are native Montréal," Caryn said. "My grandmother's bi-lingual but will only speak Parisienne French. Drew practiced for hours with me before he met her the first time."

Lauren smiled. "Madame Martineau. I'll never forget your wedding. You know how bad my French is, Caryn. When we went to the brunch she hosted the morning after the wedding, I panicked when she spoke to me. Luckily, Marty was beside me—his French is flawless." She bit back a laugh. "As hungover as I felt, I doubt I'd have been able to stand upright, much less speak French without him."

"So, what's his name, Dave or Marty?" Amelie asked. "You speak of both, and I'm wondering if you have two husbands."

Cassie watched Lauren shake her head and attempt to suppress laughter. "One is plenty for me, thank you. Dave is his given name, but I started calling him Marty when I heard his teammates in St. Louis use that nickname. I'm about the only one who uses that anymore—the Suns christened him Martini."

"I love nicknames!" Amelie gushed. "Some are hilarious." She looked at Kelly. "When I hear someone call your husband 'Captain Jack,' I picture him just like Johnny Depp."

"Yeah, he's not fond of that one…but it could be worse, I guess." Kelly helped herself to another piece of chicken. "Compliments to our chef."

"Do you deliver?" Amelie asked Tom, an inviting smile crossing her face.

"Sorry, no time for that." Tom returned the smile when he responded.

Cassie couldn't resist interrupting the flirt fest. "So, Amelie, I meant to ask you. Anything new with Chance?" She caught Lauren's smirk from the corner of her eye, even as she tried to cover it by sipping her wine.

"Are you seeing that gorgeous man?" Terri's eyes widened. "Just looking at him lights a fire...he's got that smoldering French thing going."

Amelie shot a look—*irritation?*—at Cassie. "Chance is fun…if you like bad boys." She locked eyes with Tom as she spoke, a smile flirting at her mouth. "Nothing serious. Just fun."

Cassie watched Tom as he stood to clear the table. "Can I get anything for anyone? More wine?"

Terri nodded, extending her glass, "Please. As always, you prepared a fantastic feast. You're our Top Chef."

Tom laughed as he met Cassie's eyes. "Top off your glass?"

"I'm good." She stood and gestured for Tom to stop clearing the table. "I'll get this. Our chef does not clean up. Why don't you all relax by the pool? It won't take a minute." She shook her head as others offered to help. "Seriously, I've got this."

Amelie grabbed the wine bottles and followed everyone to the pool deck. Lauren hung back, waiting until they were alone to speak. "Do I sense a little irritation with your guest?"

Cassie shrugged. "She enjoys being the center of attraction."

"Tom didn't seem too impressed by her escapades," Lauren ventured cautiously as she rinsed the plates.

"He looked like he was enjoying himself, especially when she batted her lashes at him. Don't blame her for flirting. Tom's great, but she'll be disappointed to know he has a girlfriend."

Lauren looked at her in surprise. "Seriously? Who? When did this happen?"

"You know—Katie. Haven't they had a thing for a long time?"

"Eh…Katie took a job in Minnesota not too long ago. Far as I know, they never quite made it past the friends' stage." Lauren eyed Cassie speculatively. "Do I detect some interest in the resident physician?"

"Just friends," Cassie turned toward the sink, hoping that Lauren didn't see her face flush. *No Katie? So, no more guilt that I'm lusting after a guy who's involved with someone? Hallelujah! Not that it changes anything.*

"Remember, Marty and I started as friends." Lauren prodded.

"Lauren, stop! Seriously? Why even put that thought out there?"

Lauren hugged her and kissed her cheek. "Your secret's safe with me."

20

Life decisions stayed on the back burner as the days flashed by. Cassie participated in the twins' swimming lessons, and she sometimes teamed up with Tom to give Caryn opportunities to go out with her friends. She enjoyed those days especially, though she was unsure if Tom looked at her like a younger sister—or maybe, just maybe, thought about her as more than a friend? She definitely felt chemistry brewing between them, but he had yet to do anything more than flirt with her. Cassie considered making the next move but rejected that notion when she realized how uncomfortable things could get if she'd misread the situation.

Lauren and Dave invited her to join a post-game celebration at The Center Ice Lounge. Cassie hadn't gone there since that evening with Amelie, and Caryn, and Lauren insisted she needed a fun night out.

"So, we're celebrating your two goals, Mr. Martin?" she teased as they entered the sports bar.

"Nope, our fifth win in a row." Dave's grin filled Cassie with happiness. He'd become the big brother she'd always wanted, and she loved him for never giving up on Lauren.

"Don't I need an ID?" she asked as they walked toward the bar section at the back of the restaurant.

"Are you planning to drink?"

"Maybe some water."

"You're fine," Lauren said with a laugh. "Relax—I'll share my drink with you."

Many of the team wives and girlfriends had already arrived, and a wide selection of finger food, appetizers, and chips awaited them. Cassie waved when she saw Amelie across the room, chatting with Chance Gagné. *So, she really knows him. Very well, if the body language is any sign. She smiled when Amelie met her eyes and discretely flashed a thumbs up.* Dave held chairs for Lauren and her, then went to the bar to order drinks.

"Your friend likes to play with fire." Lauren leaned closer to Cassie and nodded at Gagné.

"Did you say anything to Cam?"

"He didn't seem concerned. Reminded me Amelie attended the university in Paris and can take care of herself."

Cassie sniffed. "Maybe she set him straight the last time he intervened. Remember when she came back here after I'd taken her home the night Chance took the concussion."

"Yep. Two peas in a pod." Lauren looked up as Dave placed a frozen margarita in front of her and set a glass and a bottle of Perrier before Cassie.

"Sorry, kiddo," he said. "I'd be a hypocrite if I got a margarita for you after keeping the young players on a short leash."

"Not a problem. Thanks for letting me tag along."

Lauren laughed as Dave took the seat beside her. "You're *not* a tag-along, Cass. We should have done this sooner."

"Sure, with all your free time. This is a treat." Cassie felt a hand touch her shoulder and turned to find Cam Camden pulling back the chair beside her.

"Mind if I join you?" He flashed that high wattage smile that no doubt melted many girls' hearts.

She shrugged nonchalantly. "Help yourself."

He leaned across her to speak to Dave. "Good game, man. Feels great back in first place."

Cassie noticed that he held a bottle of beer. He caught her glance and shrugged, keeping the drink below the edge of the table. He winked as if they shared a secret, and Cassie politely returned the smile he directed at her.

"Haven't seen you around. Have you gone to any games?"

"A few. The twins keep me busy, and I'm looking at options for next year."

"Yeah? Amelia trying to talk you into moving to Paris?" Cam tried again with what she thought of as his heart-flipping smile. *For me? Nothing flips, tingles, or makes me feel special...he uses that smile on every girl.*

Instead of answering the question, Cassie asked, "She decide when she's returning?"

"Hoping she'd mentioned something to you." His grey eyes met hers expectantly.

"Sorry, not a word. Why, are you two not speaking?" She felt Lauren shift beside her and knew she was suppressing laughter.

"Not about school. Amelia said not to 'pressure' her." He used air quotes to highlight the word.

"Cassie can relate to that," Lauren spoke up, turning toward them. "The bigger the decision, the less pressure tolerated. I know that from personal experience. Amelie's young—plenty of time to decide about her future."

Cam smirked. "Especially when you have no financial obligations." He glanced across the room, his eyes tracking his sister's animated conversation with Gagné. Cassie saw his jaw clench slightly before he looked away, slowly shaking his head. He returned his attention to Cassie.

"Can we get together and catch up? Maybe over dinner?"

She hesitated for a long moment. "I need to check my schedule. Call me."

He nodded before he pushed back his chair and touched her shoulder lightly. "I'll look forward to that. I've planned to call you for weeks."

"Life gets busy. Totally understand."

"Call you soon."

"Whenever you have time." Cassie hoped her smile reached her eyes. "Good seeing you again."

As Cam moved across the room, Lauren nudged Cassie. "Well played."

"Honestly? I don't care if he calls or not. His ego can't handle rejection."

Dave caught her eyes. "Do I need to have a chat with him?"

Cassie laughed. "Don't bother, Dave. I haven't encouraged him."

Lauren slipped her arm around her shoulders for a hug. "You deserve better."

Cassie smiled, wondering again if Lauren suspected she was crushing on the doctor living under the same roof.

21

Andrew persuaded Tom to stop by Center Ice before heading home. "You know Caryn, Kelly, and Terri host that meeting for the spring Monte Carlo Gala. You get back too early, and they'll decide you need to take part in the 'Date with a Suns Bachelor' live auction."

"Right." Tom didn't hide the sarcasm. "First, I'm not a Suns 'bachelor,' and second, I'll probably work that evening."

"I don't think the date's confirmed," Andrew countered.

"I'm sure I'm working, don't worry. Told you, I don't think it's a good idea to mingle with the players outside the arena."

Andrew slapped his shoulder as he opened the door. "Just one drink to celebrate the win, bro. Don't worry about the team—they probably won't even notice." He led the way to the private room at the back of the bar. "You can hang out with the Martins while I complete my assistant captain duties. Cassie's here, too."

Tom shrugged, the hesitation disappearing when he spotted the girl with light brown hair with the Suns' blue highlights. *Maybe not such a bad idea.* "Go take care of your responsibilities. I'll grab a beer and hang out in friendly territory."

He picked up a couple bottles of beer at the bar and offered one to Dave when he reached their table. "Mind if I join you?"

"Of course not. Good to see you, doc."

"Lauren, Cassie, can I get you anything?"

Cassie patted the chair beside her. "I'm good."

"Lauren?"

She pointed at the second margarita before her. "I'm more than okay. Sit down and relax."

"I didn't know you went to the post-game celebrations," Cassie commented as he pulled his chair beside hers.

"I don't. I grabbed a ride with Andrew, and he said he needs to make an appearance." He rolled his eyes as Cassie laughed.

"So, he dragged you in here?"

"Pretty much."

"Can't shirk those Assistant Captain duties," Dave joked. "You won't see me wearing an A on my uniform."

"So, he says." Tom glanced around the area, focusing a moment on Chance Gagné. "Example. I come in here and see a player several weeks post-concussion tossing back beers. Do I find a subtle way to remind him he shouldn't be drinking, or do I pretend I didn't notice?"

"Okay, why don't you and Cassie take those seats across from us?" Dave suggested. "Then you won't see anything you shouldn't. Problem solved."

Tom shook his head as he pushed his beer across the table and helped Cassie stand. "Out of sight, out of mind. Whatever."

"You really don't want to be here?" Cassie spoke quietly as they walked around to the other side of the group of tables.

"The present company makes that a difficult question to answer," Tom said with a smile. "But, overall, no, I don't believe in socializing with players I might have to remove from a game."

"But what about Dave, Steve, John…"

"We've been friends long enough, and they get the importance of erring on the side of caution if there's a chance of concussion. Most of the others, I don't normally socialize with—and I don't want to muddy the waters."

"Like don't socialize with people you supervise in any job. I get that."

Cassie loved the way his hand rested against her back. *He must know how he affects me...there goes my heart skipping a beat again. What if I just turn around, step into his space, then just show him what he does to me?*

She saw his lips hint at a smile as Tom pulled back the chair for her. *Did he sense what I want to do...a neurologist mind reader?* Cassie saw Lauren watching them with a pensive expression as they sat at the table.

When Cam Camden called the following day, Cassie tried to mask her surprise. "Cam? What's up?"

"Just wanted to tell you I enjoyed seeing you last night. I honestly don't know why I haven't been in touch before." Cam's tone projected sincerity.

"Busy schedule," Cassie commented. "No problem."

"That's not an excuse. But I'd like to change that—Amelie and I are hosting a small get together tonight. Casual. Mostly younger guys on the team and friends."

"Tonight? Don't you guys leave town tomorrow?"

"Tomorrow afternoon. Really, this is a casual gathering, nothing special."

Cassie hesitated, "I don't know if Caryn and Andrew have plans."

"It's last-minute and spur of the moment, but that's the way we roll." He paused a moment. "I think you'll enjoy the evening."

That voice—sounds so persuasive...but sincere? Should I give him a chance? Do I even want to? What if Tom's not working tonight? I'd rather see him...

"I'm not sure, Cam. It's last-minute...I need to check with Caryn. Can I call you or Amelie back? What time does this start?"

"We're flexible. Come early and beat the traffic, or late and miss the traffic. Everyone else lives in this area," Cam said. "Or, I could pick you up. Amelie wants to see you."

"If this works out, what can I bring?"

"Just yourself."

"Okay. Let me talk with Caryn. I'll let you know." Cassie ended the call and thought about the unexpected invitation. Her mind took her back to the day she met Cam at the kickoff for the anti-bullying campaign. *Can't deny the instant attraction. Then no contact for six-seven weeks until the wedding reception. Said he'd call...Then radio silence until now. Do I even want to go to his party?*

Cassie wandered to the pool deck to watch the twins' swim lesson. She laughed quietly as Danny resisted Andrew when he tried to steer him back toward the steps. *No fear in that boy. Jenna doesn't allow Caryn to step one foot away from her.* Even with the life vests providing plenty of support, Jenna clung to Caryn's arm and resisted putting her face in the water. Danny had mastered blowing bubbles in one lesson. The instructor had predicted he'd swim like a fish before long. *Maybe this week?*

She snapped some photos with her phone after she sat on the edge of the pool. She AirDropped an adorable shot of Andrew and Danny to Caryn. Mr. Stubborn resisted all efforts to return to the steps until Andrew whisked him out of the water and held him like an airplane as he walked back to the sloped entry. Danny laughed and demanded more, pointing toward the water.

"Not now, bud. Swim lesson's over."

Cassie scrambled to her feet, grabbed a towel, and reached for Daniel. "I can take him. He's a little fish, isn't he?"

Andrew shook his head with a smirk. "More like a baby shark."

Wow, he looks so much like Tom with that smile. Makes my heart beat more quickly, just thinking about Tom. Do I really want to go to a party when I might see him? She wrapped the towel around Daniel, containing his attempts to resist and avoiding the kicks from his chubby legs.

"Hey, tiger, you don't want to hurt Miss Cassie." Andrew wrapped a towel around his waist and took the squirming bundle from her. "Did he kick you?"

"No, I'm learning his moves. Though, you may have a future martial artist on your hands."

Caryn laughed slightly as she carried Jenna from the water. "That, we don't need."

Cassie reached for a towel for Jenna and wrapped it around her as Caryn spoke with the swim instructor. Cassie pressed her lips against the cheeks peeking from within the fluffy wrap. "Did you have fun, Jen? Let's get you changed while Mommy's busy." She glanced at Andrew as she walked past him. "Give me a few minutes, and I can give him a quick bath along with Jenna."

22

"What would I do without you?" Caryn asked fifteen minutes later after Jenna and Daniel settled in for their later-than-normal afternoon nap.

"They're adorable. The difference in their strength is noticeable now—especially over these last few weeks."

"He's more than compensated for being the runt at birth. Can you believe Jenna weighed a pound heavier than Danny at birth? Their next checkup should be interesting. I think he'll jump to the ninetieth percentile in both weight and height, while Jenna remains around the sixtieth." Caryn chuckled as they walked from the darkened room. "And I worried Danny would always be smaller."

"No worries now, that's for sure. Takes after his dad, I think."

"Let's hope so." Caryn glanced at Cassie. "Did you make plans with Lauren or Amelie tonight? Take advantage of the last quiet evening before the road trip begins tomorrow?"

"Not yet. Surprise—Cam called a little while ago and mentioned a party at his place. That was unexpected."

"Do you want to go?" They walked toward the kitchen as they spoke.

Cassie shrugged. "Not sure. I said I needed to check with you

Actually, I hope I can take the twins, and you and Andrew can plan a romantic evening?" A teasing smile crossed her face. "Is this that long road trip?"

"Five games. We're not going anywhere tonight, Cassie. Andrew wants to spend as much time as possible with our love bugs," Caryn said. "When you're married a few years and add children to the mix, a quiet evening at home together is our idea of romantic. So, make some plans."

Cassie laughed. "Lauren says she and Dave chose a romantic evening at home, too. I wouldn't want to be a third wheel with the newlyweds."

"I'm not pushing you out the door, Cassie. But I can promise you a quiet night around here. Tom's meeting a friend of ours for dinner—the nurse who helped me during my pregnancy emergencies."

Cassie felt her heart fall with a thud. "That's Katie, isn't it? The one who moved?"

"Yes, I'll see her tomorrow. She's just in town a few days to get some paperwork processed at the hospital. She will not believe how big our little angels have grown." Caryn touched Cassie's arm. "Make plans if you want to go out—or enjoy the evening with us. You're part of our family."

"Thank you," Cassie said, wishing she could capture the warmth washing over her. "I love your family." She paused for a moment. "Maybe I'll go to the party for a while…I don't know. I haven't seen Amelie in a while."

"Cam asked you as his date?"

Cassie shrugged. "Don't think so. 'Come early, come late, just an informal gathering.'"

"If you feel any hesitation, don't go. We may take advantage of some time without Drew's peanuts," Caryn encouraged. "But, if you want to go, take an overnight bag in case you and Amelie want some girl time. Just don't go because you think you need to give us privacy. When we close the bedroom door, that's our special time."

"Thanks, Caryn. I'll think about it and check-in with Lauren. I'll let you know once I figure it out."

Cassie lay back on her bed and debated if she wanted to accept Cam's invitation. *He suddenly wants to see me. Why now, after all this time? Just because he saw me last night? Has he forgotten the rude accusations when he thought I'd taken Amelie clubbing and encouraged her to drink? Is this "typical Cam" attention?*

But no need to hang around here tonight. Tom's out with his ex—they'll probably realize how much they miss each other. There goes that fantasy. That's all it is, really. Tom knows I'm still trying to decide "what I want to do when I grow up." Wake-up call? Time to stop fantasizing about my hot hockey doc?

Impulsively, she grabbed her phone and pressed Amelie's number. Her friend's greeting lessened her disappointment...*make that reality check.*

"Cassie! Cliff said he invited you to our get-together tonight—can you come?"

"Who will be there?" Cassie asked. "He said you just decided to have a few friends over?"

"Yes, we used to do this all the time at home. You'll know a lot of the guys—some rookies on the Suns, their dates, oh...Chance is coming, too!"

"Seriously? So, he's going to...chaperone...the young guys?"

"Highly unlikely," Amelie giggled.

"Everyone's coming with a date?"

"It's not like that, Cass. Just a bunch of friends hanging out. Please say you'll come."

Cassie asked, "What time?"

"As soon as you can get here, Cassie. I could use some help to get things ready. Cliff thinks all he needs is a cooler filled with beer and bags of chips. I told him we needed to up that game. We just placed a ginormous order, and I sent him out for mixers, beer, and wine."

"So, *you're* the one putting this party together? Casual?"

"Definitely. Please come as soon as you can. Bring a bag in case you stay overnight. Then you won't need to worry about enjoying a few drinks!"

Cassie had already pulled a pair of skinny jeans from the closet to pair with a crop top. She didn't plan to spend the night but packed a change of clothes and toiletries in her backpack, along with one of Dave's Suns T-shirts—just in case.

Cassie touched base with Lauren to fill her in on her plans.

"That sounds like fun, Cass. About time you went to a party!"

"Sounds like Cam invited some younger players…Guess who's Amelie's date?"

She heard Lauren's quiet laugh. "Don't suppose it's that sexy French dude she was…let's say very cozy…with the other night."

"Could be the same."

"Can we give you a ride?"

"You guys going out tonight?" Cassie tried to keep the skepticism from her voice. Lauren's laugh proved her correct.

"Eh…no. We will enjoy our private spa."

"So…why are you asking if I need a ride? I have my car."

"Cassie, we'll gladly take you—and pick you up. I know you don't enjoy driving at night. Plus, relax and enjoy an adult beverage or two…just like everyone does in college. Seriously, Cass."

A rush of love for her aunt filled Cassie's heart. "I know you would, Lauren. I'll be fine. Not planning to drink. If I do, I'll stay over with Amelie."

"If you change your mind and you need a ride home, call me. Promise, Cassie."

"Promise, but please don't worry. I'll be fine. It's just a casual get together."

23

Hours later, Cassie watched the constant stream of people crowd into the large condo. *So, this is casual, Chez Camden? Just a "few" friends? He's barely spoken to me since the first guests arrived and obviously takes his role as host seriously.* He set up a bar on the huge kitchen counter, and Cassie thought he may have missed his true avocation as a bartender. She raised her eyebrows and cocked her head when he walked toward her, a red Solo cup in hand.

"Let me know what you think." His lips quirked slightly as he handed it to her. "Prepared especially for you."

She sniffed the strawberry-scented drink. "Smells yummy. What's in this concoction?" So far, she'd drunk only soft drinks and water, but the festive atmosphere had pulled her under its spell.

"I call it a CassieRita—heavy on the strawberry mixture, very light on the tequila." His silver-grey eyes reflected mischief. "I know you're not a big drinker—hope you like it."

"I guess I need to try it, then?" Cassie sipped the liquid. "Hmm… yes, very good. You sure this isn't plain strawberry punch? A Virgin-Rita? My compliments to the bartender."

"Extra punch for your drink." He rested his hand against her lower back and urged her forward. "Let me introduce you to some guests."

She knew many from the occasional games she'd attended in the suite or had met in the family gathering area afterward. Others worked with Caryn and Lauren on their promotional schedules and social media, and Cassie remembered meeting them when they stopped by the house. She stopped to chat with Amelie and Chance.

"Enjoying your free evening? Chance, Cassie is Lauren and Dave's niece—and Andrew and Caryn's nanny. They have the cutest twins ever," Amelie said. "I hope you're enjoying our party?"

Amelie's smile shone brightly, and Cassie guessed that she'd enjoyed at least a few of the strawberry margaritas. "You need to give me your brother's secret recipe. I could drink these all night."

Cam peered into her nearly empty cup, then drew her closer to his side. "Refill?"

Cassie swallowed the remaining liquid and handed the cup to him. "Yes, please." Her borderline anxiety in the crowded room lessened. Perhaps she'd relax enough to enjoy the party after another of Cam's special drinks? *Can't hurt. Couldn't taste any tequila, maybe just a splash. Tastes like strawberry punch.*

Cassie perched on a stool near the counter, content to people watch while she sipped yet another "special margarita." She suspected Cam had upped the tequila in this one and reminded herself to drink slowly. A water bottle sat beside her also, so for every few sips of the margarita, she drank water. Content, she felt a slight buzz, but nothing more. Amelie and Chase had disappeared a while ago. She didn't see them leave, but they could have slipped out or gone back to Amelie's bedroom.

She shivered when Cam came up behind her and dropped a kiss on her shoulder. "Having a good time? Still enjoying my 'CassieRitas,' or would you like to try something different?"

"No, these are perfect." She cut her eyes toward him. "I think you forgot who you were making this for—it's stronger than the others?"

Cam took the cup from her hand and took a sip. "Maybe. Why

don't I get you another?" His silver-grey eyes flashed as a teasing smile hinted at his lips.

"No, thanks. This is just fine."

Cam rested his hand on her lower back when Cassie retrieved her cup, his fingers dancing lightly against the skin left bare by the crop top. She glanced at him, noticing his eyes scanning the room. *Wonder if he's aware that Amelie and Chase left?* His fingers playfully tickled her side, and Cassie jumped from the stool, nearly dropping her drink as she laughed.

"Not fair! No tickling." She saw the mischievous gleam in his expression.

"Ah, good to know." He hooked his arm around her shoulders and drew her closer. His lips brushed against her forehead. "I'm happy you accepted the invitation."

Cassie tried to tamp down her body's reaction to his touch. *Just the alcohol making me sensitive.* He felt the involuntary shiver and turned her toward him. "Cold?" His smile bordered on a smirk. "Maybe this will help." His lips grazed against hers, pulling her against his chest. "Mm, strawberries. Sweet, just like you."

Cassie's slipped her arms around his neck, the full Solo cup forgotten until it tipped sideways, sending cold liquid down his neck and under his shirt. He jerked back at the sensation.

"I'm so sorry, Cam. I forgot…"

His eyes locked with hers. "You respond to my kiss with a dousing of frozen margarita?" He couldn't contain the laughter and eyed the half-empty cup. "I'll hold on to this for you." Without thinking, she handed it to him, immediately regretting the move when his eyes gleamed with mischief. He raised the cup over her head.

"You wouldn't?"

"I might."

Cassie stepped back suddenly and sprinted away from him, weaving her way through the crowded room, trying to maintain her balance. She glimpsed the hall bathroom and ran inside it, locking the door and leaning back against it. She giggled so hard she couldn't catch her breath. She realized then that she'd had one—*maybe two?*—margaritas too many. *You're in so much trouble, Cassie Johnson.*

Someone knocked loudly against the wood. "You can't hide out all evening, Cassie."

"I might." She looked around the room for a bath towel to protect her from a frigid margarita shower. She grabbed one, then noticed the door at the other end of the bath. *An exit? Through a bedroom maybe... Amelie's room?* She crossed the room and pressed her ear against the door. *Nothing. Quiet.* Holding her breath, she rapped lightly against the door before opening it slightly. She knocked again before looking into the room. *Empty.* She slipped into the adjoining room, carefully closing the door behind her. The full moon provided all the light she needed to tiptoe toward the kitchen.

Half-way across the room, she saw movement from the corner of her eye. Before her brain could process the action, she felt a hand cup her mouth and an arm close around her. Cam maneuvered her to the bed, playfully lifting her up and letting her drop in the middle of the mattress. He claimed her mouth when he joined her, and Cassie giggled against his kiss. He pulled back, an annoyed expression crossing his face.

"Don't go anywhere. I need to say goodbye to my guests."

"No problem," she whispered. Sudden dizziness caused her to lay back on the pillow. The room spun, and she closed her eyes, hoping to avoid nausea. Sleep. That's what she needed. Sleep.

The alcohol-induced slumber produced tangible emotions and sensations as dreams unfolded...Tom beside her, his arms holding her against him as he peppered her face and neck with light kisses. Her head spinning, her mind hazy, she swallowed a moan when he gently nibbled on her bottom lip. Opening her mouth slightly to accept the kiss, she slipped her arms around his broad chest.

Cassie drifted in a dimension filled with Tom's gentle kisses and soft hands skimming her skin. The kisses grew intense, more demanding, and her soft cotton top did little to mute the heat his touch generated. Intoxicated with these sensations, a small moan escaped her lips.

"Cassie." She barely heard the whispered words as the growing desire carried her on a fluffy soft cloud of sensuality. She wanted to drift on these clouds forever. Caught in the swirling cyclone of emotions, Cassie couldn't find—*didn't want to find*—the will to remain in control.

She focused only on the man she never believed would desire her…How did such a sweet kiss suddenly morph into two half-dressed people exploring each other's skin, sending waves of desire to her core?

She heard her name again and murmured a response. Her eyes met his, and she read desire mirroring her own. She shut her eyes and opened them again, slowing grasping that her dream had transformed into a very different reality. Cam, not Tom, leaned over her, and his fingers played with the edge of her jeans.

Cassie jerked away and scrambled away from him on the bed. "Cam, what the hell are you doing?"

"Enjoying an exquisite and responsive woman." He flashed a smile.

"I was sleeping!"

"If you say so." His flippant tone infuriated her.

"Cam, my head was spinning…I lay down to stop the dizziness. That's the last thing I remember until I opened my eyes." Cassie breathed deeply to calm her emotions. "I thought I was dreaming."

"Oh, your kisses are so much better than a dream." Cam reached to touch her face, and Cassie pulled away. She felt the edge of the bed and quickly stood up.

"I can't believe you got in bed knowing I was asleep," Cassie accused. "I didn't know you were here. How could you?"

Cam shook his head. "Cassie, you acted like you were very much aware."

"Is that your game? Serve supposedly alcohol-light drinks, then take advantage when the girl falls asleep?"

"I don't need to 'take advantage' of girls."

"Then what do you call what you just did? Never mind, I'm getting out of here."

"Save it." Cam pushed to his feet and turned away. "You shouldn't drink if you don't know when to stop."

Cassie's head buzzed as she watched him stride toward the bathroom, slamming the connecting door shut behind him. She adjusted her clothes and ran her hand through her tangled hair. *What were you thinking, Johnson? Or not thinking? You know you shouldn't have had more than one drink. How could you make such a stupid mistake?* Thank God she woke up in time.

She looked around, realizing she was in the room where Amelia had stashed her bag earlier. She spied it by the bed, grabbed it, and flipped on the lamp on the dresser. She groaned when she saw her reflection in the mirror…smeared lipstick, mascara-streaked cheeks, her hair a matted bird's nest.

She heard laughter on the other side of the door, and Cassie dug into her bag for her face wipes and a brush. Her face remained flushed, even after cleaning her skin, and she frowned as she quickly brushed her hair.

She squinted at her watch. *One in the morning. Craptastic. Drink too much, lose track of time.* She needed to get home.

24

After changing into Dave's oversized T-shirt rather than her crop top, Cassie spotted several bottles of water on the nightstand. Quickly drinking two, Cassie grabbed her bag and opened the door.

She nearly ran into Amelie. "Cassie, I thought you'd left."

"I was dizzy, so I took a short nap." Cassie tried to laugh it off. "I need to get home."

Amelie grasped her arm. "Just stay here. You don't want to drive home this late."

"I'll be okay. I need to get home by five in the morning. My munchkins are up before dawn." She glanced nervously toward the living room. "Has everybody gone?"

"Yes, I saw my brother take a girl into his bedroom, but no one else is here. The guest room is made up for you. Don't take a chance—you might get pulled over at this hour."

Great. The icing on my cake. Who knows how much alcohol's still in my system? "Are you sure you don't mind? I guess I could sleep for a couple of hours."

Amelie turned Cassie toward the guest room. "Go. I'll get you some ibuprofen and water." With a gentle push, Cassie walked into the room.

She set her phone alarm for four, thankful that she'd stuck a charger in her bag. Confident that Caryn muted her phone at night, Cassie sent her a quick text to assure her she'd see them by five a.m. She'd text Lauren in the morning—when she reached the Chadwick's. Lauren would be awake, then and she wouldn't disturb the newlyweds. Cassie set the phone on the bedside table and slipped under the covers. She fell asleep before Amelie returned with the water.

Cassie jerked awake to her phone blasting a song about a hummingbird. *Lauren's ringtone.* She quickly silenced the sound, then slid her finger to accept the call. "Hey…Lauren," she said, her voice thick with sleep. "What time is it?"

"Almost five. I couldn't sleep. I took a walk and saw your car wasn't in the driveway. Everything okay?"

"Crap!" Cassie croaked. "My alarm didn't go off! Or I didn't set it correctly. I stayed over at Amelie's."

"You're okay?" Cassie heard amusement in her aunt's tone.

"Okay, except I should be on my way to Caryn's now. I need to go, Lauren. Can I call you…"

"Yes, when you get home." Lauren's tone relaxed Cassie's jangled nerves. "I'll stop by and see if Caryn needs any help. No need to rush. Drive carefully—don't speed, okay?"

Emotion threatened to overwhelm Cassie. "Thanks, Lauren."

Cassie took a deep breath, flicked the tears from her cheek, and then scrambled to strip the bed, freshen up, and dress. She swallowed the ibuprofen with the first water bottle, then slipped the second into the side of her backpack. She quietly crept from the room and tiptoed toward the door.

Pausing in the living area, Cassie's conscience tugged at her to clean up the disaster remaining from the party. *Amelie will get stuck with all the cleaning. I should help her a bit. Help Cam? Not in his dreams? But Amie deserves some assistance.* She glanced at the counter dividing the room from the kitchen and cringed when she saw the pink liquid on the floor. The margarita she'd accidentally spilled all over Cam. *I should clean some of this...*

As if on cue, her cell phone pinged an incoming text.

Caryn: Don't hurry. Very quiet here.
Cassie: You sure? Thought I'd take a minute to clean some of this post-party mess.
Caryn: Take your time. Just don't do everything by yourself.
Cassie: No way. See you soon.

She shoved the phone into her jeans and walked to the kitchen in search of a garbage bag. Thankfully, they sat in plain view on the counter—best intentions derailed. Quietly, she walked around the condo, collecting red Solo Cups and empty beer bottles, securing each bag and setting it by the door. Next, she tackled the paper plates and half-eaten food. After collecting the plates, she glanced at the remaining refreshments in the kitchen. *Keep or toss?*

Anything that required refrigeration hit the bag. Cassie held her breath when she neared the leftover boiled shrimp. *Already smells nasty.* She quickly secured that bag, then dropped it into a second trash bag. *Eau de leftover shrimp—lovely!* Combined with the smell of strawberries and tequila, Cassie fought the urge to gag. She looked for some floor cleaner without success, so grabbing a roll of paper towels, she placed some on the floor to soak up the liquid. The sound of someone clearing his throat caused Cassie to look up. Cam towered above her, his expression amused.

"The cleaning service is coming this morning. You're not Cinderella, Cass." He held his hand toward her, but she ignored it and pushed herself to her feet. He nodded at the garbage bags by the door. "Thank you, but unnecessary."

"I wanted to help Amelie." Cassie's voice sounded cold and indifferent, even to her own ears.

"Thank you." His grey eyes met hers. "I'm sorry about the misunderstanding last night."

"Misunderstanding? Yeah, sure, I've put it out of my mind."

"So, we're okay?"

"Okay, as in you understand that you made a mistake? Or, okay, don't tell my aunt what happened?" Cassie asked.

"Maybe a little of both?" Cam's charming smile had no effect on Cassie's mood.

"Don't worry, your secret's safe. I'm embarrassed I got myself in that situation by trusting you to make my drinks." She reached for the door. "Don't bother speaking next time our paths cross."

Still fuming, Cassie tossed her bag into the trunk of her car. *And to think I believed his nonsense! Stupid. Everyone warned me, but I didn't listen. I can handle him...Delusional. Didn't you learn anything from Lauren's experiences? How could I even think he was Tom? Dreams versus ugly reality.*

Swiping tears that ran down her cheeks, Cassie paused before pressing the car's start button. *Thank God, I opened my eyes. I could have added one more notch on Cam's hockey stick. Gag.*

By the time Cassie reached the Chadwick's home, she'd shoved all thoughts about Cam, the embarrassment and regret to the back of her mind. *Concentrate on the reason you're here. To decide on your future, not find a hot hockey player or a doctor who clicks all the boxes for my perfect dream man.*

She combed her fingers through her hair and then leaned against the side of her car to quell her emotions. *Stupid, stupid, stupid...no wonder Mom wants to control my life. If Amelie hadn't seen me in the hallway, I'd have gone to my car, and probably attempted to drive home. Would I have gotten behind the wheel? Even after Lauren told me to call if I needed a ride? You screwed up, Johnson. You're not a responsible adult.*

She scrubbed her face with both hands, brushing aside the tears. *Get it together.*

"Cassie, you okay?"

She looked up and saw Tom. *Where did he come from? Can today get any worse?* She shrugged as he waited for her response. "Not really."

He held out his hand. "Let's go inside."

Cassie shook her head. "I don't want Caryn…"

"No, I meant my entrance."

Cassie walked silently beside him, her thoughts spinning out of control. *So wasted you thought Cam was Tom? Idiot.*

Once inside the apartment, Tom guided her to the kitchen. "Hot tea? Coffee? Soda?"

"No, thanks." She felt her lips quiver in an attempt to smile.

"Come here." He wrapped an arm around her shoulders and walked her to his living room. He didn't speak until they sat side by side on the sofa. "Do you want to talk about it?"

Tom saw Cassie take a deep breath before looking at him. "Don't you need to go to work?"

"I arrive long before my shift. I'm okay, time-wise."

Cassie averted her eyes as she shook her head. "I made a stupid mistake."

Tom immediately thought about Camden but kept that to himself. "What was the mistake?"

"Allowing someone to make drinks supposedly light on alcohol."

"So, you didn't realize how much you'd had to drink?"

Cassie's laugh held no humor. "Yep, I was wasting away in Margaritaville before I noticed." She pushed her hair behind her shoulders. "And I thought Amelie was the clueless one that night at the club."

Tom slipped his arm around her shoulders and encouraged her to move closer beside him. "What happened?"

Cassie leaned into him. "Nothing, really. I lay down in the guest bedroom Amelie showed me. My head kept spinning, like the room was moving. I thought I was dreaming…about a guy making out with me. It felt magical until I opened my eyes. My dream morphed into a huge nightmare."

She glanced at Tom, and he read embarrassment in her expression.

"Someone was with you?" His voice was soft, gentle.

"Yeah, definitely not the person from my dream…actually the last person on earth I'd want touching me."

Tom's heart clenched at her words, and he pushed the sudden anger aside. "Did he…?"

"No," Cassie interrupted. "I shoved him away and accused him of taking advantage of me. Things got ugly—verbally—but he left." Cassie's tone mixed bitterness and sarcasm. "If I never see a strawberry margarita again…" Her voice trailed off.

Tom pulled her closer. "I'm sorry you had to experience that. Unfortunately, there are too many jerks like that guy. You said things got ugly—did he accuse you of encouraging him?"

"How'd you know?"

"We see too many women who've had non-consensual sex while inebriated, and then worry about STDs, sometimes pregnancy. Most won't file a complaint because they think they somehow encouraged the guy."

Cassie pressed her face against his chest. Tom strained to hear her speak. "Luckily, he didn't get that far before I 'woke' up. Should have known that dream was too good to be true." She pushed back. "You need to head to work. I'm okay. Just embarrassed, full of regrets, and thankful for my guardian angel."

Tom gently wiped a tear from her cheek with his thumb. "You're gutsy, too, Cass. Stood up for yourself and made sure you regained control. I suspect you would have busted his ass if he hadn't left."

He smiled when he heard Cassie's giggle. He placed his palms on her cheeks and looked directly into her clouded eyes. "Believe in yourself. You did nothing to deserve what happened. Just the thought of someone taking advantage of you…" He saw her large trusting eyes and without thinking, lowered his face toward hers and brushed his lips against hers. "You deserve so much more, Cassie." She opened her mouth slightly, inviting his kiss, and Tom accepted that invitation…He wanted to replace the nightmare from the previous night and show her she should feel cherished…that her dreams still existed.

Time stopped, both lost in the embrace…until Tom's phone pinged with an incoming text. They reluctantly pulled away from each other, Tom letting his palm rest against the side of her face. "I'm sorry, Cass. I've thought about that first kiss so often…I shouldn't have. The last thing I want to do is take advantage of you."

Cassie shook her head as she pressed her fingers against his lips. "No, you didn't…that's what I'd call a dream." She paused, then continued in a subdued tone. "I know we can't do this, Tom. Working for Caryn and Andrew…"

"And you're Lauren's niece," Tom added. "I know all the reasons I shouldn't kiss you…and then I look at your eyes, and those intentions cease to exist." He hugged her and pressed his lips against her forehead. "I'll walk you in, then head out."

"Thanks for listening. I really needed that."

"Anytime, hon." He took her hand and guided her toward the door. "So, you going to tell me who starred in your dream before it turned into a nightmare?"

Cassie laughed, and he saw her blush. "Nope, that stays my secret, doctor."

25

Several days passed before Tom's shift—shifts—ended. The flu had hit staff and as the ER found itself under-staffed, Tom stayed until there was adequate coverage. He paused when he entered the house and saw Cassie seated at a table on the pool deck, papers spread across the surface. He hadn't seen her since they'd shared their second "forbidden kiss" that stuck on replay in his brain.

He barely remembered his last free evening—the catch-up dinner with Katie. He'd returned home early, only to find Cassie had taken the evening off to go to that party over at Camden's.

He suspected Cam had purposely given Cassie stronger drinks than he'd promised. She didn't need to tell him. He also "knew" Cam was the man who'd tried to take advantage of Cassie. He experienced the same burst of anger he'd felt when she'd confided in him. *Luckily for both of us, he's out of town for a while.*

He pushed through the door to the pool, returning Cassie's bright smile when she saw him.

"Hey, stranger," she greeted. "Where have you been hiding?"

"Long nights at the hospital. I signed on to back up the residents this week, plus staff shortage. Thankfully, that ended today." He nodded toward a chair at the table. "Can I join you?"

"You have to ask?"

"Where are your hair colors?"

Cassie shrugged. "Too time-consuming. I need to concentrate on plans after this gap year."

"Well, I officially lodge a protest. It's definitely worth the time." He saw the sparkle in her eyes as the faint flush crept on her face. "Are these the universities you're considering?"

"Just the one in Tampa. Lauren and I visited it a few weeks ago. Looking at their Early Childhood Education or Communications majors."

"Both sound good. I've heard it's a top school. I'm sure Caryn hopes she can keep you at least part-time."

Cassie sighed as she leaned on her elbow. "I'd be happy continuing full-time indefinitely. Just trying to keep my mother happy."

Tom squeezed her shoulder. "Parental pressure is tough. Just remember, it's your life, you're an adult, and you don't need to conform to any arbitrary timeline. As much talent as you have, I can see you doing anything you want."

"Thanks, Tom." Cassie glanced away before she asked the question that had stuck in her mind over the past few days. "So, how was your reunion with Katie? I forgot to ask when I had my meltdown."

"Not a meltdown, Cassie, just a talk between...um…friends. Anyway, It was good to catch up with Katie. She's happy living close to home and reconnected with a former boyfriend from high school."

"Oh…Sorry?" A slight questioning smile crossed her face.

Tom shrugged. "Why?"

Cassie averted her eyes. "Weren't you guys in a relationship before she moved?"

"I'm not sure what to call it. Yes, we got together when our schedules allowed; I guess you'd call it exclusive. Honestly, neither of us wanted to try the long-distance thing." He smiled when her eyes met his. "I think Caryn was more disappointed than either of us. They became close when her doctor hospitalized Caryn with bed rest."

"Match-making?"

"Nah, we were already friends. But relationships are tough when both people work in medicine." He leaned back in the chair and glanced at the papers strewn across the table. "Can I help you with anything? Do you have what you need to apply?"

"Don't know. Lauren said she'd help me with the student VISA. I need to check if I have to take those SAT or ACT tests." She made a face. "Hate thinking about it."

"Don't until you know for sure. Your tests from secondary school may be all that's required." He paused a moment. "If you need to take either of those tests, I can help you study. I had a friend in Toronto who wanted to go to Boston College. She got the study guide, and I worked through it with her."

"Girlfriend?"

"That was a long time ago."

"I'll welcome help if I need test scores." He saw her rueful smile. "Not a terrific test-taker."

Tom watched as she gathered the papers and organized them in a folder. He pushed aside his desire to kidnap her to his apartment. *Maybe it's worth the risk? Maybe we're missing out on something special. Or I could quickly screw up her plans, her job, and her future.* He pushed back his chair to stand. "Let me know if you need my help, okay?"

He thought he caught a gleam in her wide hazel eyes. *Could she read his thoughts?* But Cassie merely replied, "Count on it…friend."

Ouch…Friend-zoned…I should feel relieved, right? He swallowed the disappointment—irrational; he knew—and returned to his apartment.

Amelie persuaded her brother to leave the keys to his car with her during a long road trip and offered to help Cassie and Caryn with the twins. Cassie felt irritation that she called Caryn first instead of checking with her, but Caryn told her she could decide.

"I don't have a problem with it, so long as you don't feel Amelie will cause a distraction," Caryn said.

"She might, but my focus is on the twins only." Cassie made a face. "Though, she said yesterday that this road trip really makes her feel lonely. Guess with Cam and Chance out of town, her social life has taken a huge hit."

"It's up to you, Cassie. I can tell her I don't think it's a good idea," Caryn said.

Cassie caught Caryn's eyes. "I hate Amie's home alone, and I have you, Terri, Kelly, and Lauren. Selfish of me?"

Caryn hugged her with a laugh. "Don't guilt-trip yourself. With the guys gone, I expect we'll see more of Lauren, Kelly, and Terri."

"I'm okay with whatever you think's best."

"How about this–I'll invite her over tomorrow. Lauren and I are slammed with work, so perhaps an extra pair of hands will come in handy. We can see just how much Amelie's willing to help? Are you comfortable with that?"

Comfortable? Can I see her interacting with my love bugs...or am I just worried she'll start flirting with Tom if he's around? Selfish much, Cass? Remember who kept you from driving after that party...

"Okay," she answered finally. "I have some reservations, but as long as you're home, we can try it."

"Cassie." Caryn waited until Cassie looked at her. "I have no problem playing Mama Grizzly. Take that off your worry list."

Cassie giggled at the thought. "I hope you never go Mama Grizzly on me! Okay, sure, why not? I'll try to share Jenna and Danny."

"How much you share's totally up to you, Cassie. The twins may raise their own objections. The pediatrician said they may start rejecting new faces—common at their age. I'll call her back and set a few ground rules. First and most important, she needs to clear it with me before dropping in. Neither Drew, nor I want anything to distract you when you're running after two stubborn speed-crawlers!"

This time Cassie hugged Caryn. "I agree, definitely. Thank you—you're the best, Caryn."

"Blame me if it ever comes up." Caryn met Cassie's eyes. "You know, I always wished for a large family—brothers and sisters. Lauren's been a sister for a long time. Now I feel I have two with you."

Cassie blinked back the sudden tears. "I've always wanted a sister. Thank you."

Daniel and Jenna had mastered crawling and now darted across the floor in a flash. They both pulled themselves to a standing position and then cruised along the side of the couch. Cassie enjoyed the determination on both of their faces and tried to comfort them when they lost their balance and plopped to the floor. Caryn told Cassie that their stubbornness and determination was all Andrew and warned that impatience would soon follow.

Those thoughts ran through Cassie's mind as she played on the floor with the twins the next day. Unusually active—even for them—both kept her busy, giggling when they tried to venture past their play area. When they began crawling in separate directions, Cassie suspected they'd invented a new game. She almost called Caryn to watch but remembered the conference call that had started an hour earlier. Her office door remained closed, indicating the call had continued longer than expected.

Cassie spread out on the floor, enticing the escape artists to use her as a climbing wall. It didn't take long for them to discover how to make Cassie laugh, and the three giggled so hard no one heard the quiet knock on the door. Suddenly Amelie joined them on the floor.

"What are you doing, Cassie?"

"Trying to distract them. Danny and Jenna learned some new escape skills this morning. They're a hoot. How are you, Amie?"

"Good. I hate these road trips. Really miss my guy."

"How is Mr. Gagné?" Cassie asked as she grabbed Daniel before he could make a break for the kitchen.

"God, I miss him, Cass. We talk every day, but it's not the same. Although, FaceTime's providing some interesting evenings." Amelie grinned, watching Cassie's attempt to corral the twins.

"Can you hand me that box of teething biscuits on the counter? That should settle them in one place for a while." Cassie glanced at Amelie once Jenna and Daniel sat quietly, gnawing on the thick biscuits. "So, you say FaceTime's entertained you?"

Amelie leaned back against the couch. "Chance is just as sexy and gets my body responding just listening to him. *Almost* as good as having him right beside me."

"Sexting?" Cassie guessed.

"OMG, yes! When he tells me to do something…it's like he's the one touching me."

Cassie laughed and slipped her hands over Jenna's ears. "TMI! Don't corrupt my little angels."

"I doubt they understand a word."

"Still, G-rated around them, please! I don't want their first word to be 'sexting.'"

Amelie laughed, shaking her head. "You're nuts, you know that?" Without waiting for an answer, she nodded toward then pool. "Mind if I catch some rays by the pool?"

"Help yourself. I need to feed these guys lunch."

"So maybe you can join me when they nap?"

"Maybe." Cassie got each squirming baby settled and strapped safely in a highchair and then gave each a handful of Cheerios to keep them happy while she prepared the lunch. Caryn joined her shortly and began assisting her.

"Where's your extra set of hands?"

Cassie nodded toward the lanai. "Working on her tan."

Cassie heard Caryn's sigh. "So, not much help with Jenna and Danny?"

"Not yet. Amelie's watched but hasn't interacted with them. That's okay. Danny and Jenna have a new trick—they take off in opposite directions. I swear they pre-plan it!"

"I wouldn't doubt that. Sometimes, I think they already have that twin communication thing going."

"I can ask Amelie if she and Cam had their own secret language."

"With those two, nothing would surprise me."

After she and Caryn put the tired and cranky duo in their cribs for a nap, Caryn handed Cassie the baby monitor. "I've got another conference call. But with any luck, they'll sleep a couple hours. Why don't you relax by the pool, too? Help yourselves to whatever you'd like for lunch—or order out. My treat." Caryn pointed to the credit card on the counter.

Cassie asked Amelie if she would like a sandwich or salad. "Caryn's chicken salad is super delicious. Everyone wants her recipe."

"Sure, that sounds good, Cassie. It's just perfect out here. Could you grab a Coke or water for me?" Amelie flipped on her stomach and closed her eyes. "So relaxing."

Cassie didn't comment as she walked back to the house. *Wow, she and Cam must have grown up with cooks and maids. No offer to help. Sure, she's a guest, but she could at least volunteer.* Sighing, she quickly put together a platter of sandwiches, fruit, and fresh brownies. She gathered utensils, paper plates, napkins, and a selection of cold drinks and took them to the deck, setting up the table at the end of the pool. Amelie didn't move while she brought out the food and drinks, so Cassie allowed the tray to drop a few inches to make a sound. *The monitor!* Cassie returned inside to grab the monitor, smiling when she heard the babies softly snoring as they slept.

She called Amelie when she reached the table. "Lunch is served."

Her guest looked over her shoulder. "Be there in a few. Don't wait for me."

Cassie rolled her eyes. *Don't worry about that.* She smiled in surprise when the door opened, and Tom stepped into the lanai. "Lunch break?" she greeted. "Perfect timing." She waved her hand toward the table. "Hungry?"

"Always…is that chicken salad?" His brown eyes met hers speculatively.

"Caryn's specialty. Plus brownies."

"It will be worth doubling my laps today." Tom's smile caused Cassie's heart to beat faster. *Hope he can't hear it.* Tom nodded at Amelie in the corner at the end of the pool. "Is she not joining us?"

"She said not to wait, she'd be over in a few."

"In that case…" Tom pulled back a chair for Cassie, then sat beside her. "Wasn't expecting this when I walked in."

"Tom, you know I'd make lunch for you anytime…so long as you handle breakfast and an occasional dinner."

Tom recounted a humorous story concerning an intern that set off Cassie's giggles. "How did you keep a straight face, doctor?"

"Sometimes, it's difficult. I had to take a break—though, I remember being in the same situation when I was an intern." He looked up to see Amelie standing behind Cassie. "Ready to join us?"

"You bet. I didn't think you'd start without me, Cassie."

Tom watched as Cassie bit her lip and forced a smile. "I'm sorry, Amie. I misunderstood. Please, join us. Caryn's chicken salad is famous."

"Oh, this really looks good." Amelie placed a sandwich on her plate and opened a bottle of water. She turned her attention to Tom. "Day off?"

"Worked last night. Full moon, which meant a crazy night in the ER."

"That's not an urban myth?" Cassie asked. "Do weird things really happen when there's a full moon?" Her hazel eyes reflected mischief. Tom responded with a wink.

Amelie laughed. "No vampires—or is that the wolfman?"

"Not that I've seen, but you can google and read many supposedly true full-moon ER stories." Tom sipped his water as he watched her reaction. Amelie pouted just a bit.

"So, no fun stories from your experience, doctor?" She cocked her head with a teasing smile.

"Nah, most of the patients I see have some kind of head injury. What's on your agendas today?"

"Staying one step ahead of my munchkins," Cassie said. "Hey, Amelie, did you and Cam have that secret twin language? I swear Danny and Jenny are communicating." She told Tom about their sudden "escape" plan.

"We do, actually. Sometimes it's more like I tune into Cam's thoughts and vice versa. That was *not* helpful in secondary school," Amelie said and laughed. "Even in Paris, he always knew when I was having a rough day, homesick, or out with a hot guy." She shook her head. "I did *not* appreciate him jumping into my head whenever I kissed someone. Major mood destroyer."

Cassie joined her in laughing. "Is he still bugging your mind here in Tampa?"

Amelie smiled coyly. "I found if I just jump into his head once or twice, he's ready for a truce. I know it sounds bizarre, but it's hard to explain."

Cassie looked at Tom. "I think your nephew and niece have that gift. Watch out."

He smiled at the animated sparkle in her hazel eyes when she talked about the twins. *Anyone can see she loves them like her own—and the feeling's definitely mutual.*

On cue, two squawks sounded on the monitor. Cassie jumped up. "I need to get them before they disturb Caryn's conference call."

"Need a hand?" Amelie asked.

Tom watched as Cassie hid her surprise. "Come on."

He stood to clear the table. It didn't take long, and after he'd put everything away, he returned with a cloth to wipe the table. He moved the monitor, pausing for a moment to listen to Jenna babble. *Wonder who will speak first? And that first word? "Dad," if Andrew has anything to say about it.* He'd caught his brother frequently trying to coach them. Not at all embarrassed, Andrew had shrugged with a grin. "You don't think Caryn does the same thing?"

Amelie's voice caught his attention. "Cassie, before we take them out, can I ask you a question?"

"Sure."

"Tom—is he…"

Tom quickly muted the monitor, not wanting to eavesdrop, hear the question, or Cassie's answer. He placed the monitor back on the table and returned inside the house. *Just give Jenna and Danny a kiss and catch up on sleep.* He pretended not to notice Cassie's flushed cheeks and took Daniel from Amelie when he held his hands out toward his uncle and squealed.

"I got you, little buddy." He laughed when Jenna immediately mimicked her brother. "Mind if I get her, too?" he asked Cassie.

"Hey, I know where I land on their order of preferences." She gently placed Jenna in Tom's other arm. "They love their Uncle Tommy."

They all walked to the play area. “Here you go, tigers. Don’t play any tricks on Cassie or Amelie.” He caught Cassie’s eye. “Sleep calls. I’ll catch up with you later. Nice to see you again, Amelie.”

He may have imagined it, but thought he heard Amelie sigh as he walked toward his apartment. He wanted to chat a bit with Cassie, but not with Amelie vying for attention. A beautiful woman, but he preferred the spunky hazel-eyed girl with a rainbow of colors highlighting her hair.

26

Christmas suddenly loomed on the horizon when Cassie's mother mentioned flying home for the Christmas holidays. She wanted a Christmas with both parents—like they used to enjoy before the divorce. Cassie knew those holidays would never reappear. With her mother in Vancouver and her father taking a Disney Cruise, Cassie didn't want to choose between her mother and father…again. "I'll try to figure things out, Mom." She ended the conversation, then sought Lauren's input.

"I know I sound like a horrible daughter, but I'd rather just stay here for Christmas, Lauren." She watched the rain splash from the screen porch, quickly forming running streams outside. "This weather depresses me, and you know how much worse it gets at home."

"Aren't Caryn and Andrew flying up to Toronto with the twins?" Lauren asked.

Cassie nodded. "Are you and Dave going to Vancouver? That could change my perspective."

"We thought about it, but really it's too much travel for a three-day break. The team plays at home right after the break, so we'd barely have time to drop off presents and head back." Cassie saw Lauren studying her face. "You know you're welcome to stay with us. You can help decorate, we can bake Christmas cookies, and stay up late to wait for Santa Claus."

"But it's your first Christmas with Dave. I don't want to crash that."

"Hush, Cassie, we'll have time to ourselves. Have you spoken with your dad? Are they doing the Disney Cruise?"

Cassie grinned. "Taylor will so love it! Dad invited me to come with them…" She shrugged as her voice trailed off. "Mom would never forgive me if I chose the cruise over coming home. And ten days is too long to stay away."

"Divorce is hard, even when you're an adult child. Are they flying into Orlando? Maybe if they're not jumping right on the ship, we can meet for dinner." Lauren paused a moment and then sighed. "I could invite Amanda and Allyson to come here. Maybe that way, you can enjoy time with both your parents separately?"

Cassie made a face. "Why would you want to do that? And what about Dave's family?"

"We invited his family to visit during the Suns' bye-week after the All-Star Game." Lauren shook her head with a laugh. "We'll have a houseful if everyone comes."

"You don't think they will—why not leave Vancouver and warm up in this beautiful Florida sunshine? I sure would." Cassie watched as the rain continued to pound the roof. Melancholy descended with the rain, though she could not think of a reason.

"Why don't I ask my sweet husband about inviting Amanda and Allyson? I can tell them it's too far for any of us to travel for just one full day in town. Then, if they decline, you're off the hook." Lauren reached for her hand and squeezed it. "Would that help?"

"Honestly, I don't know. I just hate being in the middle. It never stops." Cassie tried to read the expression in her aunt's eyes. "Please don't do this just for me. It's time to take myself out of the middle and not visit either. I'd rather celebrate Christmas with you and Dave."

"Stop worrying, Cass. I'll talk to him—if he has *any* reservations, we won't invite them. Either way, you can't please both your parents, so don't fret. It's not your fault they created this situation."

Terri and Steve Rogers hosted a traditional American Thanksgiving Meal. They invited any of the Suns who were not celebrating locally to join them for the day. Cassie had forgotten Canada's Thanksgiving Day until her father called to share holiday wishes. Now she eagerly anticipated experiencing her first American Thanksgiving. She asked so many questions that Terri invited her over when she met with a caterer to plan the meal.

"Are you planning to hit the malls for the Black Friday sales?" Caryn grinned when she caught Cassie looking at advertised sales on her iPad.

"Heck, no! There's no way I'd stand in that crowd to shop in the middle of the night—everything's probably on sale online, anyway."

"Well, if you want the authentic American Thanksgiving experience, Black Friday shopping is a must." Caryn smiled with a wink to show Cassie she was teasing.

"I'll stick with the meal, thanks." Cassie turned her iPad off and changed the subject. "Did you and Andrew decide when to celebrate the twins' first birthday?"

"We're looking at the first Sunday in December when the team's in town for ten days. We don't want their birthday to become part of Christmas celebrations. The party may be two weeks early, but I don't think Jen or Danny will mind."

"Can I help you with the party? Address invitations, get decorations, really anything," Cassie said with a chuckle. "I missed out on that with little Taylor—it wasn't my weekend with my dad, and Mom said I could celebrate when I saw them the following week."

Cassie felt the warmth from Caryn's smile. "I'm counting on your help! Promise you'll stop me from getting OCD about making everything perfect."

Cassie crossed her fingers and held them up. "Promise."

Thanksgiving morning, Cassie enjoyed bonding time with Jenna and Daniel. Andrew had morning skate, and Caryn joined Kelly in helping Terri remain calm as the tent, chairs, tables, and a zillion other things descended on the house. She hoped Tom didn't have to work. He'd mentioned that he wasn't scheduled for Thanksgiving but would work the following two days. As always, he remained on call.

*Haven't run into Cam since that party. Just hope he doesn't speak to me...awkward. Every time I think about how close I came to adding my name to his hockey stick...*She shivered in disgust and focused her thoughts on the twins. As quickly as they scooted around holding on to the furniture, she saw first steps in the near future. *By their birthday? Please let Caryn and Andrew observe their first steps, not me. I'd feel so guilty—that's a milestone parents should witness. Ditto for first words.*

She looked up when she saw Danny squeal in delight and hold out his arms. Tom greeted her and then scooped Daniel into his arms.

"Happy Thanksgiving, Cassie." His cinnamon-brown eyes met hers, and Cassie felt that little flip in her heart. She noticed he wore a dress shirt and tie.

"Are you on your way to the hospital?"

"Just to check on a few patients." He tossed Danny slightly in the air, and Cassie laughed at the baby's delighted giggle. "With luck, I'll be back for the feast and football."

"I hope so. You won't believe Terri's menu! I'm glad I have these two to help me burn the calories I plan to consume."

"Save a plate for me if I don't make it, okay?"

"Don't even put that thought out for the universe, Tom! I'm sure there's more than enough food." She paused and smiled. "I can deliver if you have to stay."

He winked as he set Daniel on the floor. "That would definitely take the sting out of working. See you soon, I hope."

27

"Cassie, remember you're officially off the clock," Caryn said as the family crossed the street for Terri's Thanksgiving celebration.

"But what about my munchkins?" Cassie glanced at Andrew, who held the thrashing Daniel. "How do we keep them happy and not on a seek-and-destroy mission? Look, Danny can't wait to begin."

Andrew met her eyes with a grin. "I'll take this squirming bundle of energy. You have a strong son, Cary."

Caryn winked at Cassie. "*My* son. With all the people, I think they may crash earlier than usual. Sensory overload, then the constant attention—either it will make them hyper or exhaust them. Remember, Andrew set up the portable cribs this morning in one of the guest rooms."

"At least that's the plan," Andrew added.

"Just remember I'm here if you need me." Cassie entered the Rogers home, then followed Caryn to the backyard. The festive white tent transformed the lawn, and Cassie marveled at the creative decor, combining traditional fall colors with a splash of the tropics.

"Terri's an amazing decorator," Caryn said. "We've told her she should become an event planner."

"I can see that." Cassie scanned the crowd for people she knew. Lauren waved to get her attention, and Caryn nudged her.

"Go. I'll find you if we need your help."

With a murmured thanks, Cassie walked across the lawn and hoped she'd dressed appropriately. She'd chosen linen shorts and a bright floral shirt—just in case she played with the twins. Lauren looked beautiful with an autumn-green sleeveless sheath dress, and Dave… *Well, it doesn't matter what he wears. His eyes capture you, and that smile leaves you breathless.*

Lauren greeted her with a hug. "Happy Thanksgiving!"

She chatted with them for a while, and Lauren mentioned that she and Dave had extended an invitation for Cassie's mother and grandmother to visit at Christmas.

"Amanda wouldn't commit on the spot, but she'll let me know as soon as she can so we can get the airfare." Cassie saw the doubt in her aunt's eyes. "Either way, you're off the hook and spending Christmas in Tampa with us."

"Mom angry?"

"No reason to be. I explained that the break was just three days. You could think about visiting Vancouver during the Suns bye-week. With any luck, you'd split your time between your parents."

"Yeah, about that…I'll have to see. Andrew and Caryn asked if I could go to the Virgin Islands with them." A smile quirked the edges of her lips. "Tough duty, I know, but then they could get out and enjoy some time without the twins."

"Nice," Dave commented.

"Hey, you're an adult, Cassie," Lauren added. "Make your own decisions and don't worry about which you choose. If you need to work, you need to work." Cassie watched Lauren bite back a grin. "Don't let anyone play the guilt card on you."

After dinner, Cassie offered to look after the twins when they awoke from their naps. "I ate enough for three people. I need to chase them around."

Caryn laughed and placed the monitor in Cassie's hands. "Still sleeping—Drew just checked on them. Thanks, Cass."

"I'll listen for their wake-up babbling. Or maybe just relax in the bedroom and watch them sleep."

"Crowd overwhelming?"

"I've met so many new people, my brain's scrambled. I'd love some peace."

Caryn took her hand. "Let me show you where they're sleeping. I'm sure Terri wouldn't mind if you'd like to sit out by the pool. Take a glass of lemonade or mimosa and relax."

After enjoying the quiet and watching her munchkins sleep for about thirty minutes, Cassie decided that she'd get that mimosa Caryn mentioned and enjoy the late afternoon sun. *Danny and Jenna won't wake up for a while,...guess all the people exhausted them. I know the feeling...Wonder if Tom will make it. Got to remember to ask Terri about putting together a meal for him. Special delivery for my hockey doc.*

After stopping by one bar for the mimosa, Cassie walked across the lawn toward Terri's back door. She turned around when she heard her name. *Cam? What could he want?*

"Happy Thanksgiving. I wondered if you were joining the festivities." The corners of his mouth hinted at a smile, and she saw the teasing spark in his eyes. "You look beautiful."

Cassie scrunched her face as she sipped her drink. "Cam, no need to flatter me. Did Amelie come with you? I've looked everywhere for her."

Camden shook his head, his expression suddenly neutral. "She spent the day with Chance."

"He didn't want to join the group?"

"That guy's a loner. Except for my sister, whose company he evidently enjoys." He shrugged. "I think they were heading to the beach with a picnic lunch."

"Nice." Cassie sipped her mimosa again, not inclined to encourage the conversation.

Cam, however, did not notice her reticence. "About that party...I sincerely apologize for the misunderstanding. I didn't mean to embarrass you the next morning."

"Misunderstanding? Is that what you call it? You tried to take advantage of me, Cam…I told you not to talk to me. I have no reason to feel embarrassed."

"How about we start fresh? We both had a bit too much to drink. I know I made some stupid decisions."

"Don't give it another thought. I haven't."

She saw the spark in his eyes. "You'll give us a chance for a fresh start?"

"Eh…no."

"You can't deny you're attracted to me? I thought we connected." Cam's eyes darkened.

"You're delusional." Cassie's tone was flippant. "If I ever felt *any* attraction for you, it disappeared after you served me supposedly light margaritas. Don't waste either of our time. You have plenty of other girls waiting to go out with you." She turned to leave and took a step toward the house. The hand on her shoulder stopped her abruptly, and her drink splashed against her shirt. She whirled around, confronting him angrily. "I said, 'not interested,' Cam." She jerked away when he grasped her arm.

"Just talk to me, Cassie. I really want to make things right with you. Give us a chance to see if anything develops." Cassie stifled a laugh at the sincere expression Cam projected. *How stupid does he think I am?* She glared as his hand brushed against her cheek and quickly stepped back.

"Don't touch me, Cam."

"I'm just trying to…"

Cassie shook her head, "Don't bother."

She felt a hand press against her lower back and glanced to see who had stepped beside her. *Tom.* She saw his brown eyes flash and heard the harsh tone. "I believe she said, 'No.'"

Cam looked at Cassie, then Tom. "You could have just told me you're in a relationship. I wouldn't have wasted my time."

Cassie knew her face and neck had erupted in red splotches. She poured the rest of her mimosa onto the grass, not looking at Tom.

"You okay?" he asked quietly.

She nodded. "Fine. Thanks for the backup."

Tom hooked a finger under her chin and coaxed her eyes to look at him. "Can I get you another drink? What did you have?"

Very much aware of the heat generated by his hand pressed against her lower back, Cassie took a deep breath. She pointed at her soaked shirt. "Thanks, but I already look like I've had more than enough to drink." She attempted a small laugh.

"Why not grab a fresh shirt at home? Then you can enjoy your…"

"Mimosa," Cassie supplied. "It's okay. I'm just listening for my munchkins to wake up—they've had a long nap."

Tom held his hand out for the monitor. "Show me where they're sleeping, and I'll cover for you."

"You need to enjoy some of this feast," Cassie protested.

She saw the hint of a smirk on his face. "Not as much as you need to change." He dropped his hand from her back but leaned to press his lips against the top of her head. "Besides, I can manage both. Just don't take too long." His smile prompted her heart to skip a beat. "I'll watch for you."

28

Cassie reminded herself not to read anything into Tom's actions. *He's just looking out for me.* She smiled at the memory of his hand pressed against her back, and the no-nonsense tone he directed at Cam. *He'd do that for anyone. Like Lauren says, Tom's one of the good guys. Not a big deal...but he made me feel so secure...so safe...and he didn't seem to worry about anyone watching us.*

Hope this doesn't cause any problems for Tom with the Suns. Cam could be a jerk about it...but I doubt he'd want to explain himself to Dave or Andrew. Wish he'd just stay out of my way—or I may smack that smirk off his face.

Cassie silently cursed Cam as she changed clothes, noticing that her shorts also received a good dousing of orange juice. She took a minute to freshen up and brush her hair, wondering if Tom had noticed the fall colors she'd chosen for highlights. A swipe of lip gloss and Cassie was ready to go. She shoved her clothes into the washer and started the small load, hoping that orange juice with champagne didn't leave stains.

Tom sat with his brother and Caryn after he'd filled his plate with the mouth-watering feast. Caryn noticed the monitor he set on the table.

"Did Cassie leave?"

He shook his head as he decided which food to try first. "She spilled her drink, and I told her I'd listen for my niece and nephew if she wanted to change."

Andrew caught his eye. "I saw Cam following her when she left the tent. Did he have anything to do with the drink spilling?"

Tom shrugged, wondering what exactly Andrew had witnessed. "I didn't see how the drink ended up on her clothes."

The unmistakable sound of the twins babbling came through the speaker. Tom began to stand, but Caryn placed her hand on his arm. "I'll get them. Eat your dinner."

"I'll help you in a minute," Andrew told her.

"Don't worry. I saw Kelly go up to the house. I'll call you if I need you." Caryn brushed her lips against Andrew's cheek. "Keep your brother company."

Andrew waited until Caryn was out of earshot before he said. "I saw you…shall we say…have a conversation with Cam. What's that all about?"

"He wouldn't take no when Cassie told him she wasn't interested. I interrupted when he grabbed her arm." He watched his brother's expression. "Unless he's ignorant, he got the message to leave her alone."

A smile hinted at Andrew's lips. "Ready to go all caveman on him, as Caryn likes to say? You looked a tad possessive and pissed off."

"You saw that?"

Andrew laughed. "Oh, yeah. Caryn had her back to you, so she didn't see. Cam came back into the tent like a whipped donkey."

"Just an ass." Tom noted Andrew's scrutiny. "You have something to say?"

"Nope. I'm good. Just checking to see if I need to follow up with Camden."

"No need. He's on notice. Don't jeopardize team unity."

Andrew barked a laugh. "If he brings an attitude to the clubhouse, he won't leave with it. Trust me." He leaned back in his chair, a speculative smile crossing his face. "Something you want to talk about?"

"Not that I know." Tom cut up a piece of turkey and took his time savoring the taste.

Andrew reached over and slapped Tom's shoulder. "Hypothetically… if you've thought about asking our nanny for a date, there'd be no objection from either Caryn or me." A knowing smile spread slowly across his face.

"Hypothetically speaking? Appreciate it."

Cassie hesitated as she approached the tent. Tom sat with Caryn and Andrew, the twins on their parents' laps, eating bite-sized pieces of turkey and sweet potato from paper plates. Her stomach dipped when she looked at Tom, remembering how she felt with his hand against her back—and his tone when he confronted Cam.

Caryn waved her over and invited her to join them. "Hope your cute outfit didn't stain."

Cassie shrugged. "It's washing right now. Fingers crossed."

Tom pulled back the chair beside his. "Would you like a refill on that mimosa?"

"Thanks, I'm good." She looked at Caryn. "I got my break while changing clothes. So nice and peaceful in your home."

"It's your home, too," Caryn replied with a soft smile. "I don't remember what it was like before you came."

"Oh, I do," Andrew said. "My stubborn, beautiful wife was beyond exhausted. So, thank you, Cassie—consider yourself part of our clan."

Unexpectedly, Cassie blinked back tears. "That means a lot. Thank you."

"Now, if we could just get you to agree to a long-term contract," Andrew said, his blue eyes teasing her.

"Where do I sign?"

Tom held up his hand. "Sign without representation? Not advised."

Cassie giggled. "Are you volunteering?"

He shrugged. "I know how my brother negotiates. Just run any offers by me before you sign."

"Of course!" Cassie fought more laughter. "You guys are too much. Besides, you know I'm not leaving. You're stuck with me until you kick me out. I love my munchkins."

When the twins got antsy, Cassie volunteered to take them home for some playtime.

"You don't need to do that, Cassie. This is a day off for you," Caryn said.

"Honestly, I could use some quiet time with these two."

"Quiet time—with my peanuts?" Andrew laughed. "I think that's an oxymoron."

"Never…I'll thank the Rogers and tell Lauren I'm leaving, then come right back for my munchkins."

She found Lauren and Dave standing in a group of players and their families. She hesitated when she realized Cam stood near Lauren but straightened her shoulders and approached her aunt.

"I'm taking the twins home," she said.

"Oh, you need some help?" Lauren's green eyes brightened.

"Stay and enjoy the party." She leaned close to Lauren and whispered, "I'm all partied out."

She watched as Lauren tugged Dave's hand to get his attention. "I'll be back in a few. Just going with Cassie and the twins across the street."

Dave flashed a grin at Cassie. "Had enough socializing for the day?"

Cassie smiled and shrugged in response. Out of the corner of her eye, she noticed Cam watching them. "I've had no play time with my munchkins."

"Another reason Caryn loves you," Lauren said, and then rose on tiptoes to brush her lips against Dave's.

Once back in the Chadwick's home, Cassie consciously released the tension she'd felt all afternoon. She laughed when she stepped into the play area, and Daniel immediately reached for the toys.

"Hold on, tiger. Let's get you safely on the floor." Cassie laughed as she looked at Lauren. "He gets stronger every day. The way he kicks, he may have a future in soccer."

"Not surprising." Lauren placed Jenna beside him as Cassie lifted the basket of toys from its shelf. "Do you mind if I'm a nosey aunt for a minute?"

Cassie met her gaze. "You're not nosey. What's up?"

"Just something Cam said."

Cassie sighed as she rolled her eyes. "Forget anything he says. I probably pissed him off earlier."

"What did he do?"

"The guy just won't or can't believe I want nothing to do with him."

Lauren nodded. "Saw you two having a 'conversation' earlier. You looked angry or frustrated. I thought about coming over, but Tom stepped in and, shall we say, defused the situation."

"You could say that." Cassie bounced a small ball toward Daniel, while Jenna placed all the stuffed animals into a pile. "What did Cam say?"

"He asked me how long you and Tom were 'exclusive.'"

Cassie caught the speculative look in her aunt's expression. "You know there's nothing to that. Tom's like a brother." She tried to stifle a sigh.

"You'd like something more than friendship?" The corners of Lauren's mouth twitched.

"Doesn't matter, Lauren. Nothing will happen."

Lauren raised an eyebrow. "You didn't see his expression when he spoke to Cam…looked like he feels more than friendship. Just saying."

"He probably thinks of me as a kid."

Lauren hugged her before she stood. "Maybe not. He has Cam believing you two are more than friends. If you like him, be open to the possibilities. Maybe flirt a little?"

Cassie tossed a ball at her when she headed for the door. *In my dreams...*

Despite what she said to her aunt, Cassie floated on a cloud the rest of the day. The memory of Tom's hand pressed against her lower back, and that unexpected kiss—even if it was just on the forehead—held her aloft. She'd never had someone act protective on her behalf—even though she *knew* Tom had slipped into a big brother role. *It's just the way he makes me feel...safe...I can handle Cam—but I love that my doc delivered the message for me.*

She could still feel the heat of Tom's hand and the little electrical surges that had pulsed through her body. Sometimes she thought she saw something in his eyes that hinted at more than friendship…and those kisses that left her wishing the roadblocks didn't exist. Despite what Lauren said, Cassie knew that anything beyond friendship wasn't possible…or probable.

29

Andrew's hypothetical comment replayed on a loop in Tom's mind. *Did he and/or Caryn notice my attraction to Cassie? Or did that comment stem from my face-off with Camden? Maybe not as subtle as I thought.* Objections or not, Andrew's "blessing" didn't address his own reservations about getting involved with Cassie beyond the "friendship" they now maintained. *Though we've already strayed beyond strict friendship…can't put a label on this. I don't see her as a friend. I look at her differently than Lauren, Kelly, or Terri. They've never played a role in my fantasies, but Cassie—a frequent visitor.* He thought she shared some of the same feelings, but she'd voiced the same reservations he had about acting on their mutual attraction.

He smiled when he thought about her feisty attitude. She could handle Cam on her own, no doubt about that. *But when he grabbed her arm, I reacted without thinking. Camden gets under my skin with all that cockiness and little respect for women. He's not the only "player" on the team—not by a long shot—so, why should I let him push my buttons? Because it involves Cassie? Absolutely.*

Deciding exercise might clear his brain, Tom changed into his swim trunks and grabbed a towel. Forty-five minutes, or even an hour swimming laps…an excellent place to start.

The twins crashed earlier than usual after the full day's activities, and Cassie brought her iPad to the pool deck. *Time for a fun romantic comedy...jump into another world. No more obsessing about what Lauren said, Cam's annoying persistence, or Tom's actions. I can't read anything into that other than Tom acted as a friend, a gentleman. But just thinking about it gives me goosebumps.*

She settled comfortably on the chaise lounge and placed her water bottle on the table beside her. Within minutes, the story completely drew her into its world. The awkward heroine and the clueless sexy, hot hero had her flipping pages on her iPad. She didn't notice anyone's presence beside her until Tom's voice interrupted her thoughts.

"Good book?"

"Tom, I didn't hear you come out here." Cassie pressed the digital bookmark and set the tablet beside her. She nodded at his swim trunks. "Planning to work off your Thanksgiving feast?"

"I need to. Hey, I hope I didn't overstep things during your 'encounter' with Mr. Camden today. I don't want to imply you can't handle him or need help."

Without thinking, Cassie placed her hand on his arm. She caught the questioning look in his darkened, cinnamon eyes, plus something else she couldn't decipher.

"You kept me from making a scene. That means a lot to me—I would have embarrassed myself in front of many people when I slapped him." She watched the relieved smile cross his face. "I kind of enjoyed that a knight in shining armor had my back."

"When he grabbed your arm, I didn't think…just reacted. I'm sorry if I made you uncomfortable."

Cassie laughed. "The only one you made uncomfortable was Cam—I hope! I'm fine, truly. Thanks for a timely assist."

"I'd say anytime, but I hope that guy gets his act together."

Cassie watched as Tom looked at the pool and stood. He glanced at her before walking toward it. "Would you be interested in going out some night when we're both free? Dinner, a movie, something fun?"

"I'd love to." Cassie suppressed her excitement and eagerness. "You mean, like a…"

"Like a date, yes," Tom finished her thought. "I'd enjoy sharing some of my favorite places in Tampa with you." Cassie saw the corners of his mouth quirk in a smile. "Do I need to clear this with Lauren?"

Cassie shook her head with a chuckle. "I'm an adult. Besides, I don't think Lauren will have any objections."

Although their schedules hadn't meshed, Tom and Cassie began exchanging texts several times a day. Cassie looked forward to her phone pinging…nothing earth-shaking, just questions about her day and sharing bits and pieces of his. Then they started playing twenty-questions, such as favorite song, Marvel or DC, Star Wars or Star Trek, favorite all-time book, Top Chef or British Baking Show, Fixer Upper or Property Brothers, Disney Plus or Apple TV+.

Random text questions arrived at free moments, and they'd compare answers. Cassie learned so much more about Tom through this game. They'd agreed that nothing was off-limits, but Tom had yet to pose a question that Cassie was reluctant to answer. Rather than bombard him with questions, Cassie started a list on her iPad, adding to it whenever a thought crossed her mind.

Finally, the stars aligned after the twins' first birthday party. Just a small group of friends gathered for a quiet celebration. Kelly and John, Terri and Steve, Lauren and Dave, Tom, and the proud parents reminisced about the surprise birth six weeks before Caryn's due date. Caryn and Andrew had hoped that the mandated bed rest, first at home then at the hospital, would successfully postpone labor until the thirty-sixth or thirty-seventh week. The twins stubbornly refused to go along with the plan and entered the world at thirty-four weeks.

Although they joked about it now, Cassie imagined Caryn experiencing premature labor—so frightening. She and Andrew then learned the babies needed delivery via C-Section because Caryn's blood pressure had spiked. Cassie didn't know both babies had spent a week in the NICU or that while Jenna weighed only five pounds, Daniel was a tiny four pounds, six ounces. Not that anyone would believe that a year later. Danny outweighed his sister, and his height had reached the ninetieth percentile.

Everyone shared baby pictures, including many Cassie had not yet seen. She held a photo taken in the NICU the day they were born, then leaned toward Tom so he could see it. "They were so tiny."

"Tiny, but both had great lungs. That was the biggest fear—that their lungs might not be ready to function on their own." He met Cassie's eyes. "Lung function and capacity has never presented a problem."

On cue, Daniel squawked loudly, followed a second later by Jenna.

"Time for some birthday cake?" Andrew asked Caryn.

"Sure, I'll get it." Caryn passed Jenna to Kelly's arms. "We can sit in the sunroom."

Cassie stood. "I'll help you."

Two small cakes, decorated with bright balloons and a family-sized sheet cake coordinated with the paper plates and napkins. "I need to enjoy every minute of this," Caryn commented. "In a couple years, we'll be entertaining playgroup friends."

Andrew had moved the highchairs near the table, and Caryn placed the small cakes in front of each. She and Andrew had followed the Chadwick family tradition and let the one-year-olds self-serve their cake. Cassie had seen the photos of young Andrew and Tom covered in cake, both sporting delighted expressions. Andrew had covered the floor beneath the highchairs with a drop cloth and joked that the twins could rinse off in the pool afterward.

Cassie had Caryn's camera and stood aside as everyone took seats around the table. Tom caught her eye and nodded toward the seat beside him. That simple gesture warmed her heart. They had yet to enjoy an evening together—still, Cassie soaked up all the affectionate gestures, private comments, and thoughtful actions. No one noticed—or if they did, said anything. She wanted to enjoy every second of this party, but she couldn't wait for their evening together.

30

Tom mentioned their plans for the evening to Caryn and Andrew, to avoid any awkwardness when he and Cassie left for dinner. He suggested she dress casually, as he hoped they could walk on the beach following dinner.

"Tell me you're not on call," Andrew commented when Tom wandered into the kitchen. Although the twins had crashed early after the day's excitement, Andrew and Caryn were still finding pieces of cake and icing as far away as the kitchen.

"Back-up to the back-up." Tom tried to suppress a smile. "Which one has the pitching arm? My bet's on Jenna."

Caryn shook her head. "That didn't go exactly as planned. Just wait until your parents see the photos. They out-did both of you mashing their cakes." Tom saw her cut her eyes toward Andrew, taking in his not-so-disguised smirk.

"At least the icing complemented my highlights today," Cassie said as she came up behind them. Tom sensed nervousness behind the bright smile and reached for her hand.

"You're such a good sport," Caryn said. "That was above and beyond, letting them smear cake and icing on your face."

"I just hope I didn't miss any remnants." She laughed when Tom pretended to check her hair.

"You're good. And you look gorgeous," Tom added, taking in the skinny jeans and a camisole top under a robin's egg blue shirt. He watched the color rise in her cheeks, even as she replied, "You clean up very well, too, doctor."

Tom offered Cassie his arm. "Don't wait up for us."

"Like there's a chance we could," Andrew retorted. "As soon as we remove all cake residue—hopefully in the not-too-distant future—sleep is calling."

"I'll help double-check tomorrow," Cassie promised.

"No, you won't," Caryn said, her voice stern. "You have a great time. You both earned it."

"That was relatively painless," Cassie said as Tom opened the car door for her. "Did you tell them about our plans?"

"I mentioned something about it." She watched as a smile hinted at the corners of his mouth. "Neither seemed surprised nor had any objections."

Cassie watched as he walked around to the other door. The black polo shirt hugged his body in all the right places. She'd seen him in swim trunks and frequently had appreciated his six-or-eight-pack abs, broad shoulders, and the chest she knew was rock-solid. But the shirt sleeves only accented his biceps in a way that made her heart beat a little faster—but not as rapidly as it raced whenever he touched her.

"Do you enjoy seafood? Any allergies?" Tom asked as they drove toward town.

"Yes, I love seafood and no allergies I know of. If I discover a new allergy, what better than being with my personal physician?"

"Let's hope you don't," Tom said with a laugh. "No trips to the ER tonight, please."

Cassie felt relaxed with Tom. *Because we know each other so well? Friends first? And I thought I'd find a hot hockey player like Dave in Tampa...total bust. But crushing on a doctor? Never in my wildest imagination...Though I know I'd like Tom, no matter his career. No pretenses or cocky ego like some people. Just a down-to-earth, genuinely nice person...who checks every box on my "perfect guy" list.*

"What are your plans for Christmas?" Cassie asked as they passed several houses already decorated for the holidays. "Going home like Andrew and Caryn?"

"Nah, I put in my request too late. It's a busy time in the ER, and I can't take much time off—not enough for a trip to Toronto."

"Is it the busiest time of year for hospitals?"

"In my experience, yes. Between now and January, too much drinking, too many people driving impaired, kids not wearing a helmet when trying out new bikes…I could list dozens of bad decisions that end up in the Emergency Room."

"So, Christmas is no holiday for doctors and nurses. New Year's also?"

Tom smiled as he quickly took his eyes off the road to look at her. "Unfortunately, the same. But we try to work it, so everyone has at least one of those two-day holidays off."

"And you picked which to work?"

"Christmas Eve and Christmas, usually the hardest shifts to fill. I'll back-up the residents those two days, and another neurologist took New Year's." Tom glanced at the GPS. "Did you decide what you're doing?"

"Staying here. Lauren and Dave invited my mom and grandmother to visit Tampa, but they keep going back and forth about it. I doubt they'll come. My dad's taking his family on a Disney cruise, so I think it'll be just Lauren, Dave, and me. And I'll bring you Christmas dinner while you're working."

Tom caught her hand and squeezed it. "I won't discourage that." His smile caused her heart to skip a beat, and Cassie hoped the darkened interior hid the flush she felt warming her face. *Please don't let this be a dream.*

They dined at a small restaurant, Bistro by the Bay. Besides a stunning view of Tampa Bay, the intimate decor created a casual French ambiance. The cuisine featured traditional French food and American favorites. Tom recommended the Coquilles Saint-Jacques, but Cassie declined until he assured her that scallops, not oysters, were the main ingredient.

"Have you had it?" Still not convinced, Cassie looked at him with a skeptical smile.

"Yes, the house specialty. Promise, if you don't like it, we'll stop for pizza, okay?"

Cassie couldn't resist the persuasive golden-brown eyes or disarming smile. "Just because you recommend it." She set the menu aside as she beamed at him. "I trust you not to lead me astray."

"Not knowingly." His wink made her stomach flutter.

They chatted about everything and nothing as they took their time savoring the food. The evening was perfect, beyond Cassie's wildest hopes. She almost confessed her crush to Tom, but then decided that discretion dictated otherwise.

The phone call came as they left the restaurant and discussed plans to drive out to the beach. Cassie saw the frown cross Tom's expression as he fished for his work phone in his pocket. He touched her shoulder apologetically when he answered it.

Cassie watched the gamut of emotions cross Tom's face as he listened intently and asked succinct questions. Cassie realized that an emergency required Tom's skills at the hospital. She tamped the disappointment that tried to flood her mind. *He's a doctor and responds to emergency situations.*

Tom sighed as he shoved the phone back into his pocket. Cassie immediately read the remorse in his eyes.

"You're needed at the hospital," she said.

He nodded, and she could see him processing thoughts. "Yeah. Massive wreck on the interstate…expecting at least two dozen casualties. They need me ASAP."

"You need to go. I'll call Uber."

Tom's arm closed around her shoulders. "I'll call a car to meet us at the hospital. I'm not sending you home from here. You okay going to the hospital with me?"

"Whatever's easiest for you." She closed her eyes as he hugged her and felt his lips kiss the top of her head.

"Raincheck on the beach walk?"

"Any time." Cassie pulled back and flashed a bright smile. She took his arm. "Let's get you where you're needed, doctor."

After Tom helped her into the car, she saw him on the phone as he walked in front of the vehicle to the driver's side. *Wish he wouldn't go to all that trouble. If not Uber, I could call a cab.* His eyes reflected disappointment when he slid into his seat.

"I'm sorry—this doesn't happen often, but it's always a risk."

Cassie smiled. "And you control what happens on the interstate?"

"I wish." He brushed the hair away from her face, then gently cupped her chin in his hand. Cassie held her breath as he leaned toward her. "Just in case it's too crazy at the hospital."

She met him halfway and closed her eyes. Although gentle, the kiss held so much promise. She parted her lips and turned herself over to his kiss. Better than she'd remembered. Cassie leaned into Tom, as electric pulses shot sparks throughout her body. She tried to contain a sigh of disappointment when he pulled away.

"You don't know how much I've wanted to kiss you again," he said as his fingers traced her lips.

"Raincheck?" Cassie ventured in a tiny voice.

He nodded as he kissed her forehead before securing his seatbelt. "Absolutely." As soon as they were on the highway, he reached for her hand. "One of the 'perks' that comes with a physician."

"I understand. That's why you're a doctor—when there's a need, you respond. I'd want someone like you in the ER if I was involved in an emergency." She squeezed his hand. "Not someone who complains as they drag their…behinds…to report to work."

She heard Tom's soft chuckle. "Unfortunately, there are some who don't have that sense of urgency—or ignore the call. Though once they understand the situation, most do a one-eighty. Few need a kick in the 'behind,' as you so delicately put it."

Cassie bit back a giggle. "I've had to consciously work on my vocabulary around the twins…I don't want the first word that comes out of their mouths, something I didn't censor!"

"Agree. We've all had to clean our mouths. Euphemisms work just fine, and the crazier the better."

"Like 'what the puck?'"

"Maybe too close for comfort."

"How about 'fudge?'" Cassie suggested. "Fudge *that.*"

"Good one."

"You know, once I went to a Vancouver game with a bunch of friends…I got frustrated that the defense couldn't clear the zone and yelled, 'Get the puck out of there.' The lady in front of me turned around and told me to watch my mouth." Cassie giggled in memory. "My friends thought that was hilarious."

"In that case, you really meant 'puck'—correct?"

"Back then, I would have used the other word if I meant it."

Too soon for Cassie, but not quickly enough for Tom, he pulled into the staff parking lot next to the ER. She spotted Andrew standing by his car.

"You didn't need to call Andrew," she said as he held his hand out to her.

"I didn't want you to wait for a cab. My comfort zone, okay?" He grasped her hand as they walked toward the SUV.

Andrew spoke softly. "Looks like a war zone with all the ambulances arriving. It's all over the news—massive pile-up, including a tanker that jack-knifed."

Cassie saw Tom take a deep breath and close his eyes for a moment. "Thanks for meeting us, Andrew."

"No problem. Good luck in there."

Tom stopped Cassie when she moved toward the passenger door. "See you whenever…" His hug was brief, but Cassie reveled in the embrace that brought her against his chest. He brushed his lips against hers, then opened the door for her.

"Go," Cassie said, trying to keep her voice steady. "Take care of yourself."

31

Cassie watched as Tom quickly entered the emergency room, then turned to Andrew. "Thank you for coming all this way. I planned to take a cab."

"No way, especially not after this catastrophe on the interstate. I can take back roads to avoid it."

Cassie shivered. "So, he just walked into a nightmare situation?"

"Something like that. Don't know what caused it, but this time of year—too much traffic and too many people rushing to get somewhere. And speed's not a concern…until there's a horrendous accident."

Cassie looked out the window, silently praying for the crash victims and the doctors and nurses treating them. She thought about the times she and her friends had taken risks—driving too fast, ignoring snow and ice, talking on the phone or even texting while driving. She'd only gotten into a car once knowing the driver should not be behind the wheel—and the memory of that ride home kept her from ever considering it again. If either of her parents had known, she'd have been grounded her entire final year in secondary school. Thankfully, her guardian angel looked out for idiot teens.

Caryn smiled sympathetically when Andrew and Cassie entered the house a while later. She patted to the seat beside her on the couch before looking at Andrew. "I had to turn the TV off. How's the hospital handling all the injuries?"

"I think some have routed to other hospitals, but the worst are definitely going to Tampa's trauma center. Never seen a battle zone, but that's the thought that keeps popping into my head." Andrew opened the refrigerator and looked over his shoulder. "Water, soda, wine, tea?"

"Water, please," Cassie said.

"I'll make some hot tea," Caryn added. She hugged Andrew when she met him in the kitchen. "Thank you for bringing our girl home safely."

Andrew met Cassie's eyes as he held his wife. "We took a very safe, scenic route—right, Cass?"

"Yep. If you'd been a cab driver, I might have thought you were planning to ditch me in a swamp…filled with alligators. I had no idea where we were." Her attempt to sound light-hearted felt off. "Thank you again, Andrew."

Although Tom worked through several shifts, he and Cassie exchanged a few texts. The aftermath of the multi-vehicle collision left too many head injuries. Besides the neurology staff and residents, private physicians affiliated with the hospital volunteered their time. Whenever he had a break, Tom opted to grab a few minutes' sleep and fast food rather than drive home.

Cassie: Can I bring you anything? Food? Clothes? Whatever?
Tom: Yes. Pls. ask Andrew 2 bring me a set of fresh clothes for 2nite's game.
Cassie: You're coming home afterward?
Tom: Yep, unless I get a call, or we have an injury during the game. R U coming?
Cassie: Caryn's sorting through Christmas decorations. May need to distract munchkins.
Tom: LOL. Ping me if you come, OK?

She set her phone on the counter and asked Caryn if she could help her with the decorations. Seated on the floor, surrounded by boxes, Caryn laughed. "I don't even know what I'm doing anymore. I get so caught up with memories, nothing gets accomplished."

"Where do you set up the tree?"

"Actually, this will be the first year we'll have a Christmas tree in this house. Andrew's injury happened before Christmas, then last year with the bed rest and then the early arrival of the babies, we didn't think about decorating." Caryn smiled as she opened another box of ornaments. "These we bought together in Toronto and St. Louis. Lots of memories."

Cassie looked up when Andrew joined them. "Decide where you want the tree?"

"What would you think about the sunroom? I'd like it under this vaulted ceiling, but little hands may find it irresistible. We can close the doors to the sunroom, but still see the tree from here."

"Just let me know the size, babe. I'm heading over to the arena in a few. You need anything?"

"Nope, just a plan," Caryn said with a laugh.

"We could take the boxes to the sunroom," Cassie suggested. "Then, you can use the table for sorting."

"I should have thought of that! Thank you for the back-up brain." She stood and brushed the dust from her shorts. "We can easily move these."

Andrew grabbed a couple boxes before Caryn or Cassie could reach them. "I've got this. Just set aside anything you decide you won't use."

Cassie relayed Tom's request as she followed with a small box in her arms.

Andrew nodded. "I'll get his bag on the way out."

"Cassie, why not go to the game?" Caryn suggested.

"I thought I'd distract my munchkins while you're working on Christmas."

"I think I'll start fresh in the morning. Go ahead, call Lauren for a ride."

"Are you sure?" Cassie hesitated.

"One hundred percent certain. I'll probably doze during the game after Jen and Danny go to bed." Cassie watched as Caryn looked at Andrew with a spark in her eyes. "I'll see you score goals, Drew. I'm always alert when you have the puck."

"I'm sure." Andrew set the final box on the table and shook his head. "How did you accumulate so many decorations?"

"You mean 'we' don't you?" Caryn countered. "I didn't buy all of these."

"That's right—maybe one or two ornaments."

"I can't wait to see where everything will go," Cassie said.

"Please call Lauren while I help my husband pack Tom's bag." Cassie watched as Andrew shook his head, and Caryn pulled him down the hallway toward Tom's apartment. *Maybe someday, I'll find a love like theirs. Nothing like my parents. Just love…true love.*

She'd never admit it, but Cassie hadn't slept well since her date with Tom. Anxiety about the crash victims combined with worry about Tom filtered through her dreams. She refused to watch the news or read about the crash online—as did Caryn—but her imagination conjured images that led to nightmares. She considered not going to the game, but the prospect of seeing Tom trumped her anxiety and exhaustion.

She caught a ride with Lauren, happy for the chance to chat.

"Haven't seen you since you went to dinner with Tom." Lauren glanced at Cassie with a smile. "Enjoy? At least until he got called to the hospital."

"Exceeded my hopes, Lauren! Still can't believe he asked *me* out."

"Oh, I can. I've seen the way he looks at you."

Cassie felt her neck grow warm. "Seriously, Lauren?"

"And I've definitely caught you looking at him with stars in your eyes. We wondered how long it would take for Tom to ask you out!"

"We? As in…"

"Caryn and me…but also anyone who saw you two together on Thanksgiving." Lauren couldn't resist teasing Cassie.

"I'll confess I've crushed on him since the first time I saw him—please don't tell anyone, Lauren. But I never thought he'd be interested in me. He's older…"

"Just a few years." Lauren smirked. "Remember, age is a state of mind."

"And he's a doctor…I thought he looked at me like a kid sister. Why would he want to get involved with the twins' nanny, your niece? If my age didn't scare him off, the rest should have. You don't mind?"

"Not a bit. I know you hoped to get involved with a hockey player—but guys like Cam, the younger players—tend to try to sample every willing woman who comes their way. I'm so thankful you saw through Cam. But, when I noticed the chemistry that neither you nor Tom acknowledged, just figured it was a matter of time." Lauren looked briefly at Cassie. "Tom's one of the good guys—like Dave and Andrew. I don't worry about you dating him."

"One date, Lauren. Just one wonderful evening…until that horrendous wreck." Cassie shuddered. "He hasn't been home since. Not sure he's had much sleep."

"Such a nightmare. All those innocent people…" Lauren's voice trailed off. "Will Tom work the game tonight?"

"He said he is…I just can't imagine how he deals with something like this." Cassie looked at Lauren with a small smile. "I just want to see for myself he's okay…and maybe give him a hug."

32

After Cassie sent Tom a text that she had arrived at the arena, he asked her to meet him after the game near the Suns' family gathering room.

Tom: Took Uber here. Beg a ride home?

She showed Lauren the text. "No problem. Wise decision—told you he's one of the good ones."

Cassie relaxed and wandered over to the buffet, her appetite suddenly returning. She waved at Amelie near the bar, happy to see her friend.

"Feels like a century since we've talked." Amelie greeted her with a hug.

"I looked for you at the Thanksgiving meal, but heard you and Chance had some quality time at the beach?" Cassie teased Amelie as she handed her a plate.

"Oh…that day was *magnifique!*"

"Couldn't get him to come to Terri's?" Cassie selected some fresh fruit and cut veggies.

"I tried…he's really a private man. Never talks about himself or his family. When I ask him questions, he never answers. Says he lives in the present."

Cassie waited until Amelie filled her plate. She led to a high-top table and didn't speak until both perched on stools. "Does that bother you? Not telling you anything?"

"He's given me the basics. Has an older sister in Québéc City, parents deceased. He won't talk about past relationships, but said he's not married 'at this moment,'" Amelia laughed as she accented his words with air quotes.

"At this moment…what's that supposed to mean?"

Amelie shrugged. "Who knows? Not married right now. Maybe divorced? Maybe not in a relationship with anyone else? He wouldn't specify, except to say he expects us to be exclusive if we will be together."

"Serious?"

"Who knows? I just go with the flow. I dislike juggling two guys, and if exclusive means he isn't hooking up with random puck bunnies when he's on the road, I'm good for now." Amelie grinned as she looked at Cassie. "I hear you and the hunky hockey doc got together."

"Where did you…? Never mind…Cam told you."

"You know, Cam really likes you, in his way—even though he can't stop flirting with every female he sees. He came home bummed after that Thanksgiving celebration. Said that I should have told him you and the good doctor had gotten together." She raised an eyebrow, silently waiting for Cassie to give details.

"Did he tell you about what he termed a 'misunderstanding' the night of your party?"

Amelie shook her head. "Not a word. What did he do this time?"

Cassie lowered her voice to a near-whisper. Amelie shook her head as Cassie recounted the evening's events. "He doesn't understand why I told him 'not interested.'"

Amelie laughed. "I love my brother, but he needs to grow up. And yes, I've told him…many times. Even sent him a few mind messages."

"One of these days, some woman will change his thinking," she predicted. "He'll clean up his behavior to prove he no longer lives up

—or down—to his reputation. Whoever it is will knock him off his feet."

"Just hope it's sooner than later. You wouldn't believe the girls I've run into looking for coffee first thing in the morning."

"TMI—I think the warmups are about to begin. Want to sit with us?"

After the game, Cassie followed Lauren and other players' families to the gathering area near the Suns' locker room. Not interested in the variety of drinks and snacks offered, she leaned against the doorframe, watching the locker room door. *He should come out before any players, right? Unless there's an injury he needs to address...or something with the visiting team. Hope not.*

She didn't wait long. A bag slung over his shoulder, Tom's gaze fell directly on Cassie as soon as he exited the locker room. Despite the exhaustion etched in his face, Tom's eyes warmed her like the sun. Without thinking, Cassie dashed to his side and hugged him tightly.

"I'm worried about you," she admitted in a whisper.

Tom dropped the bag to the floor and hugged her. "No need to worry about me. I'm fine."

Cassie pulled back to meet his eyes. "Define 'fine.' You don't look *'fine.'*"

"Just tired, babe. An intense...what? Sixty hours? I don't know anymore."

Babe. Cassie's heart swelled when she heard that word. *Like a girlfriend "babe?" Or exhaustion speaking? Don't read anything into it... it's just an expression.* She stepped aside and held his arm. "Lauren drove Dave's car, so you don't have to worry about trying to squeeze into the Mustang—or rather *Lauren and me* squeezing into that back seat." She offered a small smile.

"Good thought. My other transportation option would require an appearance at Center Ice...or Uber."

"Your personal ride is waiting, doctor. You call, we come."

They walked to the family room, and Lauren met them in the hallway. Cassie watched as her eyes examined Tom, then handed the car keys to her.

"Go out to the car—you look like you'll fall asleep standing up, Tom. Dave shouldn't take too long—he just sent me a text."

"No argument. Thanks, Lauren."

The fresh air revived Tom. He felt he'd fallen into a time warp where all sense of day or night vanished. He'd have to concentrate to name the date or even the day of the week. He looked at his hand locked with Cassie's, fingers intertwined. *My breath of fresh air...the one person I wanted to see when I opened the door.*

Cassie beeped the SUV's locked doors open, but he stopped her before she opened the back door.

"Let's enjoy the cool breeze." He leaned against the car and pulled her beside him.

"Feels wonderful after freezing my tush in the arena." Cassie looked at him, and he read some hesitancy and concern in her expression. He brushed a stray hair away from her face.

"I could use that beach walk about now. Don't forget, I owe you." He saw the look of reproach that flashed across her eyes.

"That's the last thing I'm worried about, Tom. You look super stressed and exhausted."

"At this moment, you're right. I just need some uninterrupted sleep." His fingers lingered on her chin. "Not the first time, nor will it be the last. It comes with the territory."

"I don't know how you do it."

"Adrenaline. When you're constantly moving from patient to patient, you're not aware of time..." Tom kissed her forehead. "Caffeine helps. And texts from a special girl help even more." Tom watched Cassie's cheeks redden. "My bridge to the outside world. Thank you for that."

Tom watched Cassie's eyes blink rapidly, then she cleared her throat before she spoke.

"How many people did you treat? I haven't turned on the news or looked at anything since you and Andrew talked about the accident. Andrew said the driver of the truck may have been texting?"

"That's what I hear. We had forty-to-fifty people come through the ER. Many children, families. Victims with severe burns were immediately routed to a different trauma center...Too busy to even process everything. Or think beyond a patient's current status...Later, I'll go on a tirade about distracted driving...So many children involved."

Cassie turned toward him and held him as she leaned her head against his shoulder. "Not the time to think about that, Doctor Tom. Just the ones you helped."

After only one date and the tragic days that followed, Cassie felt a definite shift in her relationship with Tom. Neither spoke directly about the change, yet Tom and Cassie had become much more than friends, more than two people testing the waters between them. She felt a deep connection to him, and she knew he sensed it as well. *Just like we jumped off a cliff and swam to shore together. Does that mean we're soulmates? Too much emotion packed into that evening and the days that followed? Don't read too much into it—what we feel now may fade as quickly as it wrapped around us.*

Tom said nothing—he didn't need to. His eyes, affectionate gestures, and time spent with her spoke volumes—and no one else seemed surprised. Had they recognized the emotional pull between them before even she and Tom realized it? Though, she could wake up one day and find that their bubble had evaporated. Despite her fear that everything was an illusion, Cassie embraced the possibilities and shoved aside any hesitation. At that moment, she could not imagine a future without her doctor.

33

"Yes, I've explored all options for next year, Mom." Cassie tried to keep the exasperation from seeping into her tone as she talked with her mother. She didn't want to think about school. Not while her thoughts centered on her growing relationship with Tom. She released a sigh and continued, "I'll study either communications or early childhood education in Tampa and continue working for Caryn and Andrew."

"Cassie." Her mother's tone conveyed her disapproval. "That's not our agreement. One year to determine what you want to study. Not one year plus part-time student while you continue to enjoy the perks of a gap year."

She took a deep breath and concentrated on keeping her voice steady. "I plan to take a full schedule of classes. Caryn said they'll work around my class schedule. If I can get the classes I need on Tuesdays and Thursdays, those will be my days off. If not, I'll take early morning or evening classes. Lots of options."

"Have you spoken to your father about this? Just because he bought that car, don't assume he'll pay the costs of studying in the states."

"I'm not assuming anything. I'm saving money, a lot of money.

Enough for at least two semesters right now. I'll pay my own expenses." Cassie glanced out the window, the blue sky above the pool beckoning her.

Her mother didn't speak for a long moment. "You're planning to do this independently?"

"Isn't that the whole point of becoming an adult? To become independent?" Cassie paused for a moment. "Dad can start a college fund for Taylor."

"Have you told him this?"

"Not yet, but I will. I'd wanted to surprise both of you once I started classes—but I'll tell Dad next time we talk."

Her mother chuckled softly. "Congratulations, Cassandra. You became an adult when I least expected it."

"Um…thank you?" *Was that sarcasm or sincere? Hard to tell.*

"I'm proud of you, Cassie. Just focus on your goal." Cassie heard her mother clear her throat. "And don't let your father off the hook so easily. You deserve the money."

As usual, bitterness leaked into her mother's tone. "Mom, please let it go. I don't want to be in the middle any longer."

"You're the only thing your father and I have in common. You'll always be in the middle. That's just what happens after divorce…So, you're definitely *not* coming to Vancouver for the holidays?"

"I'm not choosing one of you over the other. Not any longer. I'm not going on the cruise with Dad, and I'm not going to Vancouver. I'll visit when I can spend time with both of my parents."

Any good feelings Cassie experienced when her mother praised her "adulthood" evaporated. *Nothing ever changes...probably never will. But I can and will remove myself from the negativity.*

With the Suns in town for an extended December home stand, Tom tried to include Cassie in his post-game plans. If she stayed home with the twins, he arrived soon after the game with some food they could share—dinner for him; snack for her. When Cassie attended a game, they either had dinner at a restaurant between the arena and home—or picked up food and enjoyed it in Tom's apartment. Occasionally, their schedules matched, and they enjoyed a movie, a drive along the coast, and once, even, that promised beach walk under a full moon.

He knew they had skipped right over the usual first dates and getting-to-know-each-other process. *Went straight from maybe-more-than-friends to a couple...after just one official date. Maybe it's because we live in the same house and I see her almost every day?* Sometime during the past eight months, he'd stopped thinking of her as Jenna and Daniel's nanny. He noticed the good-natured, optimistic, and down-to-earth woman...who just turned men's heads wherever she went. He loved the untamed mass of hair that often cascaded over her shoulders, painted different colors of the rainbow according to her mood. She wasn't a girlie girl, equally at home in cut-offs and T-shirts or brightly colored dresses and sandals. She didn't care if the twins' sticky hands grabbed her hair or flung a spoonful of food at her face, never showed a hint of frustration or irritation over Jenna and Danny's games.

They double-teamed the twins one afternoon while Caryn and Andrew tackled Christmas shopping. During their nap, Cassie checked the pool before the scheduled swimming lesson. Despite the lanai, bugs landed in the pool drains regularly. Cassie used the net to skim the pool and check the drains.

"I can picture Danny popping one of those flies in his mouth," Cassie said as she made a face.

"He'd probably swallow *that* instead of spitting it out." Tom rose to help her, but Cassie waved him aside.

"I've got this. I always wanted to be a lifeguard and skim the pool."

"Don't let me get between you and your dreams," Tom smirked, then ducked as she aimed the net toward him. Holding up his hands, he backed away, content to enjoy watching her. When she reached toward the middle of the pool, her cut-offs revealed more than she realized—*probably?*—and her tank top stretched across her chest. *She has no clue how sexy she looks.* He itched to slip his hands around her and "help" her move the net. *Not a great idea when we're taking care of the twins.* He glanced at the monitor to distract his thoughts.

Cassie yelped, then laughed when she opened a drain cover. "You poor thing!" Tom stood, ready to remove the invader, but Cassie gently scooped a frog into her hands and returned it to the yard. "You thought I was afraid of a frog?" She laughed when she saw his expression.

He shrugged. "Guess not."

Cassie walked around the pool to check the other drains. "Now, if I find a snake, come to my rescue." Tom could see her shiver. "I hate snakes."

"If we found a snake inside the lanai, Andrew and I would be double securing all entryways. Not Caryn's favorite, either."

"Exactly! And there are so many poisonous snakes in this area, I don't want *any* near this house." She checked the last drain, then returned the strainer to its hook. "You don't keep an anti-venom supply in your apartment?"

"Eh…no. That's something best treated in the hospital. Still, it's highly unlikely you'll encounter a poisonous snake or get close enough for it to bite. Most snakes don't want to be near you any more than you want to see them."

"Promise?"

"To my best knowledge. Stay away from the brush, especially near a lake…"

"Alligators in lakes, I know."

"That, too. If you go rock climbing, wear gloves…"

"Not likely unless it's indoors," Cassie responded.

"And wear shoes. No running around the yard barefoot."

"Seriously? That ruins my day—I love going barefoot." Cassie tried to maintain a straight face, but when Tom raised an eyebrow skeptically, the laughter burst from within her. "Too many of those tiny thorns in the grass, anyway."

Tom grabbed her as she walked past him, sweeping her into his arms. "You know what I think?" He stepped closer to the edge of the pool.

Cassie looped her arms around his neck. "You're seriously not thinking about tossing me into that pool?"

"And if I am?"

Cassie tightened her arms around his neck and leaned to kiss him. "I can think of a few dozen better things to do."

"Oh? Care to enumerate?" Tom murmured against her lips.

Cassie's response was lost in the sudden burst of chatter from the monitor. Tom shook his head with a wry smile. "I call for a raincheck."

"Me, too." Cassie wiggled from his grip and slowly slid to the ground. "We have two munchkins waiting."

34

Suddenly, it was the day before Christmas Eve. Caryn, Andrew, and the twins got up before dawn to fly to Toronto. Although both told Cassie she didn't need to see them off, she threw on some clothes and met them in the great room. Caryn frowned at her while she completed her checklist.

"You didn't need to be up this early, Cassie."

She shrugged. "I wanted to kiss the twins and wish you all Merry Christmas. I'll miss my love bugs." She kneeled beside the two restless toddlers who surfed the edge of the sofa. "You have their winter coats and hats in your carry-on?"

Andrew pointed to the bag on his shoulder. "Next year, we'll worry about snowsuits."

"Please take a picture of their reactions to snow."

"You bet." Andrew focused on Caryn. "You're convinced you brought everything you need?"

"Think so." Caryn didn't sound too sure.

"Remember, there are plenty of stores in Toronto in the unlikely event you forgot something."

"You're right," she answered with a sigh. "This is one time I'm glad my dad has a private jet. I couldn't handle the crowds at the airport."

"Just keep that in mind the next time you feel they're interfering." Andrew spoke with a smile.

"Remind me." Caryn walked to Cassie and hugged her. "Merry Christmas, Cass. We'll probably look for you seventy times a day, but please just relax and enjoy the holiday with Lauren and Dave. You'll find a few presents under the tree."

"Call us if you need anything," Andrew added.

"Everything will be fine," Cassie said as Tom joined them. "Enjoy your Christmas."

"You need help packing the car?" Tom asked.

Andrew looked around. "I think we've got most of it…just what you see here."

"Why don't you leave Jenna and Daniel with us?" Tom suggested with a straight face. He laughed when he caught the dark look Caryn directed toward him. "That would be a 'No,' I presume."

"Maybe a 'Hell, no,' if you consider two sets of angry grandparents," Andrew said.

"Can we take Jenna and Danny and get them settled in the car seats?" Cassie offered. When Caryn nodded, she gathered Jenna in her arms while Tom picked up Daniel. Cassie showered kisses on the sweet girl as they walked to the car. "I'll miss you big time."

Tom opened the back door and strapped Daniel in his car seat, then reached for Jenna. Cassie watched him plant a kiss on each forehead before backing away and making space for her. *Didn't think it would be this hard to say goodbye for three days. Just three days, Cassie…no need to get teary-eyed.*

She kissed each a second time while Andrew stowed the stroller in the back of the SUV. She backed away and concentrated on keeping her smile bright.

"Have a safe trip," she said as Tom moved behind her to close the car's back door. "Text us when you get there."

Tom looked at Cassie as they walked back inside. Her hair was beautifully disheveled, and he noticed that she flicked tears from her eyes.

"I will miss Danny and Jen," Cassie said. "I didn't think I would get so emotional."

Tom slid his arm around her shoulders and pulled her against him for a quick kiss. "They squirm their way into our hearts." Tom glanced at his watch as he opened the door. "Are you going to get back to sleep?"

Just the mention of the word caused Cassie to bite back a yawn. "Hopefully…what about you?"

"I thought I'd check in on my patients, then clear my schedule for the day. Do you and Lauren have plans?"

"Not today. Dave's planned some kind of surprise for her. They'll be out all day, maybe overnight. Big secret."

"So, we're home alone?"

"As it appears." Cassie's eyes danced with mischief. "Any plans for *your* free day?"

"I may have some ideas—if you're interested in an adventure?"

"Tell me more, doctor."

Tom shook his head. "Nope, this would be a surprise adventure. You trust me?"

Cassie giggled. "Do I have any reason not to?"

"Hope not," Tom allowed a smirk to cross his face. "I should be back in about two hours—can you be ready?"

"Depends. Anything particular I need to know? What to wear? Do I need to pack a cooler? Make some sandwiches?"

"Comfortable shoes, comfortable clothes, definitely casual." He cupped her chin in his hand. "Maybe a change of clothes." He punctuated his answer with a sweet kiss. "Two hours?"

Cassie nodded. "I'll be waiting."

Her imagination piqued by the upcoming adventure, Cassie cleaned her room and bathroom, tidied the twins' play area, and took her phone to the sunroom. The beautifully decorated Christmas tree sparkled against the sun, and she saw the reflection from the pool just on the other side of the glass wall. If she didn't see decorations everywhere she went, Cassie would not even think about Christmas. *Eighty degrees and sunny on Christmas Eve? That's July in Vancouver—if we're lucky.*

She called Amelie to wish her a Merry Christmas. She knew her friend was flying to Montréal soon to spend the holidays with her family.

"*Joyeux Noel,* Cassie," Amelie chirped in greeting.

"*Toi aussi?*" Cassie guessed. *You too?* "I hope Christmas is incredible with your family."

"Er, I just looked at the weather forecast. Freezing rain turning to snow. And I'm leaving Tampa, why?"

"You'll love seeing your family—you know that." Cassie shoved thoughts of her fractured family aside. "It can't be that much colder than Paris."

She heard Amelie laugh. "Paris gets plenty cold, but it's so magical this time of year, with all the sparkling lights around the city. I'd walk up the boulevards every evening, even the Champs, if it wasn't too congested with tourists." Amelie sighed. "Ten days home feels like an eternity."

"But will you return to Tampa? Or did you decide to head back to Paris?"

"Oh, definitely coming back to Tampa, Cassie. I'm thinking about applying to the college where you'll take classes."

"Seriously? What about Paris?"

"Can I share a secret with you? No one knows. I don't want *anyone* to know."

"You can trust me." While Amelie paused, Cassie's mind raced through scenarios. *Giving up her dream for mystery man, Chance? Too homesick to return to Paris? Pregnant?*

"They asked me not to return to the university."

"What? Did you break some rule?"

Amelie forced a dry laugh. "You'd have to do something terribly scandalous to get expelled. My grades—after my first year, I thought I had it under control when I got high scores. Second year, not so good. I didn't hit the required minimum in most of my courses. I had too much fun to study."

"Amelie…" Cassie felt her friend's regret. "I'm so sorry. Can you get reinstated?"

"Oh, if I tell my parents and they pay for private tutors…I could repeat the year."

"They don't know?"

"Not even Cam knows. Their disappointment's worse than failing. I can't handle that, at least not now. That's why I'm hiding out here in Tampa. Trying to get my priorities in order—so far, not doing so well, am I?"

"Maybe enrolling in courses here will help that," Cassie said.

"Hopefully. Please keep this between us. I just need someone to talk with. I've felt like a phony around you. I'm sorry."

"Amelie, I won't tell a soul…and I'm always here to listen. At least you have Tampa to figure things out—and a mysterious, sexy man to distract you when you need it."

"Yes, Chance. Another story for another day. *Merci* for listening to my sad tale. You have a wonderful holiday with your personal physician. I'll want details when I get back."

Amelie's news cast a shadow on Cassie's spirit, but she felt confident that her friend would land on her feet. *We may have more in common than I thought.* Cassie recognized the reasons Amelie did not want her family to know the truth about Paris. She understood too well the desire to please parents—how many times had she felt the same pressure? And yes, maybe choosing Tampa had provided the distance Cassie needed to escape the constant emotional tug-of-war between her parents? But the stress never eased.

Cassie called Lauren to share the plans for the day.

"So, you have a mystery adventure today, also?" Lauren's voice teased her. "That sounds like fun! No clues?"

"Nothing, other than dress in comfortable clothes. Have you had any hint for yours?"

"Not a word. But Mr. Martin's definitely ready to roll. Enjoy yourself, Cass. We can compare details tomorrow!"

35

Three hours later, Cassie still did not know their destination as they passed unfamiliar sights along the expressway. "Farms? There are farms in this state?" She pointed toward rows and rows of artificially shortened trees.

"Not all beaches and cities, babe." Tom nodded to his right. "Citrus groves. You can get the best oranges in the world here. Just about a year-round growing season with the weather. Think vegetables, fruit, meat, eggs—you could easily go farm-to-table."

"That's a great concept. Don't think I could eat a cow I saw in a pasture, though." Cassie made a face.

"That most likely would *not* come directly to you from a farm," Tom replied with a grin. "Maybe we can pick up some oranges and strawberries on our way back."

"Are we visiting one of those pick-your-produce farms?"

"Nope. That sounds like fun, though. Maybe another time?" Cassie caught the wink he directed her way.

"I'm game to try anything. I'll probably eat all the strawberries as quickly as I pick them—blueberries, too." Cassie leaned back in the seat and smiled as the sun hit her face through the open roof. "Never dreamed I'd ride in a convertible on December twenty-third."

She closed her eyes and relaxed in the warmth. She must have dozed, because the next thing she heard was the sound of traffic and felt the slower pace of the car.

"Did I fall asleep? I'm sorry…"

"You looked relaxed. It's fine."

"Where are we? So much traffic."

Tom pointed toward the upcoming road sign. "Near Orlando."

Cassie sounded out the word. "Kiss—a—me?"

"Close enough."

The next sign caused Cassie to turn toward her handsome doctor, who tried to hold back a chuckle. "Disney World? Is this the surprise destination?" Her voice betrayed her excitement.

"It could be." Tom merged into the designated lanes, then looked at Cassie as traffic slowed to a snail's pace. "We could go to Disney, Universal Studios, Sea World…" He pushed his sunglasses back for a moment, and Cassie caught a hint of the same excitement she felt. "Your choice."

"Where do you want to go?" She tossed the question back to him.

He shook his head. "They're all incredible. You just need to decide before we come to the exits…"

Cassie thought for a moment. "Wow…I never ever thought I'd visit any of these. I've been to Playland in Vancouver, but nothing like this."

"I promise you can't make a mistake with any of these."

"Surprise me?" Cassie beamed a smile toward Tom.

"Nope. You decide."

Cassie saw the smirk hinting on his face. "Okay, how about telling me something I don't know about Disney and Universal?"

"Here's one—Harry Potter or Star Wars?"

"Definitely Star Wars." Cassie bit her lower lip in anticipation.

"There's your answer, babe. Are you prepared to fly the Millennium Falcon?"

"Sure…maybe?"

Tom laughed. "Let's find out together. We're headed to Disney World."

With the Park Hopper Passes, Tom and Cassie explored as many attractions as possible. Cassie felt like a kid again, gawking at Cinderella's Castle and laughing delightedly whenever she spotted a Disney character. Of course, they stopped to watch the special Christmas Parade. The children's innocent screams of delight and frantic waving caused Cassie to imagine Jenna and Daniel acting the same in a few years.

"Have you volunteered to take Danny and Jen for their first trip to Disney World?" Cassie looked at Tom with a grin as they strolled through the park.

"Not in your dreams, Cassie. Can you imagine trying to keep up with them in these crowds?" Tom nodded toward their hands. He'd held hers securely from the moment they entered the park. The intertwined fingers provided comfort as they made their way through the crowded sections. "No, thank you. That experience definitely belongs to Andrew and Caryn."

Cassie laughed as she leaned her head against his shoulder. "Best. Surprise. Ever."

"You like roller coasters?"

"Love them. The faster, the better."

"That's my girl. Let's head this way—a special treat for you." Cassie caught his devilish smile.

"What's the catch?"

His eyes radiated sincerity. "Just a little warm-up for your Millennium Falcon excursion. And a great rollercoaster."

When they reached the tall silver structure, Cassie's eyes narrowed. "Space Mountain? I've heard horror stories about that!"

"Care to share?" He slipped his arm around her waist as they waited in the FastPass lane.

"No, all I know is that it's fast and dark. Just be sure you don't lose me, okay?"

"Not a chance."

By late afternoon, both felt the effects of the heat and sensory overload. Tom took a phone call as he watched Cassie sit on a bench in the shade, sipping a bottle of cool water. *She didn't exaggerate—she never flinched on the roller coaster-type rides, physical or digitally enhanced.* Her laugh captivated him…as did everything about the girl with rainbows in her hair. *We'll come back to Universal with all those mega-coasters. Soon.*

He wandered toward her after returning the phone to his pocket.

"Work?" Cassie offered her water bottle when he sat beside her.

"Nah, just Andrew letting us know they've arrived safely in Toronto—quiet time at Caryn's townhouse near the university."

"Everything okay so far?" she asked

"Charmed the grandparents, of course. Luckily Caryn realizes when they are on the verge of a meltdown, so they retreated to the condo."

"Snow on the ground?"

Tom laughed. "On the ground, falling from the sky—Toronto's supposed to get about a foot by tomorrow."

Cassie shivered and leaned against him. "I'm sure it's beautiful, but right now, I'll take a pink flamingo Christmas." She laughed, and Tom could see the specks of green in her sparkling eyes. "That's how I'd decorate my Christmas tree."

"With pink flamingos?"

"You bet, plus shells, starfish, Nemo—maybe pastel sparkling lights. Not too tacky?"

"Sounds perfect to me. When in Florida…"

"Oh! Definitely add Suns ornaments too." Cassie giggled. "Can you imagine?"

Tom slipped his arm around her shoulders and pulled her closer to him. "A friend at work has a condo just outside the park. We could stop there. Cool off, freshen up, maybe take a nap?"

"Mm…sounds perfect. My kingdom for a shower."

"No kingdom necessary, Princess Cassie. I have the gate pass and the key. Showers are complimentary."

Cassie reached to kiss his cheek. "Perfect idea…perfect day."

Refreshed by the shower and comfortable in jeans and a turquoise tank, Cassie wandered around the condo as she waited for Tom to change. A recliner in the main room called to her…she curled up on the soft leather and pulled her feet under her. *Heaven. This whole day's magical. Wish we could stay longer. So much more to see. Perfect if we could stay until tomorrow, but my hunky prince most likely has to report for his shift early…Am I imagining this connection between us? So sudden and almost overpowering.*

Too quick? You just don't go from friends to…this much more…overnight, right? Though my feelings have developed over a long time. Never dreamed Tom might want more than friendship. Talk about going from zero-to-sixty in seconds…He can't think about me the way I do him. No worries that he might lead me on or pull a "Cam-style" move. He's not that kind of guy…a gentleman. But I wouldn't say, "No," if he wants more than a kiss. Not likely.

She fell into a light sleep and awakened with a start when Tom perched on the edge of the chair. He gathered her into his arms as he slipped into the seat with her. His hair still damp from the shower, Tom had dressed only in his jeans.

"You looked so enchanting, I couldn't stop for my shirt," he said as he peppered her cheeks and neck with light kisses. Cassie saw the devilish gleam in his eyes and directed his mouth toward hers. She met him halfway and couldn't resist pressing her hands against his chest, her fingers tracing the solid wall of muscles. Cassie wanted to lose herself in his arms, the kiss overwhelming her senses.

Aching to press her skin against his, Cassie struggled to pull off her shirt. Tom finally moved her hands and slipped it over her head. Cassie moaned quietly when flesh met flesh. Tom kissed his way across her cheek and then discovered a place behind Cassie's ear that caused her to arch her back and wrap her arms around his chest. He playfully nipped her earlobe, and Cassie shook her hair to the side to give him better access to her neck. Her hands traced his spine until his jeans stopped her progress. She playfully slipped her fingers beneath the waistband.

"Cassie." His tone uttered a warning.

"Hmm?" Her lips sought his, lost in emotion. Tom lifted her, and suddenly she was straddling his lap. Each time his hand grazed her flesh, lightning flashed through her body, straight to her core. Never had her body responded this way. She ached for more.

Tom pulled away; his darkened cinnamon eyes slowly skimmed her body. "So beautiful," he murmured. Her breath caught in her throat as his fingers traced her bare flesh, stopping at the edge of her jeans. He hooked fingers inside the low-cut waist and pulled her against him and then wrapped his arms around her. "Princess Cassie, what will I do with you?"

"Anything my handsome prince desires," Cassie purred.

He cupped her face tenderly in his hands. "You know we need to slow down."

"What if I don't want to?"

Cassie watched the grin spread slowly across his face. "I might not want to either, but not today, not here. Not before we talk about what's happening between us."

Cassie nearly blurted her feelings for him but bit her lip and nodded instead.

"You understand what I'm saying?" His eyes searched hers, looking for understanding.

"I get it, Tom. Today's a magical dream. But here is…reality, not Fantasyland."

Tom brushed his hand across her hair. "I spend a lot of time in Fantasyland where you're concerned."

Cassie giggled and placed her hand atop his. "But Tomorrowland always dims those fantasies."

"Not necessarily. Fantasies can lead to reality when both in the same…galaxy?"

"Good analogy." Cassie swatted at his chest as she pushed away and reached for her shirt. She glanced at him as she slipped it over her head. "Word of warning. If you come walking in all sexy-like with your wet hair and half-naked body, I can't promise I'll ignore Fantasyland."

"Duly noted."

Cassie walked to the bedroom and came back with a shirt she tossed to him. "No more temptation, please."

36

Returning to a quiet, empty house produced an eerie feeling for Cassie. No sign of her munchkins, no toys spread across the floor, no warm greetings from Caryn and Andrew. Only the beautifully lit Christmas tree and decorations in the sunroom lightened the gloomy atmosphere.

"Thank heavens for the timer on the lights." She hugged Tom's arm as she dropped her bag on the counter. "Very strange to come home to such silence. Spooky—except for the sunroom."

"Agree, babe. I miss the sound of the twins babbling." Tom rested his hand on her shoulder and nodded toward the sunroom. "Let's sit in there for a while. Soak up some Christmas cheer."

"Do you want anything to drink? OJ, water, Coke…?"

"I'm good. Can I get you something? A glass of wine?"

Cassie laughed. "I'll probably have nightmares tonight about falling elevators or spaceships colliding. I better not get my imagination any more active."

Tom slipped his arm around her waist as they walked into the sunroom. "You okay with staying alone, Christmas Eve and Christmas?"

"Lauren and Dave invited me to stay with them. I'm not sure I'd get any sleep otherwise. I know the neighborhood's super safe with the gate access and patrols…and then the security system at this house. But I'd likely think every bump in the night's a stormtrooper breaking in or Darth Vader." Cassie giggled at the mental image.

Tom pulled her against his side as they sat on the wicker sofa. "Glad you're staying with Lauren and Dave. Christmas Eve and Christmas—best spent with families."

She leaned her head against his shoulder. "What about you? Do you wish you were in Toronto?"

"Yeah…but I have my hospital 'family.' Barring a catastrophe, we'll incorporate some holiday cheer. Lots of good food and treats." Tom kissed the top of her head. "I really enjoyed today, Cassie."

"I loved every minute of our adventure." She pulled away so she could see his face. "Thank you for today. These memories will always make me smile." She narrowed her eyes as she bit back a smile. "Especially our little 'interlude' at your friend's condo." She fanned her face with her hand. "You coming out there so sexy after your shower…what were you thinking, doctor?"

Tom laughed. "Had no idea I'd have that effect on you."

Cassie batted his chest. "Holy rigatoni, you didn't notice me self-combust?"

"My view was, shall we say, equally enticing—especially when you lost that top." He brushed his fingers through her hair, and Cassie saw his expression grow serious. "We leaped from friendship right into much more—like jumping into the deep end of the pool. If I'm honest, I've wanted to explore the possibilities for months."

"Surely you knew I wanted that, too? I thought you were off-limits—Andrew's brother, Lauren's friend, the twins' nanny…not to mention the age difference." Cassie saw the flicker of understanding in his eyes.

"I didn't want to jeopardize your job or get 'The Talk' from Lauren, Andrew, and Dave. Too much at risk."

"What changed your mind?"

"Spending time with you, getting to know you as a person, not the twins' nanny. The more time we spent together, the more certain I knew I wanted much, much more than friendship." He smiled wryly. "Took the chance and no one's looked at us sideways."

"Lauren told me she and Caryn wondered if we'd realize our mutual…*interest?*…in each other." She turned to kiss him lightly.

Tom grasped her hand and kissed her palm. "This afternoon… You're such a temptress, Princess Cassie." He winked, and Cassie felt her cheeks flush. "But we need to be on the same page…I don't do casual sex, and I don't think you're into it either?"

"Correct. One hundred percent no casual sex and ideally in a committed relationship." Her words sounded off, and she tried to explain. "I don't mean committed in a 'forever' kind of way…just an understanding…"

"That it's an exclusive relationship while exploring where the journey takes us." He kissed her forehead. "I'd very much like to see how…this…" Tom waved his hand between them. "…develops. We passed the 'Let's get to know each other' stage long ago. Shall we see where the path leads from here?"

Cassie cocked her head as she looked at him. "You really need to ask, doctor?"

"Not about to assume anything, babe. You could kick me to the curb."

"Highly unlikely." She wrapped her arms around his chest. "I'd very much enjoy joining you on this journey." She didn't speak for a moment, content to allow the happiness to swell inside her heart. *Don't make too much out of it, Johnson. He said to explore the possibilities, not commit to each other. Slow down—don't get ahead of yourself.*

She glanced at her watch, surprised that midnight had passed. "What time do you need to report for your shifts?"

"I'll leave by six, so I can check on my patients and get the status of new admissions, ER cases, etc., before shift change."

"I need to stop distracting you then. You need some sleep. Merry Christmas Eve."

Tom chuckled as he drew Cassie into his arms when he stood. "You okay with staying in the house alone?"

She shrugged. "I'm sure I can scream loud enough to wake the neighbors. Your apartment's not super sound-proofed?"

"No more than the rest of this house. You know, you're welcome to stay with me." Cassie saw the slight quirk of his mouth. "And I'm suggesting sleep, nothing more."

Cassie didn't respond as she rose on her toes to kiss his cheek.

"I'll lock up the house and set the alarm. You change into something more comfortable. Satisfactory for you, Princess Cassie?"

Cassie couldn't suppress her grin as she walked backward from the sunroom. "Beyond expectations."

Tom awakened before his alarm sounded. He reached to cancel it, then gently moved away from Cassie, hoping not to wake her. Even though Cassie had confessed it was her first "sleepover" with a man, she'd nestled comfortably beside him. She laid her head on his chest, and promptly fell asleep. Tom? Not so quickly. With Cassie's body pressed against his, he questioned the wisdom of his invitation. He tried to detach his mind from the sensations that pulsed through him, forcing his mind to think about anything besides the soft curves molded against his body. He finally fell asleep while mentally reviewing the status of every patient he followed in neurology.

Cassie murmured a protest when he left her side but fell back asleep when he kissed her temple. He showered and dressed, trying not to disturb her. His shower was cooler than usual to chase away the sleep—and the image of the irresistible sprite who defined cuddling in a whole new way. He turned the water to ice cold and counted to thirty before leaving the shower. Even the air-conditioned house felt warm as he dressed.

He quietly returned to the bedroom and gazed at Cassie. Her hair hid her face, and she now clutched a pillow against her chest. Tom resisted the urge to kiss the shoulder covered only with the thin strap of her camisole and opted to leave a note where she'd see it. *Hate not spending Christmas with Cassie. Not the first time a holiday's taken me from family and friends, but something's different this time—pretty sure it's my rainbow girl. I know where I'd like to take this relationship. Hope she's on the same page.*

37

Christmas Eve and Christmas Day passed at warp speed. Cassie enjoyed celebrating with Lauren and Dave, and she couldn't remember the last time she felt no stress during the holidays. *No splitting time between my parents, no complaints that Dad spoils me, no emotional tug-of-war.* She attended Midnight Mass with Lauren and Dave—her first—and experienced a sense of awe she couldn't explain. Even the obligatory calls to her parents didn't dim Cassie's Christmas spirit. She took Lauren's advice and ignored her mother's attempts to make her feel guilty because she'd stayed in Tampa. Her father was boarding the cruise ship, so the one call Cassie didn't dread ended much too quickly.

She and Lauren laughed their way through dinner preparations, then watched football with Dave while the meal cooked. She curled up on one of the plush leather chairs where she could watch the game and enjoy one of her favorite pastimes—watching Dave and Lauren interact. *Will I find that kind of love? Not the gooey newlywed love, but the playful bantering, the good-spirited teasing, and the many ways they find to make physical contact throughout the day. Lost count of the times Dave wandered into the kitchen to offer his help, then after receiving Lauren's "No, thank you," stole a kiss, exchanged a hug, or just touched hands. They're so cute and happy together—please, God, let Tom and me experience this.*

Still walking on clouds after Tom's surprise adventure and sleep-over, Cassie kept the note he'd written in her pocket. She tried to recapture the feeling of contentment found in his arms. *Respected, cherished, protected, peaceful.* She laughed to herself whenever she thought of his note — "No more sleep-overs…I don't have enough self-control to resist you." *Then, next time we'll do more than cuddle, doctor.*

They exchanged texts whenever Tom had a break. Dave teased her each time her phone pinged, alerting an arriving message. "Slow day at the hospital?" he asked.

"Unfortunately, no. Tom said they're seeing a lot of bike, scooter, and skateboard injuries. Most aren't wearing protective gear. Many children…"

"What parent allows their child to ride a bike or whatever without a helmet?" Lauren said.

"Probably the same type who chooses not to wear motorcycle helmets." Dave shook his head. "Hopefully, none have serious injuries."

"The only thing he said is that the hospital is providing bike helmets for the kids who come in—and anyone else who requests one." Cassie shrugged. "He said they're expecting the food poisoning and alcohol-related incidents later this evening."

"Don't know how he does it," Dave said.

"He cares," Lauren added. "That's why he's so calm and skilled."

"Well, I call dibs on this personal physician," Cassie said.

"Like we didn't know that." Lauren's knowing grin softened the sarcasm in her tone.

Cassie enjoyed cooking in Tom's kitchen. Although it didn't feature all the state-of-the-art appliances found in the house, the stainless-steel appliances were updated and sparkling like new. Cassie had asked Tom if she could spend time in the apartment while he was at the hospital.

Doesn't feel right just taking over the kitchen. Tonight's our only chance to be alone since Andrew and Caryn return first thing tomorrow…before morning skate.

She decided on a traditional Italian feast. Eggplant parmigiana—Tom had mentioned it as one of his favorite foods. Conscious of his desire to eat clean, she purchased organic produce, pasta, and cheese. While it cooked, she set the table, using the new holiday linens she'd purchased, and placed a red and white flowered centerpiece in the center.

The salad tossed and waiting in the refrigerator, Cassie had just taken the garlic bread from the oven when Tom entered the apartment, startling her. "I didn't even hear your car…"

His kiss swallowed her words as Tom swept her into his arms. "Merry Christmas, beautiful."

"Mm, Merry Christmas," Cassie murmured against his mouth. "Missed you."

"Missed you more." Tom's eyes lit a tiny spark that threatened to ignite the fire smoldering deep within Cassie. "Something smells awesome. Did you cook for me?"

"Hope you like it," Cassie said, feeling her skin flush. "It's a new-to-me recipe, so I have something else just in case."

"Smells Italian…I'll love it. And I'm starving."

Starving for you. But after the long shift, Tom might just want to crash. "I…I didn't know if you'd had dinner, but I can put it up if you planned to take a nap…go to bed…or whatever you do after working a long shift."

A smile tugged at the corners of his mouth. "Coming home to find my girl right here, with a home-cooked meal, goes straight to the top of my list."

Cassie nodded to the table set for two. "Sit, and I'll get everything on the table."

Tom glanced at the table, then at the serving dishes covered in foil. "I should serve you." He peeked under the foil of the largest dish. "Eggplant?" When Cassie nodded, he smiled. "You remembered."

"I went to Whole Foods—they gave me the recipe and made sure every ingredient's organic." She bit her bottom lip. "If it doesn't taste right, it's because I can't read recipes."

Tom persuaded Cassie to leave the plates in the sink after they packaged the leftovers and then led her to his apartment's living area. He pulled her with him as they collapsed on the sofa, capturing her mouth with a kiss he'd anticipated many times during the past two days. Tom felt Cassie relax against him as she ran one hand through his hair, while the other pulled him closer to her. He wrapped his arms around her and shifted until they lay face-to-face on their sides. He brushed her disheveled hair away from her face and sprinkled tiny kisses on her skin.

"Longest shift ever," he said. "Thought about you constantly, Princess Cassie." He kissed her forehead. "I'm happy you stayed with Lauren and Dave."

"Me, too, but I wished you could have celebrated with us. After our adventures in Disney World, I so missed you. When I woke up Christmas Eve, I wondered if everything had been a dream." Tom watched her cheeks flush. "When I realized I'd awakened in your bed…I knew then that wonderful day *was* real."

"Hardest thing I ever did, leaving you Christmas Eve. But I promise that we'll celebrate our Christmas properly tonight." He watched her eyes perk with curiosity. He leaned his forehead against hers. "And no hints, so don't ask."

Cassie's contented sigh tugged at his heart. "I love your surprises, doctor."

Tom bit back a sudden yawn and shook his head. "I promise it's not the company, babe."

She caressed his cheek gently. "Exhausted? You need to sleep."

"Not as long as you keep me entertained."

"I'll do the best I can," Cassie said.

"I just need to shower first, then we can begin our Christmas."

Cassie lightly pushed against his chest. "Go, take your shower while I finish up in the kitchen."

"Can't talk you into sharing the shower?"

Cassie's eyes widened as her face turned scarlet. "Maybe next time?"

Tom chuckled as he pushed himself to his feet, then offered his hand. "Short shower, okay? Don't spend much time in the kitchen."

"Promise."

38

When Cassie returned to the bedroom about ten minutes later, she found Tom sprawled face down across the bed. She leaned against the doorframe and appreciated the view. She fought the urge to trace the outline of his sculpted shoulders…the definition of his upper arms…run her fingers down his spine until it disappeared beneath his gym shorts.

She carefully perched on the edge of the bed. *Maybe I'll let him sleep? He's exhausted...should I just leave? Or hang out in the living area?*

She jumped and swallowed a squeal when Tom suddenly wrapped an arm around her waist. "Just going to sit there gawking?" She saw the gleam in his eyes when he pulled her against him?

"Enjoying the view." She let her fingers roam over his shoulders and back. "Impressive." She tried to swallow a giggle.

"Yeah?" He pushed her on her back and claimed her mouth. "You would deny me this?"

"I didn't…want…to…wake...you." Her words punctuated soft moans that escaped with each kiss.

"Screw sleep." He pulled back, and his eyes searched hers. "I've thought about this for two days." He lightly traced her lips. "Or we could cuddle like last time?"

Cassie offered a shy smile. "Maybe more than just cuddling?"

"Anything particular in mind?"

"Maybe swim in the pool for a while?"

Tom's eyebrows shot up. "You want to go swimming?"

"Not exactly…I thought maybe we could check off a box on my bucket list?" She saw the question in his gaze. "I've never gone skinny-dipping…Maybe?" Cassie felt the flush coloring her neck and noticed his eyes suddenly shooting sparks.

"Never?"

Cassie shook her head. "Never." She placed her hand on his bicep. "No big deal if you don't want to…"

"Skinny-dip with you? Hell, yes!" She watched as the corners of his mouth lifted slightly. He stood and held out his hand and led her to the French doors that opened directly to the pool deck. "Sure you want this?"

When Cassie nodded, he lifted her into his arms and jumped into the deep end of the pool.

Cassie swam her way to the surface, pushing her hair away from her face, laughing so hard she couldn't speak. She splashed water at him. "Your idea of skinny-dipping?"

"Nope, just getting into the water." He moved beside her. "Need some assistance?"

Cassie laughed. "I'm good—you take care of yourself." She shimmied out of her sleep shorts and tossed them on the pool deck. Her tank top quickly followed. She suppressed the urge to giggle when she caught his expression. "What's taking you so long, doctor?"

Not waiting for his reply, Cassie ducked underwater and swam like a fish across the pool.

Tom watched as Cassie swam away, her hair streaming behind her in the water. *My own irresistible mermaid. Does she have any idea what she does to me?* Tom discarded his gym shorts, then quickly swam to her side. He gently grabbed her arm before she could escape. "You want to play tag?"

"Maybe shark and minnow?" Cassie lobbed back to him. "You make a fearsome shark, Doctor Tom."

"And the rules are…?"

She pulled away from his grasp. "You're the shark, I'm the minnow. Count to ten, then catch me if you can." She plunged under the water, and Tom watched as she swam the length of the pool without stopping to take a breath. *Eight, nine, ten. Now to capture this elusive guppy.* He let himself sink to the bottom of the pool and hoped she didn't see him swim underwater. He locked his gaze on those tempting legs, lightly moving as she tread water. Staying near the bottom, Tom rapidly closed the distance between them. He reached for her leg, but Cassie sensed his presence before he could grab her. He heard her squeal, then scurry away from him. They repeated this sequence many times until Tom caught her and pulled her against his chest.

"Finally, my little minnow."

Cassie slipped her arms around his neck, taking a moment to catch her breath. "So fun! I call shark next time."

"No way I'm playing the minnow…maybe barracuda?" He felt her legs wrap around his waist, and then Cassie rested her head against his shoulder.

"Barracuda works for me. You didn't give me a chance to catch my breath."

"Then, I never would catch you. So, what's the prize, minnow?"

"Me?"

"Perfect." He boosted her up in his arms, then walked up the slope to the pool deck. "Time for dessert."

After setting her on her feet, Tom grabbed some towels. He folded one around Cassie, then wrapped another around his waist. "Cold?"

"Just a bit." Cassie reached for a towel to dry her hair. "Maybe a tad nervous."

Tom stepped back so he could see her eyes. "This isn't your first time?"

She shook her head. "I had two 'boyfriends.' Crappy relationships, both of them." She looked toward the window. "So attentive and sweet —until we had sex. Then, neither one thought to take me out for an evening. Just interested in sex." She met Tom's eyes. "I should have known better after my first ended the 'relationship' a week later. Sometimes I'm a slow learner. Or horrible in bed."

Tom noted her embarrassed expression. "Highly doubt that, princess. There's a difference between sex and making love. You deserve much better than casual sex."

Cassie's laugh sounded forced. "Actually, my mother always told me that the only thing guys want is sex. So, I had low expectations… thought that was the norm. If I'd ever talked about those 'boyfriends' with her, the first thing she'd say was 'I told you so.'"

Tom gently brushed her hair away from her face. "That's *not* the norm, Cassie. Unfortunately, some guys are selfish pricks." He hooked a finger below her chin and teased her eyes into looking at him. "You call the shots here. I'm good with cuddling if that's what you want… I'm not expecting anything."

He saw the sudden mischief transform her expression. "Maybe I'm expecting more than cuddling, doctor."

Tom slipped the towel from her shoulders. "We can arrange that." He walked her back toward the bed as they enjoyed a leisurely kiss. When her legs hit the side of the bed, he fell on the mattress, pulling her beside him. "Can't believe we're home alone," he murmured against her lips.

"We need to make the most of this private time." Cassie ran her fingers through his thick hair, encouraging him to deepen the kiss.

"Yes. Every. Single. Second."

Both overslept. Tom awoke first, and a quick glance at the clock confirmed his suspicions—it was well past Andrew and Caryn's expected arrival time. He pulled on his gym shorts and grabbed a shirt from the drawer and slipped it over his head.

"Where are you going?"

Tom sat beside Cassie on the bed. "Nowhere, sweet. We overslept…Checking to see if Andrew and family arrived home."

"Crap! I wanted everything perfect for them." She nodded toward her still-damp clothes draped over a chair. "I have nothing to wear."

Tom kissed her forehead. "Go, take a shower. I'll check things out and grab some clothes for you."

39

Suddenly the house regained its usual hectic pace—heightened by the twins' latest achievement. They took their first steps while both sets of grandparents had gathered at Caryn and Andrew's townhome.

"Daredevil Danny was the first—no surprise," Caryn told Cassie. "But Jenna was right behind him. Best Christmas gift they could give their grandparents."

"I can't wait to see them in action," Cassie said as she helped fold the toddlers' clothes. "Lots of new outfits?"

"Their grandparents spoiled them—and us—with enough clothes that we won't need to wash more than once a week. Thankfully, most are larger sizes that they can grow into."

Cassie held up coordinated outfits. "I love these. The overalls are so cute!"

"Have you made plans for New Year's Eve? Andrew and I aren't going out—It'll be a treat having a quiet night at home. So, if you and Tom want to go somewhere…" Caryn's voice trailed off with a speculative smile.

"He said he's made plans—secret, of course!" Cassie released a sigh. "I'm glad he's not working those two days…unless he gets called in."

"Don't even put that thought out there, Cassie! Your first New Year's Eve in Tampa will be perfect. End of discussion." Caryn placed the folded clothes in the laundry basket. "I predict a very romantic New Year's celebration."

"Do you know something I don't?"

"Just woman's intuition," Caryn said with a smile.

Caryn decided at the last minute to skip the game between Christmas and New Year's Eve. Daniel's and Jenna's appetite and energy had been unusually low all day. After checking with their pediatrician, Caryn told Cassie that they could be showing the first signs of a cold.

"They know I'm a worrier," she said with a laugh. "As long as they don't run a fever and stay hydrated, I should just monitor them. Drew suggested I stay home…he knows I wouldn't leave them anyway… So why not go to the game?"

Cassie hesitated. "I worry about Danny and Jenna, too. Don't you want company?"

"I'd rather you go to the game and meet up with this special doctor you've barely seen these past few days."

"I don't even know if he's on call tonight."

"One way to find out."

They left the arena hand-in-hand following the game. "In the mood for a late dinner?" Tom asked as he beeped the door locks.

"As long as I'm with you, I'm in the mood for anything."

Tom turned her and pressed her back against the car. "Yeah?" His mouth met hers with a kiss that left no doubt that he shared her feelings. Cassie roped her arms around his neck and pressed against his solid chest.

"We could get takeout," she suggested with an enticing smile.

Tom looked at her thoughtfully. "Maybe I *should* check in on my nephew and niece." He bit back a grin when her expression changed.

"You should."

"And I will…but first we'll have a quiet dinner at our Bistro on the Bay. Then after I check the twins, we can enjoy the dessert in the apartment." He watched her eyes brighten and couldn't resist another kiss. "Let's get out of here before the guys try to drag us to Center Ice." He punctuated his words with light kisses across her cheek. Cassie resisted releasing him when he opened the passenger door. *Maybe his kisses have something to do with that…just don't stop…*

Tom chuckled when he pulled back. "You don't play fair."

"Speak for yourself, Tommy. I can't resist your kisses." She placed a chaste peck on his cheek.

"We're both in trouble."

"It's so magical tonight," Cassie whispered when they sat at a table beside the picture window. "I'm so glad you found Bistro on the Bay. I love coming here." Something about the intimate French-themed restaurant enchanted her. Maybe the Bay's sparkling surface under the moonlight? The soft jazz just loud enough to set the mood? Her attentive—*boyfriend?*—across the table. Cassie couldn't restrain the giggle that escaped. *Nothing boyish about Tom…but what term works? My guy, my hunky prince, hot hockey doc?*

She saw the question in Tom's eyes. "Care to share?"

Cassie shook her head. "Just pondering something."

"Something profound, philosophical?"

Cassie swatted his shoulder with her menu. "Nothing like that, doctor." She bit her lip. "How would you introduce me to someone I don't know?"

"What do you mean?"

"Would you say I'm your brother's nanny….or the niece of a best friend…" She paused, feeling her skin flush.

Tom chuckled. "Neither of the above. What if I called you my girlfriend? Would that bother you?"

"Of course not! I just can't see myself referring to you as a *boy-friend*…"

Tom's cinnamon eyes teased her. "How about your personal physician?"

"That could work..." Cassie pretended to peruse the menu. "Don't suppose you'd go along with *my hot, hunky, hockey doc*?"

"That would be a hard no." Tom laughed as he shook his head. "Objectifying men?"

"I'm not talking about every man—just you." Cassie hid behind the menu. "Just forget I said anything…told you I was just pondering."

Tom took the menu from her and reached across the table to take her hand. "Are you having doubts about us?"

"Not really…"

"We talked about an exclusive relationship, a commitment to see where the journey takes us. Second thoughts?"

"None, but what I feel for you scares me. What if we're not on the same page?"

Tom kissed her palm. "If you knew my feelings, you might run in the opposite direction."

Cassie looked at him with a small smile. "I know we agreed to see where our relationship takes us. I don't want to get ahead of things, but I'm way past the Friendship Zone. I don't want to set myself up for a broken heart." Cassie bit her tongue, realizing she'd just admitted just how much she had fallen for this man.

"Cassie, I have no intention of breaking your heart. I know I want…*us*… " He pointed between them, "…to continue our journey." He winked as he sipped his water. "I promise I'll always be honest with you, babe, though, I suspect we're on the same page right now. Would I scare you if I said I'm falling in love with you—if I'm not already there?"

Cassie didn't expect the wave of emotions to crash over her. Her gaze blurred, and she pinched the bridge of her nose, but not before a single tear had escaped. She flicked it away and took a deep breath.

"No, those would be the happiest words I could ever hear."

Tom squeezed her hand. "I think I've loved you since the first time I saw you at the airport. I love you, Cassie Johnson. You slipped your way into my heart, and I don't want to let you go." His cinnamon eyes locked with hers. She saw the promise, commitment, and love in his expression.

She shut her eyes tightly to hold back the tears. "You know I love you, Tom. I've been afraid I'd blurt it out sometime and send you running."

She saw the flash of amusement flicker across his eyes. "Not. A. Chance. I love you; I love everything about you, Cassie. You're a breath of fresh air in a world full of phonies."

40

Cassie floated in a bubble of happiness, determined to savor every moment while praying that she'd never awaken from this dream. She didn't mention Tom when she called her mother to wish her a Happy New Year. *Not listening to her snarky comments about men or questions about how a neurologist could love me. Definitely don't need her telling me how much I'm risking by putting myself in this situation. Risk? What risk... that I might actually find happiness with a man? Risk a broken heart? Maybe... But I trust Tom—no matter what Mom thinks about men. He never pushes, lets me set the pace. If he'd just wanted a quick hookup, I probably would have been happy... but now, he says he loves me and wants to make plans for the future. Where I enroll in college. Career goals. But Mom would never believe that...I'm still just a kid in her eyes. An irresponsible, impulsive kid. And Tom's like every other man.*

She refused to give her mother a chance to dump cold water over her bubble.

No raised eyebrows greeted Tom and Cassie when they began spending their free time together. Cassie loved when Lauren spoke of them as a couple. Her heart soared every time Caryn, Terri, or Kelly referred to them as "Tom-and-Cassie"—like a single entity. She'd taken the job in Tampa hoping to decide a path for the future—and maybe date a professional hockey star. Instead, she'd discovered someone she wanted in her future and now tried to plan an educational path that would enable her to stay in Tampa.

Tom suggested she explore local community colleges for the core curriculum she'd need no matter what career she followed. Some even offered online courses that would mesh seamlessly with her schedule. She told Lauren and Dave and the Chadwicks when she applied for the upcoming semester, but hoped to surprise her parents when she presented her post-gap-year plan. With her twenty-first birthday in sight, Cassie felt a new resolve to show her independence.

Tom offered the use of the office in the apartment that he'd set up during his residency. Cassie thought her basic textbooks looked out of place surrounded by the medical tomes and journals, but she gratefully accepted the invitation. So far, her schoolwork coordinated smoothly with the evenings that Tom had to work or during the twins' afternoon naps. Her days were full, but Cassie had never felt happier.

Tom's part-time job as the Suns' concussion specialist had resulted in few mandatory removals from games, with only a handful of players referred to the hospital for further evaluation. Occasionally, an opposing team's coach or player argued the necessity of Tom's decisions. Still, with the backing of the front office and buy-in from each team's training staff, contested decisions quickly reached a resolution.

During the third period of a mid-January home game, Tom watched Andrew take a hard hit against the boards. He observed Andrew hit the glass head-first, then moved closer to the monitor to determine if his head bounced against the ice as he fell. Tom ignored the players squaring off around the boards, and scrutinized Andrew, waiting for him to move.

Andrew had pushed himself to his knees by the time Pettit reached his side. He shook his head when Jim Pettit spoke, and Tom guessed his brother would try to convince the trainer he could stay on the ice. *No surprise—he'll insist he's okay.* After watching his brother skate a few feet away from Pettit, Tom knew Andrew needed further evaluation.

Andrew resisted Pettit's attempt to skate him toward the bench until Steve Rogers and John Peterson quickly escorted him off the ice and down the tunnel to the training room.

"Where do you want him?" John asked when he saw Tom. Andrew shook off the hands helping him and entered the darkened room before Tom could respond.

"Thanks," Tom said before following his brother into the room. He clapped a hand on Andrew's shoulder.

"Dirty play. How do you feel?" Tom nodded toward a chair.

"I'm fine. Dizzy at first."

"Headache?"

"What do you think?" Andrew countered with a wry smile. "Feels like my head bounced against the ice."

"It did. You want to text Caryn before I do the exam?" He offered his phone to Andrew.

"Thanks." Tom watched as his brother swiped at the phone, finally opening the Messages app. He paused a moment before typing Caryn's name, shaking his head, and finally closing one eye to focus on the screen. He typed a short sentence, then pressed "send."

"Short and sweet," Andrew commented when he handed the phone back to his brother.

"Relax, and I'll get you through the exam." Tom glanced at Pettit, who stood to the side. Andrew had difficulty tracking the penlight, eventually shutting his eyes against the light with a sigh.

"Andrew, I'm sending you to the hospital for further tests," Tom said.

"That's bullshit, Tom. Just give me some time here. I'm okay."

Andrew opened his eyes, and Tom recognized the flash of stubbornness. "You send me to the hospital, Caryn will panic. I'm not putting her through that again."

"She's on her way down," Pettit spoke up. "She can go with you."

"You know the protocol," Tom spoke softly.

"I don't need further evaluation. I know the freaking protocol."

"Dan's waiting for you at the hospital," Tom said evenly. "You convince him you're fine; he'll send you home."

"Effing waste of time."

"You want to leave in your uniform or change?" Tom ignored his brother's outburst.

"You're giving me a choice?"

"If you can handle it." Tom watched as Andrew unlaced his skates with his eyes closed. He removed them, pulled his jersey and pads from his upper body, then reached for the treatment table to steady himself as he slowly stood to shed the rest of his uniform. When he paused for a long moment, Pettit offered to help.

"Lucas is collecting your personal items to give to Caryn. Let's just get you into these sweats."

Tom slipped out of the room and updated Harper. "He's going… reluctantly. I don't think it's anything serious, other than a mild concussion, but with his history…"

"Take no chances," the coach agreed.

Tom saw Caryn walk hesitantly toward them and met her halfway. "He's okay, Caryn. Conscious and bitching about having to go to the hospital."

"Can I go with him?"

"That shouldn't be a problem. Maybe you can help with his attitude."

Caryn's soft laugh sounded strained. "Where is he?"

Tom showed a closed door about ten feet away. "Dan will meet the ambulance—Andrew won't have time to complain. I'll come as soon as the game's over and either take you guys home or help restrain him in a hospital bed. Either way, he'll be fine, Caryn."

"Will you let Cassie know we might be late?" Caryn asked as she walked beside him toward the door.

"No worries. I'll also call Lauren." Tom hugged her affectionately before he reached to push the door open. "Good luck with him."

As soon as the ambulance left, Tom pressed Cassie's name on his phone. She answered before he heard it ring.

"Tom, what's happening? How's Andrew?"

"On his way to the hospital—just precautionary tests, nothing serious, babe." He updated her on the situation and relayed Caryn's message.

"Tell her not to worry. The love bugs are fast asleep."

"Not sure when I'll see you, Cassie…Someone will come by in case you need backup."

"We're fine. Please keep me in the loop."

"Promise. Call if you need anything."

Cassie sighed as she set her phone on the counter. *Andrew left the ice on his own—just a little help from his teammates. That's a good sign, right? Nothing like the trauma two years ago.*

She didn't know the details of Andrew's head injury, but from comments knew that it was a life-threatening situation, followed by over a year of rehab. Cassie sensed Caryn's wish to avoid those memories, and she didn't want to pry by asking Lauren. She found plenty of information on Google, but only read enough to understand the horrific accident and slow recovery. *Hope Caryn's not experiencing déjà vu… surely, some of her friends had arrived at the hospital.* Cassie hated feeling helpless and concentrated on the only thing she could—blanketing Andrew and Caryn with prayers.

41

"Any news?" Cassie asked when Lauren and Dave stopped at the house on their way home.

"Unless something has changed, Tom sounded confident that Andrew's doctor would keep him at least overnight," Lauren said. "Just for observation."

"And an 'overabundance of caution,' as Tom put it," Dave added.

"Can I get you anything? Water, soft drinks, coffee?"

"We know where to find it, Cass. Relax while you can—do Daniel and Jenna wake up during the night?"

"Not usually. I'm fine, guys. You don't need to babysit me. I know where to find you if I need help."

"Maybe we'd like to catch up with you," Dave retorted with a grin as he sat down in the living area. "We don't see much of you now that you're taking classes and spending your free time with our favorite doctor."

Cassie felt her cheeks flush. "I saw you at the game last week. School has been more difficult than I ever thought. I have to pass algebra before I can take any core classes."

Lauren made a face. "Feel your pain. Though keep in mind, your

Language Arts scores exempted you from some classes and gave you credit for core courses."

"Which does zero good until I get through algebra. Why do I need algebra to succeed in communications or early childhood education, anyway?"

"Hell, if I know," Dave said with a grin. "If it's not too advanced, I can probably help you."

"Just secondary school algebra. It left my brain as soon as I completed the course. I'll gladly take any help offered. The quadratic equation is some medieval torture device."

Both Lauren and Dave laughed. "I've never needed to use it, so I'd agree with you, kiddo," Dave said. "But I can teach you a trick to solve them. I remember when my sister Kimberl7 and brother Jake both needed a bit of assistance."

"If you can help me with that, I think I can test out of the class. I think I did okay until that section."

"Save a couple hours Sunday afternoon then. Tell your doctor you have a math emergency."

"I think he's working, anyway. Thanks, Dave."

Lauren brought bottles of water from the kitchen. "Why don't I order a pizza? It may be a while until we hear from Tom."

Tom tried to shake off his brother's anger over Dan Forster's insistence that he stays overnight at the hospital. *Dan nailed it when he said that Andrew's over-reaction and angry outburst just confirm our diagnosis of a minor concussion. If he hadn't recently recovered from the TBI, Dan would have released Andrew. Once he calms down, he'll under stand. Hope Caryn can work some magic with him.*

He recognized Dave's car in the driveway, so he entered the house through the front door. Cassie greeted him with a sweet kiss and an offer of food.

"Pizza sounds great," he agreed as he walked toward Lauren and Dave. "Thanks for hanging out here."

"So, what's the news?" Dave asked. "Minor concussion, like you thought?"

"I'd say, 'yes,' but he's so angry over having to stay overnight, I might upgrade that to a mild concussion. I told him I'd see him when Dan releases him. He may settle down with just Caryn there."

"He's not blaming you?" Cassie asked when she set a warmed pizza on the counter, along with the salad she'd added to the order.

"No, he's just frustrated. Convenient and safe target." Tom laughed softly. "Better me than Caryn. I told her not to take any crap from him."

"Should I go over there?" Dave asked.

"Nah, Peterson's there with Kelly—back up just in case. Guarantee he'll be embarrassed about his reaction once he's feeling normal."

He perched on a chair by the counter. "My niece and nephew sleeping like angels?"

"Of course," Cassie said. "What can I get you to drink?"

"No need to serve me. I'll grab something in a while." He glanced at Lauren and Dave. "Did you guys eat?"

"Yes, doctor," Lauren teased. "If you don't think you will go back to the hospital, we'll head home."

"Nope, I'm here and not on call. Dan told me to not set foot in the hospital until Andrew's released." He looked at Cassie. "So, you're stuck with me. Our first overnight assignment with the twins."

"Under control," Dave commented as he hugged Cassie and clapped a hand on Tom's shoulder. "Holler if you need anything."

"Keep us posted," Lauren whispered as she kissed Cassie's cheek. "Call if you need us to take a shift."

Cassie stepped behind Tom and felt the tight muscles in his shoulders. She squeezed them softly. "How about a massage?"

He looked at her over his shoulder. "You offering?" She loved the little smirk that crossed his face.

"That's the idea, doctor." She lifted on her tiptoes to kiss his cheek.

"Put on something comfortable, and I'll meet you at the pool. I'll check on the love bugs while you change."

"Underwater massage?"

"Hadn't thought of that. We'll have to see." Cassie ran her hands over his back. "See you in a few, hockey doc."

Cassie pulled the light blankets over Jenna and Daniel, smiling at the way Jenna clutched her teddy bear and Daniel slept with his little fist pressed against his mouth. She stopped in her room and grabbed her bottle of lavender oil plus a jar of lotion. *A few drops should relax my guy. Never heard Andrew and Tom exchange a harsh word. If Andrew went off on Tom…it must bother him. Can't imagine Lauren doing that to me, but I'd definitely feel hurt, betrayed…Can Tom step back and see it as a medical thing? Maybe?*

She picked up two bottles of water before walking to the pool deck. Tom sat on a chaise lounge and stared at the pool. She couldn't read his mood, so she opted for a teasing tone.

"You do realize you need to lose that shirt, Tommy?"

"Bossy, much?"

"I can't use my magic lotion on you." She perched beside him on the lounge. "You know I love to…explore…your muscles."

Tom pulled the shirt over his head and faced her with a challenging smile. "Now what, masseuse? You taking your shirt off, too?"

"When you give *me* a massage. On your stomach now."

Tom chuckled as he complied. Cassie scooped skin cream into her palm and added a drop of lavender oil. She heard his contented sigh as she smoothed the cream over his shoulders before climbing to straddle his lower back. Now she could lean into her hands as she kneaded his shoulders, alternating firm pressure and feathered brushes.

Neither spoke as Cassie worked the tightness out of Tom's shoulders. The lavender had a relaxing effect on her as well. She loved the ripple of his muscles beneath her hands and found her thoughts drifting to the little electrical sparks traveling to her core. She shifted slightly, and Tom groaned.

"Do you realize what you're doing to me?"

"The same thing you're doing to me? Making me feel all tingly,"

Cassie said. Tom carefully turned onto his back, his hand holding her in place.

"*Masseuse extraordinaire.*" His cinnamon eyes sparked as she shifted again. "You do realize you're not relaxing me now?"

"Seriously?" Cassie pretended innocence. "The lavender soothes me, makes me feel so…"

Tom cut her off as he pulled her to him and claimed her mouth. "… seductive?" He deepened the kiss. "Have your way with me, Ms. Johnson."

Cassie ran her fingers against his lips. "Oh, I intend to, Dr. Chadwick."

They both laughed at the twins' impeccable sense of timing when Daniel, then Jenna fussed. "Time out," Tom said.

Cassie slid to her feet and held her hand out. "Just a short rain check."

42

Cassie awoke before Tom and carefully slipped from the bed and took the monitor with her. She expected the twins to awaken shortly and hoped to shower while she had the time.

Jenna and Daniel sat in their highchairs, tossing Cheerios when Tom emerged from his apartment a while later.

"Why didn't you wake me?" he asked as he kissed Cassie's cheek.

"I wanted you to get some extra sleep…at least until I got our munchkins fed." She handed him the plates with diced bananas and one of Caryn's muffins. "Please give them this while I get their milk."

"Don't we look domestic?" Tom winked after Cassie placed the sippy cups on the trays.

"We survived our first night alone with the twins."

"Piece of cake. But I'm not telling Caryn," Tom said. "They could go away some weekend."

"Highly unlikely. I'm not sure who's more protective of Danny and Jenna." Cassie pulled back a chair and sat at the table. "Any news on Andrew?"

"Just spoke with Dan. He's sending him home but won't clear Andrew to play until he sees him in forty-eight hours." Tom opened the refrigerator and looked at the contents.

"So, you can't clear him?"

"Nope, I'm out of that line of fire. How hungry are you? I can make pancakes. Or an omelet? Scrambled eggs?"

"All the above?" Cassie said with a giggle. "I'll eat anything you cook." She caught a chunk of banana Daniel threw at her. "Does Caryn have their car to drive home? Do we need to get it from the arena?"

"Rogers and Peterson took care of that last night. Pretty sure Caryn will check in soon."

"Surprised she hasn't." Cassie laughed as she looked at the assortment of foods that peppered the floor. "Hope she doesn't walk in before I can clean the floor. She manages breakfast so much better than me."

"You mean 'us,'" Tom corrected. "Takes two of us to do what she does." He cracked eggs into a bowl. "But between you and me, I think we'll have everything ship-shape before they get back."

Tom heard Caryn and Andrew enter the house as he prepared to go to work. Tempted to walk out his private entrance rather than risk another confrontation, he grabbed his keys and walked to the main living area. He heard Caryn laughing in the nursery with Cassie as the twins babbled excitedly. Andrew leaned against the counter, his eyes shut against the bright sunlight streaming through the windows.

"You want to sit?"

Andrew shook his head, then rubbed his hand across his face. Tom guessed that he hadn't slept and was most likely dealing with a significant headache.

"Can I get you anything?"

Andrew glanced at him, his eyes revealing nothing. "I'm good."

Tom thought Andrew's smile seemed forced when the twins reached for him as soon as they spotted their dad. Caryn laughed and nodded at Daniel.

"Do you hear what your son's saying?" She sat Daniel on the counter between them and waited until Andrew deciphered the babbling.

"Da…dadada…dada…da!"

Tom caught Cassie's eyes when Andrew's expression softened. "His first word…that we recognize," Caryn laughed. "You called it, Drew."

"You're Daddy's little man, aren't you, peanut?" Andrew lifted Daniel into his arms as he sat on the counter chair.

"Cassie, we have to double down with Jenna now." Caryn reached for her daughter. "Mama…ma…ma…" she quietly prompted.

"You won't let your mama down, will you, pretty girl?" Cassie kissed Jenna's forehead before moving toward Tom. "You heading to work?"

He nodded as he stepped beside her. "Call you later."

"Tom, thanks so much for helping last night," Caryn said. "With you and Cassie here, we had no worries."

Tom pulled Cassie against his side. "It was all Cass. All I did was sweep up Cheerios this morning." He pressed his lips against her forehead.

"Not true," Cassie added. "Jenna and Danny love their Uncle Tommy."

"When do we see you next?" Caryn asked while trying to keep Jenna from grabbing a handful of hair.

"At or after the game Thursday. Did Dan give you any indication when he plans to clear you to play?"

Andrew met his eyes, and Tom read the lingering anger. "Imagine you'll know before I do."

"That's between you and Dan. He's your admitting physician."

"But, you're quick to decide who leaves a game."

"Drew…" Caryn whispered.

"I'll always err on the side of caution if there's a chance of a head injury." Tom kept his tone soft and even. "You two get some rest," he said as he grasped Cassie's hand. "Walk me out?"

Cassie didn't realize she'd been holding her breath until they stepped outside. "Tense much?" She looked at Tom's eyes for a hint of his thoughts.

"Take nothing Andrew says personally. He's pissed and frustrated —but that's an effect of the concussion. Normal and expected…Caryn knows how to deal with this."

"It doesn't bother you?"

"That he's angry with me? Not a bit. Maybe disappointed since he knows what he went through before—I'll give him a pass. If he wants to direct his anger my way, fine. Better me than anyone else."

Cassie searched his expression before sliding her arms around his neck and urging him closer for a kiss. "I'll miss my personal physician. You spoiled me last night."

Tom chuckled as he pulled her against him. "I intend to spoil you every chance I get. I hope you have a quiet afternoon with the twins so Andrew and Caryn can rest. If you need back-up, remember Kelly and Terri are just a text away. Lauren, too. Take care of yourself, okay?" He punctuated his instructions with a soft kiss. "Call me if you need anything."

Her heart fluttered when he kissed her again before walking to his car. She blew a kiss to him as he backed out of the driveway, her mind and body buzzing with emotions that continued to strengthen. *If this is a dream, please never let me wake up.*

Andrew kept to himself during the following two days. He spent most of the day in the bedroom with the blinds shut. Caryn explained the sensitivity to light and loud noises, so Cassie did her best to keep the twins occupied and quiet. They loved the outdoors, so Cassie took them on long walks in their stroller at least once a day. Lauren invited them to spend some time at their home—Cassie felt Caryn's relief and was quick to accept the invitation. She accompanied Cassie and the twins on the short walk to the house.

"You can't know how much I appreciate you going above and beyond to keep the house quiet. He'd never admit it, but I know loud or high-pitched sounds trigger migraine-like headaches. Thank you for picking up on that…it's been a long couple of days."

"When does Andrew see the doctor again?"

"In a few hours. Say a prayer he's cleared to play when we see the doctor this afternoon. I can handle a few days of this, but, please, no more." She met Cassie's eyes with a small smile. "I hope Drew's okayed for the game before he sees Tom. I've never seen them argue, much less experience Drew's attitude. He'll apologize once he's feeling 'normal' again."

"Tom said he doesn't let it bother him…just part of the concussion effect. But I hate the tension between them. Never expected that."

"Fingers crossed he's back on the ice next game…we'll know later today." Caryn looked at Cassie as they approached Lauren's front door. "I'll call to let you know if it's 'safe' to turn the kids loose at home."

43

Within a week, Andrew had returned to the first line, and everything appeared normal between the brothers. When Cassie saw Tom, he assured her they had worked through their issues. Tom joked that he'd told Andrew he'd rat him out to their parents if he ever gave him that attitude again.

"So, he doesn't want to disappoint them?"

"Never—nor does he want to listen to a lecture from Mom." Tom smiled when he met her eyes. "He's the golden son who can do no wrong. If he ever disappointed her…well, she'd never let him forget it. She always said that we were each other's best friend…no matter what, we could count on that. We grew up with that expectation. So, besides being my brother, Andrew's my best friend. Neither of us ever wants to disappoint her."

Cassie chuckled. "My mom *expects* me to disappoint her. Low expectations."

"I'm sure she's proud of you."

"She'd have preferred I never grew up."

"Well, you accomplished that spectacularly. You're working full-time, taking classes, and keeping everything organized. That's what I call exceeding high expectations."

Cassie hugged him. "Thank you for believing in me…that means more than I can explain. So, will you leave for the game soon?"

Tom glanced at his watch. "Yes, and I'll bring dinner home if you can wait?"

"Wait for you? Do you need to ask?"

Cassie's comment about her mother's low expectations gnawed at the back of Tom's mind. Did her mother really expect her to fail? *Wanting Cassie to remain a child could show that she wished to keep Cassie dependent and under her control. Twisted thinking either way. Can't imagine growing up in a divided household, absorbing her mother's negativity and hostility toward men. From what Lauren's said, her sister embraced the belief that their mother had set in motion. But Lauren had escaped her past. Her mother's attitude could be the source of Cassie's low self-esteem. If only she could see herself the way I do, and everyone who knows her does.*

Tom vowed to help mend her self-esteem. He applauded her accomplishments and supported her desire to prove her independence and ability to make her own life decisions. *Things most of us take for granted.*

He loved her optimistic nature and the hint of rebellion she sometimes displayed…a free spirit who chose positivity and whose empathy extended to everyone she encountered. Like the ever changing rainbow highlights in her hair, Cassie brought sunshine wherever she traveled.

Tom acknowledged the sense of guilt that lurked in the back of his mind. He'd completed his education and had settled into his profession, but Cassie had just begun exploring her options. Could he convince her they'd make it work, no matter where her studies took her?

He knew that Andrew and Caryn had dealt with a similar scenario. Just as their love blossomed, Andrew was traded to St. Louis from Toronto. Caryn had at least another year before she graduated from the university in Toronto. They made it work, long-distance relationship and all. Tom remembered the challenges they faced and the mutual determination that their love would guide them through those months.

Cassie Johnson. "The One" he didn't want to—*could not?*—live without? Tom sighed as he stopped at the nurses' station to look over patient charts. The intricacies of neurology diminished when he compared it to love.

Amelie returned to Toronto mid-January. She'd emailed Cassie once from Montréal. Her parents had learned the truth about her grades in Paris—and she had an edict to come up with a satisfactory plan to make up the lost credits. Cassie shared her schedule at the community college and sent her the links to apply and course selections. Amelie loved the option of online courses and only needed a year's worth of credits to catch up. She planned to accomplish this in two semesters.

"I've played the twin card with Cliff—he'll let me stay with him and will pay the tuition. One condition—I quit my job and devote the time needed to score all A's."

Cassie chuckled. "You can do that—though it may cut into your time with your hot French guy."

"We'll see. Chance didn't bother to contact me the entire time in Québéc. Not even on New Year's Eve. I may not have time for *him.*"

At Caryn's suggestion, Cassie invited Amelie over when she returned to Tampa. With the Suns out of town for a long road trip to the West Coast before the All-Star break and bye-week, Caryn felt Amelie might feel lonely at the condo. Amelie arrived the next day with a small overnight bag, her class schedule, laptop, and textbooks.

"I hope I can get ahead in my course work, so Cliff lifts my home arrest when he gets back."

Cassie laughed and showed Amelie the guest room she'd prepared for her friend. "It's easy to work ahead on the online courses. I wish all of mine were online—especially algebra." Cassie made a face. "Dave's tutored me a couple times, but when I think about retaking the placement exam, I panic. I don't want to stay in remedial algebra."

"Tom's good at math, isn't he?"

Cassie shrugged. "I assume he's good at every subject, but I haven't asked him about algebra. He's so busy at the hospital, I don't want to waste any time I can spend with him on algebra. Would you?"

Amelie quickly unpacked her suitcase while Cassie curled up on a chair near the French doors to the pool deck. "So, you and Tom—serious?"

"Well, we're exclusive and everything."

Amelie raised an eyebrow. "So, you're in love?"

Cassie felt her face and neck warming. "We haven't told anyone yet. Still feels like a dream come true. He is the best thing that's ever happened to me."

"So, he's amazing in bed?"

Cassie knew her cheeks had reddened. "I think so."

"No details?" Amelie teased.

She shook her head with a giggle. "Amazing pretty much sums it up." Cassie glanced at her wrist. "I need to check on the twins and see what Caryn wants to do about dinner. Make yourself at home. Let me know when you need the WIFI password."

Amelie hugged her impulsively. "I've missed you and spending time with Caryn and the twins. Thanks for keeping me from feeling sorry for myself at that condo."

44

Caryn caught Cassie's eye while they prepared the twins' dinner plates, then nodded toward the playroom—their former great room—where Amelie interacted with Jenna and Daniel. The twins giggled and brought their favorite toys to place in her lap.

"Attitude adjustment," she said. "Wouldn't believe it without seeing it."

"I guess facing her folks about what happened in Paris affected her more than she'll admit. She's definitely more fun to have around. Not so hung up on herself," Cassie whispered.

"I noticed." Caryn winked. "How nice for you."

Andrew's ringtone sounded on Caryn's phone, and Cassie excused herself and joined Amelie and the twins. Daniel concentrated on lining up blocks, while Jenna threw a nerf ball back and forth with Amelie.

"I can't believe how much they've changed! When did they begin to walk?" Amelie asked.

"Christmas—perfectly timed for their grandparents to see their first steps." Cassie handed a block to Danny, who carefully aligned it with the others.

"Do you have trouble keeping up with them now?"

"They keep us on our toes. Their mission is to open every cabinet or drawer within reach—I can't manipulate the childproof locks, and they somehow get passed them. Now, they've discovered how to open doors. So, we have to triple check that the doors to the pool stay locked. I'm sure a fence surrounding the pool is coming soon. Our little shark here," Cassie said, indicating Daniel, "would spend all day playing in the water if he could."

"I'll feel better when that fence gets installed. You know how I obsess over that pool." Caryn added as she walked toward them. "Let's get you guys cleaned up for dinner." Jenna fussed and reached for her mom, and Amelie smiled at Caryn.

"Could I take Danny, please? You don't mind, do you, Cassie?"

"No, I'll put up their toys. Just be careful—Daniel likes to kick when you pick him up."

Tom entered the front door just as Cassie stowed the last basket of toys on its shelf. "Too late for a snowball fight?"

"Sorry…but you're just in time for Jenna and Daniel's dinner. If they see you, they'll insist you sit with them." Cassie walked to him so she could greet him properly. "Did you have a quiet day?"

"Somewhat. Mostly follow-up visits with discharged patients. You know, we're still treating some of those injured in that massive pile-up."

Cassie shivered. "But they're recovering, right?"

"Head injuries can take longer to heal than broken bones."

"Our first date—I hate that the accident's part of the memory of that wonderful, romantic evening."

Tom hugged her and kissed her temple. "That was just the first of a lot of romantic adventures—no bad memories attached to the rest, I hope?"

"Like going to Disney? I'll never forget that surprise…or New Year's Eve…anytime we go to the Bistro by the Bay. Yeah, you're a romantic guy."

Tom brushed the hair away from her face. "Just around you, babe. You have plans for dinner?"

Cassie bit her lip with a rueful smile. "Amelie's staying here a few days. She's lonely with Cam on the road trip. And she's taking courses like I am, so she hopes to get ahead on the online courses."

"Unless Caryn has something already in the works, I'll see if she'll lend me the kitchen…"

"Tom, you have carte blanche in the kitchen," Caryn said with a laugh as she came around the corner. "I have plenty of options, but nothing planned yet. Be my guest—I'd love something from our Top Chef."

"First, we need to feed the munchkins." Cassie stepped away and rounded the counter to the kitchen. She watched as Jenna waddled toward her uncle and raised her arms.

"I think she will say 'Tom' before 'mom'—she loves her Uncle Tommy," Caryn said with an affectionate smile for her honorary brother.

"She just misses Andrew," Tom scoffed. "I'm a look-alike substitute, right, Jenna?" As if on cue, she squirmed and demanded to get on the floor. She must have sensed her twin's approach as she headed toward the corner before any of them heard or saw Daniel with Amelie.

Tom laughed as he watched her drop to her knees. She could crawl much more quickly than walk. Jenna called out what sounded like babble, but Daniel responded as he met her in the living area. "Makes you wonder what they're plotting," Tom commented.

"Mayhem," Amelie answered. "Danny is one stubborn little man."

"Double dose of stubbornness from Andrew and Caryn." Tom winked when Caryn shot a look his way. "The right type of stubborn, of course. Never give up."

"Good save," Cassie retorted with a grin. She watched Amelie greet Tom as she set the twins' plates on the counter. *A little too happy to see him? No, don't even go there. There's nothing to worry about with your hockey doc. Even though Amie's looking at him like she wants to jump him.*

She flushed when Tom glanced at her as if he'd read her mind. His lips twitched with a smile and his eyes darkened when they met hers. Goosebumps danced across her skin when he continued to hold her gaze several beats longer than necessary. She flashed a smile. *Message received, doctor.*

During dinner, Tom questioned Caryn about her and Andrew's plans for the bye-week. "Did you have to reschedule everything when Andrew learned he's on the All-Star team?"

"Lucky for us, the game's in Miami, and Drew assures me it's a quick flight to St. John's. So, we'll enjoy South Florida for a few days, but still have plenty of days in the Virgin Islands." Caryn looked at Amelie when she heard the audible sigh. "I hear it's exquisite. Though, those beaches on the French Riviera must be spectacular."

"Not when the entire country's trying to claim a spot," Amelie replied with a laugh. "It's much more beautiful in the fall after *la rentrée*, back to work and school. Fun for a few days' break during the fall."

"Still insisting on taking my niece and nephew with you?" Tom asked Caryn as he poured white wine into Amelie's empty glass. "Can I convince you with more wine?"

Caryn shook her head. "Not ready to leave Jenna and Daniel yet… even though both grandmothers keep coming up with reasons why Andrew and I need to get away by ourselves. Maybe next year." She exchanged a smile with Cassie. "So much less stress since Cassie's coming with us. Plenty of opportunities to take time for ourselves."

"So, you're just going to leave me behind like stale bread."

Cassie giggled at Tom's botched analogy. "Maybe like yesterday's news?"

"Whatever you say…you're leaving with no thought to Jenna and Danny's uncle."

"If you can get the time off, we'd love for you to come," Caryn said. "The house we're renting is huge. When's the last time you took a vacation?"

Tom shrugged but didn't reply as Amelie looked at Cassie. "How'd you get permission to miss classes? Two of mine have no cuts."

"I'm working ahead as much as I can, so my professors are on board with that. The online courses are not a problem. I just need to test out of the algebra class. Dave's FaceTimed with me a couple times to help in test prep." Cassie paused as she sipped her wine. "If I don't, I'll try again next semester. Not a big deal."

"I didn't realize you might have to drop a class," Caryn interrupted. "I don't want to interfere with your classes."

"I hadn't decided to take classes when we talked about the Virgin Islands," Cassie reminded her. "I don't mind waiting until next semester to test out of algebra. Seriously." She pretended to glare at Tom when she heard his quiet chuckle.

"But what you can take is limited until you complete that course or test out," Amelie added.

"I said I didn't care." Cassie's voice had an edge to it. "Dave thinks I'm about ready to retake the test."

"We can discuss it then," Caryn said. "We'd love for you to join us —you can't imagine how much—but your courses come first." She smiled to lighten the tone. "It's all a moot point when you ace that test, anyway."

Amelie excused herself after helping to clean the kitchen after dinner. "I need to work on homework—you don't mind, Cassie?"

"Not at all! I like to study out by the pool—nice and relaxing. Unless certain people cause distractions by swimming laps." Cassie looked at Tom with a hint of a smirk. "Present company excluded."

"Oh, of course," Amelie giggled, with a glance at Tom. "Cannot imagine who could distract you around here."

Cassie felt her cheeks warm. "Make yourself at home. I'll check in with Caryn and see if she needs help with the munchkins." Cassie glanced at Tom over her shoulder. "Want to say good night to your nephew and niece?"

Caryn had just closed the door to the nursery when Cassie and Tom approached it. "Asleep already?" Cassie whispered.

"All the excitement must have exhausted them. Not complaining, mind you." Caryn's eyes shifted from Tom to Cassie. "Do you have any plans?"

Cassie shook her head, but Tom reached for her hand. "While Ms. Amelie hits the books, let's go for a walk."

"Twist my arm."

Caryn laughed at their antics. "Good idea. I have a FaceTime date with my husband—can this road trip get any longer?"

"Just look forward to the byc-week and All-Star game," Cassie suggested. "You'll have, what, ten days of togetherness?"

"Not sure that's enough time to catch up, but we'll make the most of it."

45

"So, you really will ditch me and run off to the Virgin Islands?" Tom teased Cassie as they walked around the front of the subdivision.

"Could you possibly get the time off?"

"Maybe part of the time—like the All-Star weekend. I seriously doubt I'd get ten days approved." Tom placed his arm around her shoulders and pulled her against him for a kiss. "So, what do we need to do to get you through this algebra class?"

"Ideally, I test out. I tried once, and my score wasn't high enough. So, I'm stuck in remedial algebra for the semester unless I try the test a second time or drop the course."

"How many times can you take the test?"

"Three. After that, I must complete the course. I don't want to use up all my chances this semester. I'd rather drop it, keep working on my own, then try the test again before the summer semester—or when I feel more confident." She pulled back and looked up at him. "It stinks—I can't transfer to any of the major courses until I complete that requirement."

Tom saw the frustration in her expression. "Don't get discouraged. There are plenty of brilliant writers and creative people who struggle with math. And you, my love, are brilliant. I can help you follow-up on the topics Dave's working on with you. Yes, even including your favorite—the quadratic equation."

"I hate wasting our time together on remedial math."

Tom chuckled at her expression. "I have some incentives in mind that could take the sting out of this. We can work a certain amount of time, then enjoy an incentive."

A speculative smile crossed her face. "You going to share these incentives with me?"

"Nope—my surprise, but I can promise not to disappoint."

Tom spoke with his supervisor, Dan Forster, about taking time off around the upcoming All-Star break and bye-week.

"You set the schedule, Tom—talk it over with your colleagues," Forster said. "I have no objections. If you get creative with your schedule and swap shifts with a few other doctors, you might pull it off. You're the first to volunteer when anyone needs a shift covered, so call in some favors."

He wanted to surprise Cassie if everything worked out. And he absolutely must talk with Caryn to confirm they truly had the space available at the rented house. Andrew may not want another person tagging along…unless he decides with two adults taking care of the twins, they'll have more opportunities to go off by themselves, during the day or at night.

Would he enjoy experiencing the island paradise with Cassie? *No question. Even if we have little time to ourselves, any amount of time together trumps not seeing her for at least a week.* When Tom approached Caryn, she said she'd already spoken with Drew. He had "no reservations" and asked Caryn to think about going out on a boat for twenty-four hours or visiting St. Thomas and St. Croix on day-trips.

Caryn laughed softly when she relayed that message to Tom. "I think his new goal is to convince me that Danny and Jenna will happily survive twenty-four hours without me."

"You know they'll be in good hands. Cassie's a second mother to your 'munchkins.'"

"Yes, and they adore their Uncle Tommy…not to mention our personal physician. If I ever leave them, I'd put you and Cassie at the top of the list." Tom saw her cut her eyes toward him, a teasing glint in her expression. "So, about you and Cassie…"

"Yes?" Tom forced himself to keep a neutral expression.

"You complement each other perfectly. Do you think you're…" Her voice trailed off, and her eyes asked the question.

"An exclusive couple? Definitely."

"Have you thought about the future?"

Tom shrugged. "Somewhat, but I want her to chase her dreams. I've been there, done that—but Cassie hasn't. She needs the opportunity to chart her own course for the future. When the time comes, I plan to step back and watch her soar."

"Keep in mind that Drew and I had a similar situation. His moving to St. Louis for two seasons tested our commitment to each other. In the end, we both sailed the same course."

"We could follow in your and Andrew's footsteps, or discover our goals take us separate ways."

"Does Cassie know how you feel?"

"Yes, and we're both thinking about the future." Tom reached for his water bottle and took a long drink. "Nothing permanent yet, but the thought's planted."

"You may discover Cassie's dreams include staying in Tampa." Caryn smiled as she snacked on a cracker.

"You know something I don't?" Tom challenged, his tone light.

"Just an observation. You know—woman's intuition."

Caryn's questions about his relationship with Cassie stuck in Tom's mind. *Nothing new, but I need to get a sense of Cassie's dreams for the future. I've already followed my dream; I've taken the route I chose to become a doctor. Cassie's just beginning her journey.*

He posed the question one evening when they took a walk after dinner. "You've never shared your dreams for your life, Cassie. You have so much talent, I can see you succeed in any career you chose. When you were younger, did you dream about what you wanted in your future?"

"Besides a prince on a white horse?" Cassie responded with a grin. "I knew I didn't want to follow either of my parent's footsteps. My mother's an accountant, and my dad's the IT director for his corporation. I knew early on that neither of those would play a part in any thoughts about my future. As you know, I'm allergic to math."

"Good point. But all joking aside, you came to Tampa for a year to decide your plans for the future. I know you're taking classes, but where do you see yourself next year? Five years? Do you have a dream for your life?"

"Honestly, I don't know. I left Vancouver with the main goal of getting away from my mother's overprotective smothering so I could function as an adult." She shrugged. "I don't know what I want to do with my life…maybe teach preschool or go the communications route. I never thought about working in either area, but the more I help with the twins and watch Caryn and Lauren manage their business, the more I think about including one or the other in my future." She looked up and Tom saw her thoughtful expression. "Did you always want to enter medicine?"

"When I realized that playing hockey wasn't a viable career, I thought about medicine. Watching my mom and dad deal with Dad's health issues opened that possibility to me. If you'd asked me when I was twelve, I would have insisted that I'd play pro hockey." Tom gazed at one of the community lakes. "No, I didn't grow up dreaming about the med school route."

"Did you ever second-guess your decision?"

"At least once a month through med school and interning."

"That's reassuring," Cassie said with a soft laugh. "I dreamed of having a 'normal' family—no constant bickering between parents, no tug of war using me as the rope, and not a mother who wants to run my life. Something like Caryn and Andrew have with the munchkins and you. That gives me hope that my dream is attainable."

"It is, babe. You know, you're part of the family now."

"Eh…does that make us siblings?" Tom saw the teasing glint in her hazel eyes.

"Hardly. Let's amend that to an honorary member of our family."

Cassie turned so she could face him. "Why the interest in what I want to do when I grow up?" She cocked her head as she waited for Tom's answer.

"It's complicated," he said. "We're on this journey now to see where we go as a couple…"

"A journey beyond any dreams I had," she interrupted, her voice soft.

"I'll second that." Tom punctuated his words with a tender kiss. "But I see June approaching more quickly than I'd like. You have decisions to make. I don't want to impede you living your dreams." At Cassie's crestfallen look, he added, "Cassie, what I feel for you goes way beyond where we are now. That will not change except to grow. I want you to pursue your dreams—school, travel, whatever. Please understand that I will wait for you. I don't care how long you take or where you need to move, I'll wait for you. I promise I'm not going anywhere."

"And if my dreams include you?" Cassie ventured, averting her eyes.

"We can take these steps together. Just don't give up an opportunity because of me. I'm not going anywhere…you know, you've had my heart since I met you at the airport, and I'm not taking it back."

"I wouldn't let you anyway." Cassie placed her palm against his chest. "Are you saying you think we could have a forever kind of…relationship?"

"If that's what you want as well."

"If you only knew…I worry that if you knew how much I…dream about that, you'd run."

Tom held back a smile. "Let's quit talking around it, babe. I want you in my life now and through eternity."

"I want that, too." Cassie's smile brightened the twilight.

"Then perhaps we move forward together? Explore your options—no matter where they take us?"

"You'd really do this for me?" Cassie's eyes filled with tears.

"I'll do it for us, Cassie."

46

The end of the season's longest road trip finally arrived. With the team plane scheduled for an early evening touchdown, Cassie heard Lauren and Caryn discussing plans for a spa day early that morning. She suspected Kelly and Terri had cleared their schedules also. The four friends taking a Girls' Day Out caused tiny pinpricks of jealousy, but Cassie knew they'd included her in many other plans when possible.

"You seem more excited about this girls' day than the group going," Caryn teased Cassie as they cleaned up after the twins' breakfast.

"You all deserve this day—I'm ecstatic you guys planned this. Getting all glammed up for your husbands' homecoming. I'm enjoying it vicariously."

"I'm happy we got this scheduled before the team gets home." Caryn looked at Cassie with a smile. "Plan a spa day with Amelie. You need to pamper yourself, too…we both need hours away from our little bundles of joy who've decided that throwing food is more fun than eating it."

Cassie giggled as she replied, "The look of pure joy on their faces cracks me up. It's like they scheme and coordinate the timing."

"Nothing they do surprises me anymore," Caryn said. "*Do you* feel comfortable with the twins all day? Please tell me if you have any reservations."

"Caryn, I promise you we'll be fine. Amelie said she might stop by and help, but either way, Jenna and Daniel assured me they'll be little angels today."

"That so? So, you're learning their twin-speak?" Caryn laughed. "Please don't let Amelie distract you. I know, shall we say, how scatterbrained she can get?"

"I won't let Danny or Jenna out of my sight."

While the twins took their morning nap, Cassie surprised Caryn by switching the toys—bringing back older toys they had set aside weeks ago. When the twins saw them again, they always reacted as if they'd received brand new toys. She and Caryn had developed this system several months ago…so far neither Jenna nor Daniel had caught on.

She'd just completed the toy switch when she heard happy sounds chirping on the monitor. Delighted by the "new" toys, Jenna and Daniel excitedly examined them. Soon, each played with a different toy—Jenna stacked blocks. At the same time Daniel concentrated on lining up the stuffed animals by size. Cassie quickly opened her phone to capture the moment on video—the first time they'd shown such concentration and intent when interacting with their toys. As soon as Cassie set her phone aside, Jenna noticed that Daniel had placed her stuffed bear in his lineup and reached to grab it. Daniel voiced displeasure, then swatted his hand against her block tower, scattering the plastic blocks. Within a few seconds, the happy brother and sister morphed into two disconsolate children. Both wanted Cassie's undivided attention, and she tried to comfort both.

When Amelie opened the door after knocking, Cassie greeted her with a smile. "Just in time—help!"

Without Cassie asking, Amelie sat by Jenna and collected blocks. The tears still flowed from the toddler's eyes, but she grasped a block with a happy squeal and began to rebuild her tower.

Amelie looked at Cassie with a knowing smile. "They already know how to push each other's buttons."

"Guess I shouldn't feel surprised. Another twin thing?" Cassie asked as she set Daniel beside her and handed him the box of small cars he loved. "One second babbling happily, the next crying pitifully." She helped Daniel line up the trucks as if they were in a parking lot. "So happy to see you walk in the door. How were your classes this morning?"

"Boring. I wish I'd taken my classes seriously last year." Amelie made a face. "These classes are a joke and a complete waste of money."

"So, you think you'll be able to ace them?" Cassie handed another car to Daniel.

"That's the plan. If I score straight A's, I'll reapply to Paris." She watched Jenna take additional time as her block tower grew taller. "Maybe a future architect here—what do you think?"

"Nothing would surprise me. So, have you heard from Chance?"

"He's called a few times during this road trip. After he ghosted me while I was in Montréal, things aren't the same. He doesn't understand why I 'expected him' to contact me."

Cassie laughed. "Guys just don't get it, do they?"

"I think your doctor does," Amelie said with a smirk. "Perfect, right, Cass?"

"I have no complaints." Cassie's heart did a little flip whenever she thought about Tom. "Do you mind watching them while I get their lunch warmed up?"

"Not at all. I won't let either escape."

After lunch, Cassie took the twins outside while Amelie worked on her homework on the pool deck.

Daniel had tried to pull Cassie toward the pool when they passed the door on the way outside. She knew he wanted to swim; he was like a little fish in the water.

"Not today, Danny. We'll swim tomorrow when your daddy's home."

"Dadada," he repeated. Cassie loved the sound of his voice as he tried to say, "daddy."

"Let's bounce the big ball on the porch." Both Jenna and Daniel liked to clutch the beach ball with two hands and bounce if off the ground. If successful, both giggled and clapped their hands. Cassie retrieved the ball, then emphasized whose turn came next. It amazed Cassie how quickly both grasped new concepts—taking turns, sharing. *When they choose to cooperate.*

When they tossed the ball on the grass, Cassie moved to the lawn and beckoned them to retrieve the toy. She watched them scamper across the yard, shrieking in delight when they lost their balance and plopped down on the grass. She called their names and bounced the beach ball to get their attention. Jen opted to rush toward her using her speed-crawl skills, and Daniel tottered in her direction with a determined expression. *Looks so much like Andrew…it's as if he's mimicking his father.*

After thirty minutes, Cassie herded them back indoors and led them to the play area before fixing each a glass of juice. Daniel slurped his drink eagerly, and Jenna waved the cup around before taking a sip. Cassie glanced at her watch. A bit too early for the afternoon nap, but Cassie hoped to finish up the laundry while they slept.

"You have an amazing mama," she told Daniel and Jenna. "You keep her running around all day long, and she never gets too tired to play. I hope I can be a mom just like her someday."

"Could you watch Jen and Danny for a minute?" Cassie asked Amelia when she came in from the pool deck. "I need to freshen up."

"Sure, take your time." Amelie spread out on her side and encouraged both toddlers to climb over her. "I'll yell, 'Help!' if they tie me up."

"Nothing they do would surprise me." Cassie glanced over her shoulder as she walked across the room. She loved those children so much. She couldn't imagine life without her munchkins—or their parents. *Someday, I hope Jen and Danny understand how lucky they are to live in a home where both parents love each other and them unconditionally.* She wished she'd enjoyed such a peaceful environment. Cassie wondered if she'd have more confidence in her future if she hadn't been used as a ping pong ball by her parents. She received mixed messages consistently—her mother expected perfection and criticized her study habits each time she fell short. Her dad congratulated every accomplishment, but his expectations demanded that the grades reflect her very best work—even if a score was just "average."

She thought about her remedial algebra class as she quickly changed her T-shirt. Her mother would express disappointment that she couldn't test out of a secondary school-level math course. She'd assume Cassie didn't spend enough time on her studies. Her father would do his best to encourage her but would also expect her to at least pass the test.

Thank God, I'm taking this course on my dime. I won't feel guilty if I don't share that information... Why open myself to more criticism and unspoken disappointment?

She knew she'd made the correct decision in enrolling in the community college program in Tampa. With no one looking over her shoulder, Cassie could try new courses, risk exploring different career choices.

Cassie listened to the laughter and excited chatter as she stepped into the bathroom. Amelie constantly surprised her. A few months ago, Cassie could not imagine her sitting on the floor playing with the twins. Now Amelie sought an opportunity to spend time with Jenna and Daniel. *She doesn't care if food lands on her face or if a sippy cup "accidentally" spills its contents on her shirt. Did it take this long for her to feel comfortable with the toddlers? Or maybe it's because she's not distracted by her mysterious French hockey player?*

Cassie thought about the matching outfits Daniel and Jenna wore—the colorful overalls and the girlie details on Jenna's. *They'll soon outgrow them. Wonder if this makes Caryn sad or happy to welcome a new stage in their lives?* The twins changed so rapidly that Cassie sometimes wanted to capture them in a bubble of time so she could enjoy them just a little longer. Before she knew it, Jenna and Daniel would enter preschool.

Cassie laughed to herself. *Now I sound just like Mom. "You're growing up too fast, Cassandra...just yesterday you entered school. Now time for the university."*

As Cassie walked back to the living area, she listened to Jenna's babbling and Amelie's laughter. *Danny's strangely silent. Ready for a nap, maybe?*

She chuckled when she saw that Jenna had climbed on Amelie's back, trying to give her a stuffed animal.

"For me?" Amelie cooed as she set her cell phone aside. "Can you bring another one?"

"She must love you," Cassie told Amelie. "You're holding some of her favorite animals. Good thing she hasn't decided to give you Danny's toys…" She looked around the play area, expecting to find a sleepy, worn-out toddler. "Where's Danny?"

Amelie pushed up on her elbows and pointed toward the row of cars perfectly aligned. "He was right there…just a second ago…"

47

Cassie scanned the area, and her eyes immediately focused on the open door leading to the pool. Dread twisted her stomach as she rushed to the pool. She spotted Daniel near the deep water. He stood too close to the edge, holding out his hand, trying to touch the water. She didn't want to startle him, so Cassie sprinted toward him. Before she could envelop him in her arms, the toddler leaned too far over the water and tumbled headfirst into the pool. His arms flailed in panic, mouth open and screaming. Before she could grab him, Danny sank below the surface for a moment that felt like an eternity. He popped up, choking, his eyes widened with terror. Feeling like she was moving in slow motion, Cassie grasped his arm and pulled the struggling toddler against her. The terrified child kicked and flailed thrashed wildly, scratching her face and delivering solid kicks to her abdomen.

Holding Daniel securely in one arm, she reached for the side of the pool. Cassie tried to lift him up to the edge, but his weight plus the continued thrashing worked against her. She called Amelie for help, but when she didn't respond, Cassie began pulling him to the shallow water. She nearly lost her grip several times as Daniel struggled. When she could touch the bottom, Cassie wrapped both arms around him and walked up the sloping no-steps entry.

Danny no longer struggled or screamed, suddenly limp in her arms. Cassie grabbed a towel and gently laid him on the pool deck. *Has he exhausted himself? Did he swallow water?*

She closed her eyes as her water safety training played through her mind. *Airway, Breathing, Circulation....* "Danny! Danny!" She gently jostled him; no response. She checked his mouth and pressed her fingers against his neck. His heart beat steadily, but she did not detect a breath. Cassie grabbed the emergency medical kit Tom had installed and pulled out the child-sized respiration mask. She slipped it over his face, used her hand to seal the edges, and began blowing air into his lungs. She counted off the recommended intervals, checked his pulse, then reported the process.

"Cassie, what happened?" Amelie shrieked. Jenna began crying at the sudden outburst, and Cassie paused between breaths.

"Call 911...and please take Jenna to the nursery." Cassie continued the breaths, praying the entire time. *Please help him, God. Please...* Suddenly Daniel's shoulders twitched, and Cassie removed the mask just before he coughed up water. She turned him on his side and kept her hand under his head as water spewed from his mouth. "You're okay, Danny. You're okay." She knew she was speaking to herself but clung to the belief that he could hear her voice.

His eyes fluttered open, and Cassie watched as he gulped air and opened his mouth to scream. "That's my boy. Scream. Keep breathing."

Amelie returned with an armful of towels and helped Cassie wrap him with several to warm him. His continued screams brought a sense of relief, and Cassie held him tightly against her chest. "You're okay, Danny. You're okay." She looked at Amelie. "Is Jenna in her crib?"

"Yes, and paramedics should be here any second. I'll meet them outside."

"Please let Tom know so he can meet the ambulance. Use my phone...call his work number. And we need to contact Caryn." She heard herself speaking as if she were outside her body. Her head spun, and black specs gathered at the side of her eyes. *Deep breath. Long deep breaths. You cannot faint. Concentrate on Daniel.*

The next minutes passed in a dense fog, and finally, she heard voices as if she were deep inside a tunnel. She took another lung-expanding breath, and the fog gradually lifted. The paramedics—a woman and a man—pried Daniel from her arms and positioned him on a gurney.

"He's okay, isn't he?"

The male paramedic didn't answer as he assessed Daniel and gave the vital signs to his partner. "You the mother?"

Cassie shook her head, then looked at Amelie as she hovered anxiously. "Did you talk with Tom?"

"Yes, he said he'd alert emergency services and meet the ambulance."

"Do you know how long the child was under water?" the paramedic continued.

"Just seconds. He fell in headfirst. I jumped in immediately, but he swallowed water before I could reach him." Cassie took a deep breath. "Danny screamed, kicked, and tried to get away from me. Then, just as we were walking out of the pool, he stopped moving." Cassie pushed her fear aside. "I began rescue breathing—not long after that, he coughed up water." She looked at the gurney where Danny lay.

The male paramedic asked Cassie for Daniel's family information. The woman slipped an oxygen mask over his face.

"He's breathing. Just a little supplemental oxygen," she explained.

Cassie pushed herself to stand and watched exhaustion overtake her munchkin. *He looks like a doll on that huge gurney.* She leaned over him so he could see her face. "You're okay. Your Uncle Tommy is waiting to see you, baby." She quickly kissed him as the female paramedic gently moved her aside. "Can I go with you?"

"Jenna," Amelie reminded her. "You can't leave her. I contacted the spa and asked the concierge to give Caryn a message to call you. I'm not sure she understood."

Cassie's thoughts jumbled as she trailed the gurney to the ambulance. "Can you go to the spa and tell Caryn?"

"On my way."

Cassie choked back a sob as she watched the paramedics load the gurney into the ambulance. Her little angel nearly drowned… Happened so quickly, in seconds. *He's scared and doesn't know these people...I didn't notice the pool door had been open. I should have checked when Amie came in from studying. Can't believe I got distracted. The one thing Caryn reminded me, "Don't get distracted if Amelie stops by today."*

She realized the female paramedic was speaking to her.

"We know Dr. Chadwick. We'll make sure he's contacted when we arrive."

"Thank you. Is Daniel going to be all right?" Cassie wrapped her arms around herself, hoping to stop the trembling.

"His signs are good. Luckily, he wasn't under water longer than a few seconds. He'll get a complete assessment at the hospital."

Cassie nodded, unable to speak and trying to contain the urge to cry. "Thank you," she whispered. She watched the ambulance until it disappeared from sight, and only then allowed tears to escape.

48

Cassie fought to keep her emotions at bay while she calmed Jenna. Once she'd changed Jenna's clothes, Cassie took her to her bedroom, and sat Jenna on the floor near the dresser. Cassie tossed her wet clothing into the bathroom sink and wrapped a towel around her.

Her love bug watched as Cassie dressed and squealed her approval when Cassie showed Jenna the shirt she planned to wear. She babbled something only Daniel would understand, and when Cassie swept her into her arms. Jenna patted the brightly flowered fabric.

"You like that, little angel? You love flowers, don't you? Just like your mom."

Jenna cooed in response. Cassie carried her to the nursery and sat on the rocker. She forced her worries aside and concentrated only on the precious child she held. The rocking motion soothed her nerves, and she watched as Jenna closed her eyes in contentment. Cassie continued to rock, long after Jenna had fallen asleep, her mind drifting to the haunting vision of little Daniel falling into the pool.

Caryn's greatest fear and it happened on my watch. The door to the pool is always locked. How could I not notice? Why did I leave both of them with Amie—I could have taken Danny with me to "freshen up?"

Or put both of them in their cribs like I usually do. It's hard enough chasing one, much less two of these bundles of energy...Now Daniel's in the ambulance, probably terrified because I got distracted.

After looking at her phone for what felt like the hundredth time, Cassie slipped it into her pocket. *Two hours already*. She willed Tom to send her a text, a voice message, anything to let her know Daniel's condition. Tempted to call, she didn't want to interrupt him. *He'll call as soon as he can. Unless he's angry with me, disappointed that I allowed Daniel to fall into the pool or blames me for Daniel's condition.*

Why hadn't she locked the door or double-checked it like Caryn always did? Amelie may have accidentally left it open after she'd completed her coursework. But it was Cassie's responsibility to ensure that the door was always locked; she hadn't even noticed that it was open. Cassie had failed her most important duty—keep the twins safe—and she couldn't imagine the fear, disappointment, and anger that Caryn felt.

She walked to the pool deck and picked up the discarded towels. She saw the residue from the regurgitated water, so after throwing the towels in the wash, she cleaned the area. The spot where Daniel tumbled into the pool seized her gaze, and a rush of icy dread spread through her. What if she'd checked the kitchen first? Or if she hadn't been so close when Danny fell? What if he hadn't responded to her rescue breathing?

She flicked the tears aside and swallowed the sob that threatened. She checked again that her phone battery showed fully charged; that she hadn't missed a call or a text. Not knowing anything weighed on her mind, and as time passed, Cassie's anxiety morphed to panic.

Finally, she heard a light rapping on the front door, and Lauren and Dave entered before Cassie could reach it. As Lauren hugged her, Cassie felt her control slip and tears streamed from her eyes.

"How's Danny?"

"Stable when we left," Lauren said. "Tom said his doctor will admit Daniel to monitor him. He also said the paramedics told him you'd saved his life; you kept calm and knew exactly what to do."

"It's my fault it even happened. My carelessness could have cost his life."

"The important thing is that Danny *will* recover," Dave said. Cassie turned toward him and saw the empathy in his eyes.

"If I'd done my job, he wouldn't be at the hospital. I didn't even notice the pool door was wide open."

"You can't change what happened," Dave said. "This was an accident, nothing more. Everyone knows how much you love the twins. And you saved Daniel's life."

Cassie's gaze moved from Dave to Lauren. "How's Caryn?"

"Pretty shaken up. Thankful as soon as she saw Danny." Lauren squeezed her hand. "Now that Andrew's arrived, she'll calm."

Cassie walked to the play area and began picking up the blocks and toy cars. It felt like days had passed since she'd watched them interact with her friend. Amelie's iPhone lay on the floor amongst the toys, and the memory of Amelie setting it aside flickered in her mind. *What was she doing with her phone? Shopping? Texting? Posting on Instagram?* "Did you see Amelie at the spa?"

"Yes, I'm not sure where she went after that." Lauren met her eyes. "Was she here today?"

Cassie nodded. "She stopped by to help. Caryn okayed it—but reminded me about distractions. I welcomed the help today. She's been a different person since Christmas. Jenna loves her—she always reaches for her." She attempted a tight smile. "Amie no longer cares if she gets mauled with sticky hands."

"Sounds like she's done a one-eighty with her attitude." Lauren stepped in front of Cassie and gently grasped her arms. "Why don't you sit down, Cassie? You're going to wear a path on the hardwood if you keep pacing." Lauren guided her to the sofa. "And you look like you'll collapse at any moment."

"Have you eaten?" Dave asked.

"Not hungry."

"Pizza? Pasta? Spaghetti? Salad?" Lauren offered. "I know Mr.

Martin is very hungry, so take advantage of the offer. You can save it for later. Maybe some chicken parmigiana?"

Cassie shrugged. "Sure."

"What do you want, squirt?" Dave asked Lauren.

"Surprise me."

Dave looked at Cassie. "Don't beat yourself up, kiddo. Remember that this was an accident *and* that Daniel's okay."

Cassie nodded when she met his gaze, but her heart knew she'd never forgive herself for putting Daniel's life in danger.

Lauren persuaded Cassie to sit on the couch and brought her a bottle of water.

"Will Andrew or Caryn give you updates on Daniel?"

"Someone will contact me if his condition changes," Lauren said. "Tom said Daniel's stable…The main concern is if any water remains in his lungs."

"Has he had a chest X-Ray?" Cassie pictured Daniel's face as he'd gasped for breath. "I told them he coughed up water."

"I'm sure the paramedics put that in their report. You know our little guy will get the very best care. He's in good hands." Lauren reached for her hand. "Can you tell me what happened?"

Cassie shrugged. "Amelie came over to help, then study. The twins loved playing with the 'new' toys I'd swapped…so enthralled." Cassie flinched at the memory. "After lunch, I took them out to play while Amelie did some coursework on the deck. I guess I forgot to check that the door was closed. Then, I asked her to watch both, so I could go to the bathroom. I could hear laughter and babbling even in my room." Her voice choked and Cassie took a deep breath. "When I came down the hallway, I couldn't hear Daniel…I…I thought maybe he'd fallen asleep. But he wasn't with Amelie."

Cassie took a deep breath and sipped some water. "When I saw the pool door open, I knew where he was… I spotted him…at the edge of the pool down by the deep end. Danny…tumbled into the water before I could reach him." She looked at Lauren as tears streamed down her face. "He wasn't under water for more than a few seconds, but…he screamed and kicked until I could get him to the shallow end. Then he just went limp."

"Luckily, you knew what to do. You didn't panic." Lauren hugged Cassie. "Did Amelie say how he slipped out that door?"

"She didn't notice that Danny had moved. Jenna had climbed on her back. She may have used her phone." Cassie handed the phone to Lauren. "I found it near where she'd played with Jenna...I should never have left both twins with her."

"Amelie should have watched both babies. I just don't understand how Daniel got away without her noticing." Lauren's tone reflected her disapproval. She swiped at the screen on the phone. "Locked. But look at these notifications, Cass—texts from many people. Now you know how Daniel slipped away."

Cassie closed her eyes for a long moment. "It doesn't matter, anyway. The twins are my responsibility. I can't blame anyone else." Cassie cringed when her phone sounded. "Mom."

"Let it go to voicemail. You don't need to speak with her right now." A short time later, a beep indicated that Cassie's mother had left a voice message.

"So, your spa day completely blew up, and now you're here instead of celebrating with Dave at home…Mom would say I'm a colossal failure, and she'd be right."

"Stop, Cass," Lauren interrupted. "Look forward. Remember, Danny's okay. He didn't drown. You did not leave Amelie playing with Jen and Daniel, thinking she'd text while 'watching' them. If Amelie's attention focused elsewhere for even several seconds…you know how quickly toddlers can scurry out of sight. You're not the only person who needs to apologize and accept responsibility."

Cassie began to reply but stopped when the door opened, and Andrew entered his home. She stood, her breath catching in her throat as Andrew approached. She started to ask him about Daniel, but the look in his eyes caused the words to die in her mouth.

49

When Andrew spoke, his voice sounded controlled, too calm. His steel-blue eyes conveyed suppressed anger —*rage?*

"How the hell did Daniel get near the freaking pool?"

Cassie felt tears welling in her eyes. "I'm so sorry, Andrew..."

"Answer. The. Question." His voice chilled her like a bucket of ice.

"I don't know…I didn't notice the open door."

"What, were you distracted? Did you leave them alone? Why the hell wasn't that door locked? What was so important that you didn't notice my son was missing—talking on the phone? Texting someone? Sleeping?"

Cassie shook her head, unable to respond.

"Whatever had you preoccupied nearly cost Daniel's life. You *do realize* that, don't you? You either left them alone, or you were oblivious to what they were doing. What could possibly be more important than keeping our children safe?"

His eyes pierced Cassie like knives. She struggled to find her voice. "N-nothing," she stammered. "I didn't leave them alone. Amelie...I asked her…" She stopped to take a deep breath, Andrew's glare holding her captive.

"*She* was here? No wonder you weren't paying attention." Andrew didn't wait for her to answer. "I'm taking Jenna with me to the hospital."

"Jenna's napping. Please let her sleep and have dinner. I can bring her over then. I promise I'll keep her safe."

Andrew stared at her for a long moment. Cassie saw him glance at Lauren, then shake his head. "You'll understand that your promises mean nothing. Pack up her dinner while I get her."

"Why didn't you tell him what happened?" Lauren whispered when Andrew left the room. "He can't blame you for taking a bathroom break."

"I tried to tell him…It doesn't matter. I did exactly what Caryn had warned me about—I allowed Amelie to distract me. I didn't even *notice* the open door. I know Caryn keeps that door locked, and I didn't notice it was open."

Cassie pulled Jenna's plate from the cupboard and filled it with fruit, biscuits, and cheese cubes and then snapped the lid in place. "You heard Andrew cut me off. I know Amie can get distracted, then I trusted her with both babies." Cassie opened the pantry and poured animal crackers into a Ziplock, then filled two bottles and placed everything into an insulated container.

Lauren opened her mouth to argue, and Cassie held up her hand. "Please, Lauren, let it go. I should never have expected Amelie to watch both munchkins…At the very least, I should have taken one with me when I freshened up. I wish I could…" Her voice trailed off as she heard Andrew's voice and Jenna's excited laughter. She placed the container of food on the counter and nodded to it before he walked past the kitchen. "Jenna's dinner."

Andrew grabbed it without speaking. Cassie's eyes drifted toward the toddler she loved as if she were the mother. *Mother? That's a laugh. What mother allows her child to get near a pool? Don't deserve to think about motherhood.*

She hesitantly looked at Andrew. "Andrew, I need to tell you…"

"Not now."

"Please, I can explain…"

"Stop. I don't want excuses." Andrew snapped. He met her eyes for a long moment, started to speak, then stopped. He grabbed Jenna's bag and left without another word.

Tom had no time to think about anything besides his nephew's near-drowning and checking on his current patients. Plus, the ER had several accident victims requiring a neurologist. *Not even a full moon...don't think.* He checked Daniel's chart as often as possible, satisfied with what he read. *No water in his lungs, thank God. Fussy... sleeping. Good signs.*

When he saw the backlog of patients in the ER, he opted to stay on after his shift to help reduce the time people had to wait before seeing a doctor. Two hours later, only a few remained in the waiting area, and Tom headed for the showers and a change of clothes.

When he entered Daniel's room, Tom did not expect to see Jenna. She squirmed on Andrew's lap and protested when he didn't allow her to play on the floor. He exchanged glances with both Andrew and Caryn.

"Anything new?"

"Daniel does *not* have pneumonia," Caryn said. "Thank you, God. He's not thrilled with the IV but hasn't tried to pull at it. Just groggy right now. It could have been so much worse."

Tom walked to the bed and touched Daniel's shoulder as he checked the monitor. "His vitals look very good." He smiled when Daniel turned toward his voice, then tried to reach for him with one arm. Tom moved his hand so Daniel could grasp some of his fingers.

"As usual, he loves his Uncle Tommy," Caryn said.

"That feeling's mutual, right, little buddy?" He leaned to kiss his forehead. "Would you like me to take Jenna for a while?"

"That would make her thrilled," Caryn replied with a small smile. "She has way too much energy right now."

"I can take her home."

"You're not on call?" Andrew asked skeptically.

"Barring anything catastrophic, I'm off the next two days."

Tom watched Andrew's expression. *Does he not trust me? Do they want Jenna with them?* Andrew didn't speak for a long moment.

"If you get called in, you'll bring her with you?"

"If that's what you want. What about Cassie? You worried about leaving Jenna with her?"

"And why would you think that, Tom?"

Tom tried not to flinch at the sarcasm in his voice. "Have you talked with her?"

Andrew nodded. "I doubt she'll be there when you get home."

"Did you fire her?"

"I didn't need to. Cassie knows how I feel—I'll never trust her with my children again."

"Did she explain how Danny got to the pool?"

"No."

"Did you ask?" Tom prodded.

"What the hell does that matter? He fell in the pool and nearly drowned. How or why isn't relevant. That it happened should give you a clue why Jenna's not at home."

Caryn interrupted, her voice soft. "Drew, this was an accident. Cassie didn't panic; she *saved* Danny's life."

"And you're willing to risk another 'accident?'"

Tom saw resignation in her expression. "We'll talk about this later after Daniel's released."

"We'll see."

Tom recognized the tone in Andrew's voice. *When hell freezes. Over my dead body. No freaking way.* Rather than respond, Tom reached for unhappy Jenna.

"Call if you need anything," he said.

50

Cassie turned off her phone and dropped it along with the clothes she shoved haphazardly into her travel bag. Lauren packed a suitcase more carefully than her niece.

“You know, you don’t need to take everything now. I can get the rest later,” Lauren said.

“I’m not putting you in the middle of this. You’re Caryn’s best friend. You’re like sisters. I don’t want to be the first thing that comes to her mind when she sees you.”

“Caryn will understand.”

“I doubt it. I certainly don’t.” Cassie grabbed another suitcase and emptied drawers. “I want nothing to remind them of me when they come home. Did you tell Dave not to bring dinner here?”

“Yes, but he’ll stop by to help us load everything into his truck.”

Cassie sat on the bed with a sigh. “Please don’t let this make either of you uncomfortable around Caryn or Andrew. I don’t fault them at all. I screwed up…Please just let it go.”

“We’ll be fine, Cass. Don’t worry about us. You know, with the All-Star Game and bye-week coming up, there’s plenty of time to get past this initial fear and anger. Knowing Caryn, she’s not blaming you.

Andrew may see things differently when he has the time to process what happened. You saved Daniel's life."

Cassie didn't reply as a sob lodged in her throat. Instead, she grabbed her backpack and tossed everything in the bathroom into it. *I should check the pool area in case I left my iPad out there.* After opening the French doors, Cassie scanned the tables. The only thing she saw was Amelie's backpack. *Not my problem.* She again traced her steps to the spot where Danny fell into the pool. She felt the hitch in her heart as the vision of Daniel trying to touch the water flashed through her mind. *Oh, Danny, I'm sorry I failed you.*

She walked inside the great room and checked carefully in case she'd left something there. She followed her earlier steps, stopping in the nursery to tidy Jenna's bed. She put her favorite teddy bear in the middle of the bed, then without thinking, turned on Daniel's mobile. *I'll never hear "Twinkle Twinkle Little Star" without thinking about Danny and Jenna.* She stared at the stars and moon that circled his crib, remembering the many nights she and Caryn had rocked the twins while that song played.

She didn't know how long she stood there with tears streaming down her cheeks. She startled when a hand gently gripped her shoulder. *Dave. Thank God...I can't look at anyone else right now.*

"The truck's loaded. Lauren will drive your car, kiddo. Let's get out of here and head home."

Cassie nodded and moved away from the cribs. Would she ever see the twins again? Hold her love bugs? Watch their next amazing milestone? As she left the nursery, she couldn't quell the feeling that she'd never set foot in there again.

Lauren and Dave did not allow her to dwell on the horror of the day. Despite her protests, they insisted she sit at the dinner table with them. Pasta, soup, and garlic bread—the ultimate comfort food—tempted her. Despite claiming she had no appetite, Cassie accepted a portion of garlic bread and nibbled on it.

Dave opened a bottle of wine and poured glasses for Lauren and

Cassie. She drank hers much too quickly, but the warmth that spread throughout her chilled body dulled her thoughts. She shook her head when Lauren offered to refill her glass.

"Not just yet—empty stomach."

Lauren nodded at her plate. "The chicken is fabulous. I know Italian food is your weakness."

Cassie sampled the chicken and suddenly felt her appetite awakened. "Comfort food." She spun her fork to gather spaghetti and spoke quietly. "Thank you for this afternoon…I'd still be staring at Daniel's mobile." She caught Lauren's eyes. "Have you heard from Caryn? Any updates?"

"No pneumonia—and that's because you took care of Danny just like a paramedic. You got all the water from his lungs."

"Least I could do." Neither Lauren nor Dave acted as if they heard Cassie's muttered sarcasm.

"Just a few more days, and we have ten days free." Lauren changed the subject.

"When does your family arrive?" Cassie asked Dave.

"No one's given me their flight schedules—I have a feeling we'll have a merry-go-round with members of my family coming and going. Be prepared for a madhouse. My family overwhelms and captures all the oxygen, but I think you'll enjoy Kimberly—she's about your age, Cass. She's always wanted to swim with dolphins."

"Me, too, as long as the dolphins don't live in a concrete pool or captivity."

"If there's one around, she'll find it," Lauren predicted. "School may come as a welcome respite, Cassie."

"I no longer have to worry about completing all my coursework by the All-Star break." She looked at Dave. "I hope I can test out of remedial math next week if you think I'm ready."

"You're more than ready, kiddo. You just need to believe in yourself. We can try a practice test if you'd like?" Dave continued. "I went to the site of the company that produces these tests. They have several you can use for test prep."

"How did I not know that?"

"Your school may not advertise it, but don't worry—everything's legit." He paused a moment while he drank some beer. "We may want to try a practice test before my family descends on Tampa. I highly recommend that."

Cassie looked at Lauren. "You put my stuff in your office. You'll need the extra space for the family."

"Nothing's set in stone yet. We don't even know who's coming when."

"My nephews can sleep in the screened porch unless we get a cold snap," Dave added.

"You think you can keep them away from your secret pool off the master bedroom?" Cassie asked.

Lauren giggled. "We're hoping they don't figure out it's there. We'll take them to the big community pool and get passes. No problem."

"I think I'll apply for on-campus housing." Cassie sampled another bite of the chicken. "I'd considered it before but didn't think I could handle the commute. Now that's not a problem, so I might as well get the full college experience."

"Cassie, you're welcome to stay here. Today, next week, as long as you want," Dave said. "Don't go to the dorm because you think we don't want you—or that you'll inconvenience us. We enjoy having you with us."

Her eyes suddenly misted, and Cassie reached for her water. When she finally spoke, her voice sounded hoarse. "Thank you. If you weren't here, I don't know what I would do…where I would go."

Lauren grasped her hand and squeezed it. "We're family, Cassie. You can stay as long as you want."

Tom arrived home with Jenna to an empty house. He called Cassie's name, but didn't expect to hear her answer. He carried Jenna with him as he walked to her room. The open door revealed no sign of his rainbow girl. *Not really surprised. Andrew's temper on top of the guilt she feels…I'd want to get away from here too. I'll check with Lauren. Either Cassie's phone died, or she turned it off.*

"You hungry for dinner, Miss Jenna?"

His niece patted his shoulder and babbled words he assumed meant "Yes." He stopped in the nursery to change her diaper before allowing her to speed crawl to the great room. She made a quick turn into the play area, and Tom chuckled as she pulled out the basket of blocks, then wandered to the window overlooking the pool.

With one eye on Jenna, he scanned the deck, trying to picture Daniel by the pool. *Where did he fall off the side? Cassie told the paramedic he went in headfirst. So lucky she got to him just after he tumbled into the water.*

He took a deep breath before returning to Jenna. "Good job with the blocks, Jenna!" She held out her hand, clutching a block. "Do you want me to put this on top?"

Jenna responded with happy-sounding babble. Tom carefully placed the block on her stack, then watched as Jenna laughed and pushed the tower over.

"You trickster!" Tom picked her up and held her over his head. "Did your brother teach you that?" He settled her in the highchair and placed a handful of Cheerios on the tray. He opened her dinner plate, set it on the tray, and then filled her sippy cup with milk.

Jenna spied the cup and reached for it. "Thirsty, sweet Jenna?" Tom thought of the times he'd joined Cassie in the kitchen to help feed the twins. The Cassie he knew would never knowingly leave the pool door open. She always triple-checked that the lock had engaged. Nothing distracted her when she cared for the twins. Something didn't add up, and Tom determined to discover the truth.

51

Feeling a buzz from two glasses of wine, Cassie excused herself and returned to Lauren's office. *Time to organize some of my belongings.* She dumped the contents of one bag on the bed, then groaned at the disorganized mess. *I can't do this now. Don't even know where I put my phone. At least I won't worry about dodging Mom's call…calls? Wonder if Tom's tried to call or text? But why should he? He may feel the same as Andrew. Last thing I want is to cause a rift within his family.*

She collected her toiletries and carried them into the adjoining bath. Then she folded and stacked the clothing on the bed. She exchanged her clothes for an oversized shirt…Dave's? Tom's? She couldn't remember.

She quickly completed her evening routine, then flopped on the bed, too tired to pull back the covers. She hugged a pillow to her chest. She said a prayer for Daniel, Jenna, Caryn, Andrew, and Tom, then closed her eyes, hoping she'd wake up in the morning and find that the horrible day was just a nightmare.

When Tom couldn't reach Cassie after getting Jenna ready for bed, he assumed she'd turned her phone off or had forgotten to charge it. He called Lauren reasonably confident he'd find Cassie with her.

"Tom, hi. How's Daniel?" Lauren greeted.

"Just spoke with Andrew. His doctor wants Daniel to stay in the hospital twenty-four to forty-eight hours in case of residual problems. I think that's unlikely. The little guy's exhausted, not agitated at all."

"Thank God...How's Jenna holding up confined to one room?"

"I brought her home with me. Don't know what Andrew was thinking. She was irritated, cranky, and hungry." He stepped out on the front porch to enjoy the fresh evening air. "Just like any toddler."

"I'm glad you have her. Caryn and Andrew do not need to handle a rambunctious, unhappy child right now."

Tom chuckled. "True. Jenna collapsed right after dinner. Fell asleep as I was changing her clothes." He paused for a moment. "I'm assuming Cassie's with you? I haven't been able to reach her."

"She's here. As for her phone, I doubt she knows where it is. I saw her toss it into a bag with some clothes, but even though she started unpacking, she also collapsed—she's sleeping curled up on a bed full of clothes."

"How's she doing?"

"Devastated." He heard the emotion behind the word.

"You were with her when Andrew picked up Jenna?"

"Yes. Not pleasant for either," Lauren said. "Cassie didn't make excuses, but Andrew didn't want to hear her explanation; she apologized and accepted full responsibility."

"Did he ask...tell her to leave?"

"Not in so many words, but the implication was clear. Cassie wanted all of her belongings out before they came home—nothing to remind them of her."

Tom paused with a sigh. "After all these months, Cassie's a huge part of our family. Jenna and Daniel will look for her, Caryn understands it was an accident, and she's thankful Cassie saved Danny's life. Andrew may take some time, but I think eventually he'll accept that accidents happen. It doesn't matter who's at fault. Daniel's safety and health—that's what counts."

"Cassie didn't leave the twins…" Lauren began at the same moment as Tom heard Jenna's cries of distress over the monitor.

"Let me get Jenna settled down. I'll call you back when I can."

"No problem, Tom. If you need any back-up, call me."

"Thanks, Lauren. I think I'm good for the night." Tom paused a moment. "Please tell Cassie not to blame herself—she saved Danny's life. She needs to remember that instead of dwelling on the accident."

For a moment of panic, Cassie did not know where she'd awakened. She felt the bed and the piles of scattered clothes and then remembered that she'd taken everything over to Lauren and Dave's home. Her dreams had revolved around the twins. Images of Daniel and Jenna tumbling into the pool ran on a constant loop. Cassie desperately tried to save both, taking turns blowing air into their tiny lungs. Neither showed signs of responding, so Cassie switched to two breaths each turn. She felt her heart thud against her chest, the physical sensation causing her to wake with a start, but the dream's images hung in front of her eyes like photos on a wall.

So, yesterday really happened—not a nightmare…I hope Danny's out of danger. It's way too late to ask Lauren if she's heard anything new. Hang on, my little tough guy. Can't bear to think about the panic you felt when you fell into the water. I should have been there, Danny. I'm so, so sorry.

Cassie flipped on the bedside lamp and saw the bottle of water that Lauren must have brought in after she'd fallen asleep…*passed out?* Either way, she drank it gratefully.

After refolding and organizing the clothes on the bed, Cassie stored them in the empty dresser Lauren had indicated. Swallowing a yawn, Cassie picked up her travel bag and emptied it. *My phone. Thought I'd left it at the Chadwick's. Dead. My charger? Who knows?*

She remembered that Dave and Lauren kept an extra charger in the kitchen, so she tiptoed across the house with her phone. She plugged it in and made sure she muted the sound. *Don't need my mother's ring tone blasting everyone awake. How long can I dodge her?*

Cassie picked up another water bottle, then her stomach rumbled when she spied the covered bread from the Italian dinner. She tore a large piece, wrapped it in a paper towel, and returned to her room. She needed time to think.

Late the next morning, Cassie forced herself to get out of bed. The hot shower did not wash away the guilt, remorse, or fear for Daniel's safety. Quickly dressing in a T-shirt and jeans, Cassie wandered down the hallway toward the kitchen. She knew Dave had probably gone to morning skate and wondered who spoke with Lauren. A few steps further and Cassie stopped, recognizing Tom's voice. *What's he doing here? Does this mean Daniel's home from the hospital? Can I face him?*

She turned to retreat to her room but stopped when she heard her name mentioned. She eavesdropped for a few moments.

"Yeah, an ambulance chaser tried to give his card to Andrew. When he declined, the guy didn't give up. He told Andrew he should think about the potential medical bills and suggested a meeting to go over options."

"What options?" Lauren asked quietly.

"Lawsuit for damages, pressing charges…"

"Cassie didn't break a law, did she? It was an accident. Do we need to get a lawyer?"

"When the lawyer pushed Andrew, he told him to leave—he has no intention of suing, and as far as he's concerned, the idea of pressing charges is absurd."

"I can understand the lawsuit idea. But, did the police talk to either Caryn or Andrew?"

"No, and don't worry about either scenario. Caryn overheard the conversation and said she would call security if the lawyer didn't leave."

"That's the last thing they need. I never considered that the police might get involved." Lauren's voice sounded shaky to Cassie.

"Not unless the physician suspects abuse or neglect of any kind. Here, we all know that's a non-starter."

Cassie walked back to her room and took a few minutes to compose herself. *Even though it was an accident, I acted irresponsibly. "Negligence?" Is that the term lawyers use? "Child endangerment?" Wouldn't blame either Andrew or Caryn if they reported me.* Cassie's mind wandered to Amelie, wondering what she'd said when she found Caryn at the spa. *Maybe I'll call her later, or she'll get in touch with me.*

But Tom? She now faced her worst nightmare. Once Caryn and Andrew "gave their blessings" to their relationship, she felt confident she'd do nothing to jeopardize her job or come between Tom and his family. *But I managed to screw things up. Big time. Why did I ever trust Amie to watch both Jenna and Daniel? Caryn and I have trouble keeping up with them. Amelie couldn't be expected to handle both. Incredibly stupid, Johnson. I also didn't check the door to the pool after Amelie came inside. Andrew's right—I was distracted, obviously.*

Tom most likely regrets getting into a relationship with me. No doubt he's infuriated with me, just like Andrew. Danny's his nephew. He'll question my judgment—rightfully. Too young, too immature...a wake-up call he didn't expect. Cassie didn't want him to feel obligated to stand by her, jeopardize his relationship with Andrew's family. *Tom needs to support Andrew, not me.*

Cassie looked around the bedroom at Lauren's office. Will Lauren's relationship with Caryn suffer? What about their company? *Everything's upside-down because of my stupidity and carelessness. Maybe the best thing I can do is move away—not be a constant reminder of Daniel's near-death?*

Cassie glanced at the suitcases, still packed with clothes. Tempting to pack her car and drive away...somewhere? Vancouver? Definitely not an option. She could accept the offer at the university in Toronto—maybe visit Europe in the interim? How could she stay in Tampa—a constant reminder of how close they came to losing Danny?

52

Cassie stared at the hummingbird feeder near the bedroom window, taking deep, measured breaths. *I wish I'd taken that meditation class in Vancouver. Maybe then I could clear my mind? Escape this nightmare for even five minutes.*

Lauren knocked and opened the door a crack. "May I...?"

"Of course, come in. How's Danny? Anything new?"

"Daniel's showing no signs of any after-effects. I'm so proud you remembered your first aid training and took that lifeguard certification course."

"Maybe I can get a job as a lifeguard." Cassie's attempt at humor felt flat.

Lauren sat beside her. "You didn't eat much last night. I have blueberry pancakes ready to cook for you. Can I entice you to leave your room?"

"Daniel's home?"

"Not yet. Tom said it's just precautionary, but he'll stay another day." She paused a moment. "He's here. He said he's tried to reach you since yesterday."

"I found my phone, but not the charger. It's in the kitchen right now—I turned it off, so I don't have to talk to Mom just yet." Cassie pulled her hair back into a high ponytail. "Why does Tom want to see me?"

"Worried about you? Maybe to reassure you that Daniel's okay? I definitely know he doesn't want you to blame yourself." Lauren tried to soothe her niece.

"Why not? I know I didn't protect Danny. Tom has to feel as furious as Andrew."

"You don't know that. Don't you think you should give him the time to talk with you?"

Cassie shrugged. "I guess I owe him the opportunity to vent his anger."

"Give him a chance." Lauren hugged her, then offered her hand for Cassie to stand. "Have you heard from Amelie? I hope she does the right thing and explains what happened."

"Danny was my responsibility, no matter what Amie did or didn't do."

Lauren stopped walking and grasped her arm. She spoke softly. "Just think about it—you're not the person who lost track of Daniel."

"I'm not throwing her under the bus. I should never have asked her to watch both twins." Cassie saw Lauren's expression. "Please don't mention it, Lauren."

"Cassie, I won't promise either way on that. Trust me not to say anything—unless I need to intervene."

Tom checked his emails while he hoped Lauren could persuade Cassie to leave her bedroom. *Just want to hug her and tell her Daniel's okay. Hope she's not overwhelmed with guilt. Caryn doesn't blame her—Andrew will come around in time. They both know how much Cassie loves Jenna and Daniel.*

He looked up when he heard Lauren's voice. Leaving his phone on the counter, he met Cassie halfway across the room. His rainbow girl appeared defeated, her eyes dull, and exhaustion reflected by her entire persona. Without speaking, he pulled her against his chest and wrapped his arms around her. He felt her tremble and pressed his lips against her head. "I've worried about you since I got Amelie's message yesterday."

"Danny will be all right?"

"At this moment, he's sleeping peacefully. Give him a couple of days and 'Demo Danny' will return full force."

"Thank God. Danny shouldn't suffer because of my stupidity."

"Accidents happen. I see them every day in the ER." Tom brushed his hand over her head. "You're my hero for staying calm and remembering your training."

She shook her head. "I'm no hero."

"You don't get to choose my heroes."

"Have you eaten, Tom?" Lauren asked. "Blueberry pancakes on the menu."

"Dave actually left some?" Cassie asked with a small smile.

"I made two batches of batter. I've learned not to underestimate his appetite before a practice."

Tom guided Cassie to a seat in the breakfast nook. "Orange juice, coffee, water, Coke?"

She looked at him with a ghost of a smile. "Sit. You're the guest. I'll get the drinks." Cassie took the pitcher of juice from Lauren. "What would you prefer, doctor?"

"OJ sounds good."

Tom watched as Cassie quickly set the table. *Maybe she needs to keep busy?* He pulled a chair back for her and leaned over for a kiss when she sat beside him.

Cassie smiled when she looked at the pancakes on her plate. "You made these for my birthday all the time. The ultimate comfort food. Thanks, Lauren."

"My stress relief food, too," Lauren reminded her.

"I'll need your recipe," Tom told Lauren. "Unless it's a family secret."

"I'll share—but you have to promise to cook these for Cassie."

"Easy promise."

"Not that easy, since I'm no longer living in the house." Cassie sipped her juice after tasting the pancakes. "How's Caryn? Exhausted?"

"Hope she can catch some sleep today."

"When do you think Danny will come home?"

"Maybe today, at the latest tomorrow." Tom brushed the hair away from her face.

"Thank God." Cassie met his eyes. "What about Jenna? She can't be happy confined to a hospital room."

"I brought her home with me last night. I'm off for a couple days. Kelly's watching her now."

"I'm glad." Cassie nodded. She ate silently, the negative thoughts returning to her mind. *Just another screw-up. Had the perfect job, incredible employers, and most lovable children in the world...Then only in a matter of minutes, Danny nearly dies, I destroy Caryn and Andrew's trust, and my presence in their lives is no longer tolerated. Press the DELETE key. I've fallen short of Mom's lowest expectations —further proof that I'm unable to function without her oversight.*

A voice nagged her. It didn't have to end this way. Would they understand she only left the twins with Amelie for a few minutes? Would that change anything? Shift some blame to her friend? Could she even do that and live with herself? Probably not. But why did Amelie allow herself to get distracted with that phone?

Cassie's heart ached at the thought of not seeing the twins every day, not feeling at home in Andrew and Caryn's home. She hated accepting help from Lauren and Dave. She needed to decide where to move and how to take care of herself.

Cassie swallowed a sigh and drank some juice. She glanced at Tom beside her. *Family means everything to him—Family comes first, as it should.* Cassie promised herself that she wouldn't become a wedge between Tom and his family.

53

Later that day, Tom asked Terri and Steve if they could stay with Jenna. He invited Cassie to go for a ride with him—walking on the beach might soothe her mind. He debated sharing his belief that Caryn would ask Cassie to continue as their nanny. *Andrew will eventually come around. Once he relaxes and thinks rationally. But, if I say something to Cassie, she may get her hopes up, and then they decide to go without a nanny.*

He reached for Cassie's hand and squeezed it as she stared out the passenger window. "Outstanding scenery?"

Cassie shook her head and looked at him. "Just thinking. Couldn't tell you where we're headed."

"Getting closer to the Gulf. Would you like to walk on the beach?" He lifted her hand and pressed his lips against it. "I go there when I get stressed."

"Helps?"

"For me, just breathing the air at the beach de-stresses. Walking is a bonus."

"I need that in megadoses today," Cassie said.

Tom glanced at Cassie. "Promise, we'll go wherever we need to find it."

"Can we go back in time?"

He squeezed her hand. "Maybe not that, but we can find a way to ease your mind, put everything in perspective."

Grateful that Tom didn't engage in conversation, Cassie felt a semblance of peace descend as they wandered down the beach. The sun had just set and very few people remained. If she concentrated on the sensation of soft sand brushing against her feet and the gentle sea breeze caressing her skin, she could blank her mind. The constant movement of the sea sweeping in, then clearing the sand as it retreated, lulled her into an almost-hypnotic state. Her mind quieted after a while, allowing her to process the preceding day's nightmare.

She clutched Tom's hand as she tried to examine every act that had led to Daniel falling into the pool. *If only I'd paid more attention to the surroundings—how long had that door been open? Did Amelie forget to close it after she went out to the pool deck to study? I can't imagine Caryn leaving it open, and I hadn't stepped on the pool deck all day. Maybe Amelie thought she had closed it, but the lock didn't engage completely? Even if she had turned the lock, it wouldn't hold if the door hadn't closed properly.*

She felt the negative thoughts closing in and consciously pushed them to the back of her mind. She'd never had a problem defending herself or speaking out. Why now? Amelie hadn't called her—maybe feeling guilty herself or trying to escape any blame? Possibly she had called? Cassie remembered that she hadn't checked her phone.

Pulling it from her pocket, she unlocked the phone and scrolled through the missed calls—mostly from Tom, two from her mother… and a text from Amelie.

Amelie: U OK? How's Danny?
Cassie: He may come home today.

She didn't bother telling Amelie she wasn't okay. Did it matter? She shoved her phone back into her pocket and turned to look at Tom.

"I'm sorry I didn't check my phone sooner. Thank you for trying to contact me."

He stopped and slipped his arm around her shoulders. "I'm sorry I didn't call you sooner…things got hectic and by the time I could…" He shrugged. "Once Amelie called, I didn't think to check my phone."

"I didn't expect you to…your priority was Daniel."

Tom halted, causing Cassie to stumble against him. "Sorry, babe." He paused a beat. "Was Amelie visiting yesterday?"

"She wanted to help since everyone had planned the spa day. I appreciated her stopping by."

"Did she help you with Jenna when you discovered Danny?" Tom asked.

"Yes, and I asked her to contact Caryn. I think the spa has a no cell phone policy, so when she couldn't reach her, I asked her to go to the spa and take her to the hospital."

"Did she come back then or call you?"

"No, but I just read a text she sent. Why?" Cassie's heart raced. *What if Tom asks me to construct a timeline? Where everyone was and what we were doing before anyone noticed Danny missing. What would I tell him? That I left Amelie alone with the twins while I "freshened up?"*

"No reason, Cass. I just now remembered that she'd called me about the ambulance on route…after that, everything's a blur."

"I can understand that…I keep thinking about all the what-ifs. What if I'd double-checked the door…what if…"

Tom silenced her by pressing his finger against her lips. "No what-ifs, Cassie. We can't change what happened. Just make peace with yourself and move forward."

They walked in silence as Cassie digested Tom's words. *How do I find peace about yesterday? Where do I find it?* She knew Lauren and Dave would walk beside her, no questions asked. Tom? She couldn't put him in that position.

"Tom, will you answer a question honestly?"

His brown eyes met hers. "I will never lie to you, Cassie. That's not an option. What do you want to ask?"

"Do you think Caryn and Andrew will ever forgive me?"

"Of course, they will. How could they not? No matter what happened, you saved Daniel's life. That's the only thing that matters… to them and to me."

"Can *you?"*

"Forgive you? There's nothing to forgive, babe."

"I don't want to make things awkward for you."

"You can't."

"What if I can never see the twins again? Or if I'm not welcome in their home?" Cassie averted her eyes.

Tom turned her toward him, grasping each shoulder. "Why would you think you'll never see the twins?"

"Because of what happened…I wouldn't expect Caryn and Andrew to want me anywhere near them." She searched his eyes and read concern and something she could not decipher. He held her gaze for a long moment before he spoke.

"Cassie, Caryn told Andrew yesterday that she knows this was an accident. She knows you'd never knowingly put Daniel or Jenna in danger…Andrew? He may take time—remember when I sent him to the hospital for further evaluation? He *will* need space. He's reacting to a danger to his family he could not control. I don't know what he said to you, but I'm guessing he allowed his anger to speak…"

"He had every right," Cassie interrupted. Tom held up his hand.

"I'm not judging his actions. But I know him—and at some point, he *will* realize that the most important takeaway is Danny's health. He knows it was an accident   it may take a while for him to acknowledge that." He brushed the hair away from her face. "I think Caryn will reach out to you. I don't know when or how long it will take, but Andrew will forgive you. He'll realize he's thankful that you handled everything calmly and professionally."

"What do I do until then?"

"Just take each day, sweetheart. There's no reason to hide, go somewhere, or move away. I promise you that." He lifted her chin and kissed her tenderly. "Please don't make any decisions right away. Especially if you're thinking about leaving Tampa."

Cassie smiled slightly. "Have you been reading my mind? I'm not sure where I would go…or live."

"I hope Tampa's still on the list."

"Until I sort things out. I can't impose on Lauren and Dave indefinitely."

"Did they hint you'll be in the way?"

"No, but…"

"Like my mom always says, 'Don't buy trouble.' Please stop assuming things, babe. Let each day unroll and see what happens." She saw the hint of a smile at the sides of his mouth. "Why don't *we* go somewhere for the week?"

"Eh…your job?"

Tom stopped to pick up a perfect shell and handed it to her. "I wanted to surprise you. I swapped days and called in a few favors. So, I'm off beginning when my shift ends on Friday."

Cassie pretended to examine the shell, a beautiful shade of pink. *Tom planned to surprise me…by going to the Virgin Islands? And the All-Star Game?*

"What about the All-Star Game? Please don't cancel that because of me."

"You're the only one who knows I have time off. No one's expecting me in Miami. Caryn most likely has a back-up plan for the twins. If she doesn't, I'll go, and then we can head to Ft. Myers for the week." He pointed to the shell in her hand. "You won't believe the shells you'll find on Sanibel and Captiva Islands—enough beautiful and unbroken shells to fill a bucket."

"You've been there?"

"No, but someone at work came back raving about it…suggested a couple of places to stay." Tom flashed the smile Cassie had a hard time resisting. "Say you'll come with me on my vacation."

Cassie surprised herself by laughing quietly. "When did you plan this?"

"Uh…just now?" He grinned.

Cassie batted at his chest. "You don't need to do this, Tom. Go to the Virgin Islands like you planned."

"The only reason I planned to go was to get some—shall we say *quality time?*—with you. Come with me for the week. I can promise you days and nights of quality time you'll never forget."

Cassie leaned her face against his chest. "Caryn and Andrew may need you in the Virgin Islands."

"They don't know I got the time off. They'll manage without me." He flashed his most persuasive smile. "Quality time for us, Cassie. Please don't make me beg."

"No need to beg. You know I'll go anywhere with you."

He cupped her chin in his hands and met her lips in a soft, exploring kiss. Cassie parted her lips slightly to accept the kiss, slipping her arms around his chest and leaning against him when her legs felt like rubber. "Is this a sample of quality time, doctor?"

"Come home with me tonight?" Tom asked when they returned to the neighborhood.

"Eh, not such a good idea, doc. Andrew and Caryn could bring Danny home anytime." Cassie pulled back to look at him. "I wouldn't feel comfortable, even though your apartment is separate. If I heard the munchkins, I don't know how I'll react. Cry, probably." She rested her head on his shoulder. "It's okay, Tom. I can dream about our 'quality time' in Sanibel."

54

When he returned home from work the following afternoon, Tom walked through the front door rather than his private entry. He heard both twins babbling happily, and he followed the sound to an unused bedroom close to the master suite and the great room. The room resembled Toyland. He paused a moment in the doorway, observing Daniel, looking for any sign of the near-drowning.

The toddler's bright eyes focused on what looked like a new toy. He turned it around in all directions until he'd seen every side. He looked up, saw Tom, and tossed the plastic truck to him.

"Thanks, buddy," Tom greeted as he entered the room. "Decided to contain the damage?" He smiled when Caryn met his eyes.

"They really need a playroom. This should do, don't you think?"

"What? No toys strewn all over the great room?" Tom picked up Daniel when he reached for him. "You like your truck, Danny?" He squatted to give it to him and then looked at Caryn. "He looks great. Would never know…"

"Yes, I agree with you," Caryn interrupted.

"Have you gotten any sleep?"

"While they napped, but not a deep sleep. Everything's still crashing together in my mind." Caryn picked up Jenna when she objected to Tom holding Daniel. "Tonight should be better."

"It will. I don't think you need to worry about Daniel. He's not showing any after-effects at all."

"That's what all our doctors said." Caryn kissed Jenna's forehead, then laughed softly. "In fact, someone wanted to swim today, believe it or not. He pitched a bit of a tantrum when I told him no."

"I believe that absolutely. I'd say Danny has a lot of his dad's personality in him."

Caryn agreed with a laugh, then sobered. "How's Cassie?"

"Not good…repentant, assumes responsibility, overwhelmed by guilt. She's having difficulty trying to process everything."

"Does Cassie accept it was just an accident? I certainly don't blame her. Does she know that?"

Tom thought for a long moment. "She blames herself…Nothing I say changes her mind."

"I need to see her, preferably with the twins. I will eternally be grateful to her for saving Danny's life." Caryn's eyes filled with tears. "The house feels so empty without her."

Tom started to respond but stopped when his brother entered the room.

"Nice job, Caryn," he said. "Perfect idea to make this a playroom." Andrew turned to Tom. "I know I haven't thanked you, but I can't tell you how much it meant that you coordinated everything once Danny arrived in the ER."

Tom shrugged. "You know there's nothing I wouldn't do for you guys. I'm thankful Daniel doesn't appear to have any lingering effects."

"Not even coughing," Caryn added. "He wants back in the pool, Drew. Don't know how I feel about that."

"We'll double up on the swim lessons. I'm more concerned he'll be afraid of the water." Andrew glanced at a backpack he held. "Here are some textbooks and notes Cassie left. Will you get them to her?" he asked Tom.

"Of course." Tom gently returned the squirming toddler to the floor before he accepted the bag. He set it on top of the toy shelves and pulled out the top book. *Calculus?* He opened the cover, looking for a name. *Nothing*. He set that text aside and looked at the next. *Basics of Accounting. Obviously not Cassie's books.*

"Anything wrong?" Caryn asked.

"These aren't Cassie's. There's no name, but I know she's not taking either of these courses."

"Don't worry about that now. I'll look at the books later," Caryn said, stifling a yawn. "Are you working tomorrow?"

"Short shift. What did you decide about the All-Star Game and your bye-week plans?"

"We'll keep our plans unless the pediatrician doesn't want Daniel to travel," Andrew replied. "We have an appointment in the morning."

Caryn's voice sounded wistful. "I was so looking forward to you and Cassie traveling with us." Tom saw her glance at Andrew, who maintained a neutral expression.

"Yeah, that resort sounds amazing. I'm glad you're sticking to your plans. Take a week and just decompress," Tom said. "Why not leave Danny and Jenna with me? Then you can truly relax."

"Why don't you just come with us?" Andrew asked.

Tom shook his head. *Was that a challenge in his tone? Does he really think I'll go alone when Cassie was included in the original plans?* "Sorry, brother. A week in paradise sounds tempting, but I can't do that to Cassie."

"Of course not," Caryn replied. "We'll enjoy just having our peanuts with us, Drew. A family vacation. But now it's bedtime—for Danny, Jenna, *and* me."

Andrew lifted Danny as Caryn stood with Jenna in her arms. Tom began to collect toys, but Caryn waved her hand. "Leave them…that's the nice thing about a playroom. We just shut the door."

Tom slipped the backpack over a shoulder. "Pretty sure I can guess who left these."

Caryn glanced at him. "Amelie? She enjoys studying by the pool. Just put them on the kitchen counter, Tom. If she doesn't realize it, I'll call her tomorrow." Tom saw speculation spread across her expression. "I wonder if she stopped by to help Cassie yesterday?"

Andrew's laugh conveyed no humor. "Amelie help? More like Amelie distracts."

"Drew…" Caryn warned as she glanced at Tom. "Did Cassie say anything about Amelie coming over yesterday."

"She mentioned it."

"I assumed she did since she came to the spa to tell me about Daniel."

"Did she take you to the hospital?" Tom questioned.

Caryn shook her head. "The girls took me. Amelie was too distraught. I told her to go on home."

"I can drop these books off tomorrow on my way to work." Tom started to say something further, but after glancing at his brother kept his opinion to himself.

"I'll call Amelie and let her know you're coming by tomorrow," Caryn said.

"Warn her, please, that I'll be there early…around six."

Caryn nodded with a smile. "Absolutely."

Tom saw Andrew watching him. He waited to see if he said anything, but after a beat, Andrew turned and followed Caryn to the nursery.

Tom arrived at the condominium early and waited in the lobby. Caryn said Amelie had promised to meet him at six o'clock, so Tom took advantage of the extra time to think through the questions he intended to ask. *Maybe she'll volunteer the information that she was at the house when Daniel fell into the pool? It's the only explanation that makes sense. If she came over to help Cassie with the twins, did she use the pool deck for a study break? What could she add to Cassie's account of the near tragedy?*

Not sure what he expected, but he never imagined Amelie would emerge from the elevator, a bright smile on her face, and dressed for success.

"Hi, Tom! Thanks for bringing these—I thought I'd have to tell my professors I left them at home." Her smile came across too bright—*flirtatious?*—too happy for Tom's mindset. "Danny's fine? No after-effects?"

"Ready to take on the day."

"That's a relief," Amelie said with a laugh. "I love those children so much. How's Cassie today? She sounded overwhelmed last time we spoke."

"I haven't seen her today." Tom paused a moment. "Do you know exactly what happened? Were you there?"

"Yes...One second we were playing with the twins. We'd had such a wonderful day…Jenna pretended I was a climbing wall. The next moment Cassie screamed for me to call 911…It was…frightening," she said with a visible shiver.

"So, you didn't see him go out by the pool?"

She shook her head. "I don't know how he got out there…It's all a nightmare." She paused and look at Tom with a small smile. "I thought I'd go over today, to see if I can give Cassie a hand with the twins."

"No need. She's not working today."

"Too distraught?"

"Yesterday was hard on her."

"I know—so scary to see Danny like that." Amelie shuddered.

"But you don't know how Daniel got to the pool? That door's always locked…maybe you left it open after you did your homework?" Tom nodded toward the backpack. "Found your books on the table near the pool."

"Tom, I don't think I left the door open. Maybe I did?" Amelie shrugged. "Either way, it was unintentional, no matter who forgot to lock that door."

"Were you distracted for a few minutes? Possibly using your phone?"

She glared at him. "What are you implying?"

Tom leveled his gaze to meet hers. "That there's more to the story than appears? I intend to discover exactly what happened yesterday." He held her eyes for a long beat. "I need to get to the hospital. Thanks for meeting me at the crack of dawn."

"No, thank *you* for bringing these books. Maybe I'll see you later."

Tom didn't reply; just nodded and turned to leave. *She says the right words, but her body language disagrees. No eye contact while she spoke about what happened. Didn't seem that upset—definitely not, compared to Cassie. Maybe she doesn't feel any responsibility or remorse? Or relieved that Cassie's accepted the blame?*

55

Cassie set her alarm early to beat the traffic Friday morning and drove to the campus. She hoped to change her status to full time and apply for student housing. Her mood lifted when she opened the moonroof and felt the sun warming her face as she drove. She wanted to get her Plan B in place before she spoke to her parents, especially her mother.

Cassie hadn't decided what or how much she would disclose but wanted her plans solidified as quickly as possible. Then her mother could not insist she return to Vancouver. *Or try to insist...I won't go back now. Why should I? I'm an adult. I'm not asking for money. She can't treat me like a child forever. So, why do I worry about talking to her? I can choose what information I share...and what I keep to myself. She's my mother, but I'm not an immature teenager she needs to control.*

Cassie returned to Lauren and Dave's feeling unsettled. She couldn't switch to the full-time student classification until registration opened for the summer semester. Then she could apply for student housing. *IF*

I pass algebra. Big if... When she entered the house, Cassie found a note from Lauren. "With Caryn, checking in on our love bugs." *When will I see them again? Probably not for a long time.*

Her positive thoughts quickly disintegrated, replaced with sorrow and guilt. *How can I stay here and never interact with Jenna and Daniel...knowing that I'm not welcome in their home...that I've put both Lauren and Dave in an awkward position? And even worse for Tom...* She hoped that moving on campus would give her enough distance. Caryn and Andrew wouldn't have to look at her and be reminded of the afternoon that Danny nearly drowned.

She searched online for an apartment, but anything near campus obliterated her budget. *Maybe I should just use the money and go to Europe? See Paris, London, Rome. Maybe interview for an au pair position—I won't have any references...can't give Caryn's and Andrew's names. Choose a second Plan B—follow Lauren's example and move to Toronto for the university?*

She curled up on a lounge chair in a sunny corner of the lanai. She refused to dwell on her remorse. She made the horrific mistake...she needed to accept the consequences and move on. *Life doesn't promise second chances.*

Cassie fell asleep and awakened to the sound of voices coming from the kitchen. *Jenna, Danny babbling? Dreaming?* Then she heard Caryn's voice in a conversation with Lauren. *Caryn's here with the twins?* She hesitated to make her presence known. *I'm the last person Caryn needs to see.*

Hearing Danny and Jenna's happy voices splintered her heart; she had no expectation that she'd interact with them soon...or ever again. Cassie willed the tears not to escape and said a quick prayer that neither Lauren nor Caryn would notice her. She shut her eyes and tried not to eavesdrop on their conversation.

Reaching for her earbuds, Cassie hoped to escape within her music. She selected a playlist she and Tom often listened to and was about to insert the earbuds when she thought she heard Amelie's name. *Caryn mentioned her?* Curious, Cassie strained to listen to the conversation.

"Has Amelie seen Cassie today?" Caryn asked.

"Not that I'm aware—unless they crossed paths on campus. Why?"

"She stopped by the house, offering to help with the twins today. When I said we'd given Cassie some personal time off, she immediately volunteered to fill in as long as needed."

"Including your trip to St. John?" Cassie heard the hint of sarcasm in her aunt's voice.

"Yes, especially the trip to St. John. I told her I'd consider it, then discuss it with Drew."

Cassie's heart plunged. Amelie watching the twins at home frightened her, but the thought of her keeping up with Danny and Jenna on a beach in St. John spelled a disaster just waiting to happen. *I can't let that happen. Caryn knows how distracted Amie gets—Surely, she won't seriously consider taking her to St. John's.*

She closed her eyes, taking a deep breath. Should she interfere? Caryn said she'd discuss with Andrew; would he consider it? *Not from what he said about her after the accident...But, under the circumstances, he might.*

Cassie drifted back into a light, dreamless sleep. She gradually realized that someone had joined her. Opening her eyes, she smiled when she saw Lauren.

"Wow, I didn't mean to fall asleep. What time is it?"

"Mid-afternoon. You needed the rest." Lauren affectionately brushed Cassie's hair away from her face. "Caryn brought the twins to visit. She hopes to see you."

"She does?"

"You bet. I didn't realize you'd come home after class. You're tucked away in this corner...*almost* invisible. I just happened to look at the bird feeder and noticed you."

Cassie pushed herself to a sitting position and absently pulled her hair back into a low ponytail. Lauren held out her hand to help Cassie stand. "You don't need to ask if Danny and Jenna want to see their 'Ca-Ca.'"

Taking a deep breath, Cassie wiped her palms against her jeans and walked with Lauren toward the great-room. Her thoughts ranged from excitement over seeing the twins, to fear that Caryn would echo Andrew's anger, to hesitation. Should she mention her reservations about Amelie?

Danny spied Cassie first. His face lit up, and he babbled "CaCa" while holding out his arms toward her. Cassie looked at Caryn. "May I?"

"Of course, Cassie. Absolutely."

Cassie scooped Daniel into her arms. "Danny," she choked as tears flooded her eyes. She laughed when Daniel grabbed her hair, then patted her cheeks. She felt Jenna using her legs as a climbing wall, so Cassie sat down so she could hug both. "I love you both so much," she whispered.

Caryn knelt beside them so she could wrap her arms around Cassie. "Thank you so much for saving Danny," she said in a whisper. "I can never adequately express my gratitude."

"But I didn't keep them safe."

"Accidents happen, honey. You didn't panic. You reacted perfectly."

"Can you ever forgive me?"

Caryn smiled as she cupped Cassie's face with her hands. "There's nothing to forgive, Cassie. Please believe that. Do *not* blame yourself—it could have been me, and I would have had to wait for 911 to begin treatment." She shook her head. "After the bye-week, I'm taking the same courses you did."

Cassie brushed tears from her cheeks. "I didn't notice the door was open. I let Danny get out to the pool."

Caryn held up her hand. "And Drew should have had that fence installed weeks ago. I should have insisted he take care of it. All three of us could assign blame, but that accomplishes nothing. Daniel's alive and healthy, the only thing that matters."

"And his doctor okayed him to travel?"

"One hundred percent okay. We leave for Miami this evening."

Cassie smiled. "That's wonderful. I'm happy for you."

Lauren pointed to Daniel and Jenna—each had fallen asleep leaning against Cassie. "Adorable."

"I should get them home. Just one more thing, Cassie," Caryn said.

"I can't apologize on Drew's behalf. Whatever he said came from extreme stress, fear, and feeling helpless. I know that's not an excuse, but please try to let it go. Before long, he'll regret what he said and apologize."

"He doesn't need to apologize. I understood what he said and why. I wouldn't want to trust me with your love bugs, either."

"I have confidence in you, Cassie. In his heart, so does Drew." Caryn paused a moment. "I hope by the end of next week he processes everything and understands that despite our best efforts, accidents can happen."

Cassie shrugged. "I hope you can enjoy the All-Star festivities."

"Drew has a friend he played with in Toronto. They have teenage daughters. We might ask them to babysit. Also, Amelie volunteered to travel with us."

Cassie tried to maintain a neutral expression as she met Caryn's eyes. "Keeping an eye of both these angels might get overwhelming…" She looked at Daniel, cuddled by her side. "Maybe Tom can get the weekend off."

"I won't accept Amelie's offer. We'll meet his friend's daughters; everything will work out."

56

Tom shook his head and tried to keep any frustration from his voice. "Cassie, unless you've changed your mind, we'll head down the Gulf Coast to Fort Myers this evening or tomorrow morning, and we'll spend the week on Sanibel Island."

"How could I change my mind, Tom? A week with you—all to myself."

"So, why are you encouraging me to go to the All-Star weekend first?"

Cassie hesitated. Tom read the indecision in her expression. "I feel…horrible about spoiling Caryn's weekend. Now, she might not have the chance to attend all the activities."

"I don't think you need to worry. A friend of Andrew's plays for the Panthers and has teenage daughters. I think they've already discussed babysitting."

"She's not considering Amelie, is she?"

"I think Amelie offered to help."

"And you're asking me to babysit the babysitter?" Tom couldn't contain the smirk that crossed his face.

Cassie swatted his arm. "Hardly. If you go, there's no reason for babysitters. I don't think Caryn's seriously considering Amelie." She took a deep breath. "We talked for a while this morning—she brought Jenna and Daniel to see me."

Tom sat down on her bed and patted the seat beside him. "I know they were thrilled to see their Aunt Ca Ca. Cassie, what's up with Amelie?"

He watched Cassie bite her lip and avert her eyes. "I underestimated her, eh…distractibility."

Tom laughed softly. "Babe, I think everyone's aware of her short attention span. Anything in particular?"

"If I tell you something, will you promise to keep it confidential?"

"That would depend, Cass. Do you trust me to use my best judgment?"

"Y..yes, but I really don't want…this…to get back to Amelie. Or have it look like I'm using her as an excuse. I'm not," Cassie stammered. Her eyes held his, and Tom brushed his hand against her cheek. "She's not a very responsible person with the twins…"

"How 'bout I tell you what I think?" Tom waited for Cassie's nod before continuing. "Amelie was over the afternoon Danny fell into the pool, correct?"

"Yes, but…"

Tom held up his hand. "Let me finish. Andrew found Amelie's backpack and textbooks on the pool deck and thought they were yours. I dropped them off at Cam's condo the following morning on the way to work. When I asked her about the accident, her answers were vague… ambiguous. Has she called you since then?"

"Not today, but…"

"Hang on for a moment. Amelie's evasiveness helped confirm my thoughts." He paused and leaned to kiss Cassie's forehead. "Was Amelie watching Daniel when he got through the pool door?"

"I made a mistake—I needed to visit the bathroom and grab a clean shirt. It took maybe five minutes…"

"So, you asked Amelie to keep an eye on them?"

Cassie nodded. "I don't know how it happened, but Danny got away from her…you know the rest. I could hear them giggling on the monitor, all three of them. Then, Daniel must have scooted away…I don't know how that door was left open. I found Amelie's cell phone later. She received a lot of texts around the time of the accident. But none of that matters. The twins were my responsibility, not Amelie's. I should never have left them."

Tom's heart clenched when Cassie clamped her eyes shut, trying to stem the tears. He pulled her onto his lap and wrapped his arms securely around her. "Hey, Cass, listen to me…We can't change what happened, and I get that you don't want to assign any blame. Or look like you're using Amelie as an excuse. But, don't you think Andrew and Caryn have a right to know?"

"They already know I'm irresponsible…"

Tom interrupted. "No, maybe you made an error in judgment, but never irresponsible."

"I'd say something if they seriously planned to hire her—unless they're planning to take her with them." Her hazel eyes pleaded with him. "Otherwise, please just let it go."

"I'm not sure I can, Cassie. They need to know, so Caryn doesn't ask her to babysit—now or in the future. You understand that, don't you?"

"Yes, I guess so. I hadn't thought about that. If something happened, I couldn't live with myself."

"Cassie, I think telling them the details that led to Danny getting near the pool will help both understand what happened and why you assumed all the blame," Tom said.

"Tom, I'll always know that Danny could have…died…because of me. Whatever Amelie did or didn't do changes nothing."

He lifted her chin and kissed her gently. "Stop being so stubborn," he teased her. "I promise that soon you'll realize no one blames you, and you're beating yourself up needlessly. I also promise I plan to fill your brain with other thoughts in Sanibel."

Cassie concentrated her energy on deciding what to pack for the coming week with Tom. Her heart fluttered each time he crossed her mind—often—and a tightness in her chest signaled a new emotion she dared not acknowledge.

Lauren knocked on her door shortly before she and Tom planned to leave, then entered the bedroom/office.

"Do you need to work?" Cassie asked.

"No, I'm caught up. Unless there's an emergency, I shouldn't have to spend much time on my clients while Dave's family is here." Lauren handed a bag to Cassie. "Just a little something special for your trip."

Cassie peaked inside the bag. "Lauren, what did you do?" She pulled a soft multicolor sundress from the package. "Oh, my gosh! It's so beautiful…and luxurious…feels like silk."

Her aunt laughed. "It is silk. You can dress it up or down—just don't wear it in the pool or ocean!"

Cassie threw her arms around her aunt. "Thank you. It's the most beautiful dress ever. Don't worry, I'll warn Tom about not tossing me into any water."

"We wanted to get you something special for your vacation. You deserve some spoiling."

Cassie flicked a tear from her cheek. "I'm so lucky to have you and Dave. I can never repay you for everything you did this week."

"That subject is taboo, as of this second. Think only about your romantic week on a beautiful beach with your 'hot hockey doc'—did I get that right?"

"Almost. My red hot, hunky hockey doc."

"I can hear your heart pitter-pattering as you talk about him. He's a keeper, Cass."

Cassie felt her cheeks grow warm. "*I'm* hoping…I also hope he doesn't feel awkward about being with me because Andrew's beyond angry. They're so close—I don't want to come between them."

Lauren picked up a T-shirt and folded it before placing it in the suitcase. "Just don't build imaginary walls like I did with Dave. Tom and Andrew will work everything out. Don't push him away—I wasted so many years. If Tom had doubts, he wouldn't plan a beach week with you." She gently tapped Cassie's forehead. "Purge any doubts and allow yourself to believe Tom's sincere. Just follow your heart."

57

As Tom drove down the coast with Cassie, he felt her tension ease the further they left Tampa in the rear-view mirror. The sunset and early evening sky provided a soft backdrop for the clear blue waters and white sand beaches. He heard Cassie's sigh as she appeared to shake off the week's trauma and embrace the beauty surrounding them.

She rested her hand on his thigh. "Tom, I don't think I've ever seen anything this breathtaking. Feels like we're in another world."

Tom covered her hand with his. "I hope you'll continue to experience that once we arrive at our villa."

She turned her face toward his. "If you're in this world with me, it can only get better."

"You can count on that, babe. Our private world." He glanced at her eyes, reassured to see a hint of the sparkle return. *Hope this week heals my girl's spirit. Hate watching her drowning in a sea of guilt, self doubt, remorse...Cassie hasn't really smiled since the accident. Priority one once we're in our villa...*

"Ground control to Major Tom," Cassie softly broke into his thoughts.

Tom laughed. "You like that song, huh?"

"Seemed like your brain was maybe in the stars." He glanced at Cassie and saw the smile spread across her face. "Both my mom and grandmother like that song. Not sure I understand it, but yeah, it kinda gets stuck in your head."

"Yep, now I'm guaranteed to have it singing in my head for the next day or so," Tom said. "Did I 'space out' on you?"

"You looked like you were in deep thought."

Tom lifted her hand and kissed it. "I wanted to tell you that Andrew appreciated knowing the whole story about Danny getting to the pool. He'd already told Caryn he didn't want Amelie watching the twins… too distractible."

"It changes nothing, though."

"It just might," Tom said. "Andrew's got a lot to think about. He complimented your maturity in handling everything and not making excuses. Beyond that, he'll need to get past this All-Star weekend to think through everything and discuss it with Caryn." Tom gently squeezed her hand. "I hope that lightens your guilt, Cassie. And once we arrive at our villa, let's put everything about this aside and focus on us."

Cassie's smile made his heart soar. "I'll do my best to block it all from my mind. But I'll have no trouble focusing on you."

"Us," Tom corrected.

"Us," she repeated in a whisper.

Cassie awakened when Tom kissed her forehead and brushed the hair away from her face. "Hey, you," she said with a sheepish smile. "I fell asleep?"

"That you did. I'm glad you got to rest. Ready to check out our villa?"

"You bet." She took Tom's hand as she exited the car, then turned in a full circle to take in the resort's beauty. The valet encouraged them to check-in while the porter transferred their luggage to their villa. Tom handed off the keys, and Cassie pressed against his side as they walked to the front desk.

Opulent beauty greeted her eyes at every turn in the lobby. The lobby was an open-air structure on both sides, and if she listened carefully, she could hear gentle waves, tree frogs, and other nightlife chirping. Tom retrieved the keys to their villa, and she could see the Gulf in the darkened skies thanks to a full moon. "So peaceful," she whispered.

"Agree…Enjoying the tree-frog symphony?"

"Love it. I think I heard an owl—or my imagination heard one."

"Maybe we'll hear it again on the way to our villa—I hope it meets expectations."

"Will you stay in my room?" Cassie tried to resist a grin.

"Plan to."

"*That* exceeds my expectations. Lead on, doctor."

Following the map of the resort, Tom and Cassie slowly walked to their building—the one closest to the Gulf. She saw the beautiful white sand reflected by the moon and noticed a few white-tipped swells heading for the sand.

"I think we arrived in paradise." Cassie looked up at Tom and pointed to the beach. "Beyond perfection."

Tom drew her closer to his side and pressed a kiss on her forehead. "Anywhere with you feels like paradise."

She blinked back a sudden wave of emotion. "Thank you for this." She managed a smile while struggling to control her tears. Tom pulled her against his chest and wrapped his arms around her securely. She welcomed the scent of his cologne, the soft cotton pressed against her face, the security promised by his protective embrace. She reveled in the sudden tranquility that flowed through her soul before reluctantly pulling away.

"You always know just what I need."

"*You're* the only thing I need." He grasped her hand and showed the entrance to the group of villas. "If I listened to the instructions, I think we enter here. Our room's on the top floor."

"Perfect that it's not a high-rise; just a few stories. Penthouse, eh?" Cassie teased.

"Not promising that, babe, but hopefully a five-star experience."

Cassie sat on the deck directly facing the Gulf while Tom accepted their luggage from the porter. Thousands of stars sparkled in the sky, a masterpiece no human could hope to duplicate. Tom handed her a glass of champagne before he sat beside her.

"Compliments of the house."

Cassie tipped her glass against his. "To a magical week."

"To a magical week and making forever memories," Tom added.

Cassie sipped the glass flute, flavor bursting inside her mouth. "Oh, wow…never guessed champagne could awaken every single taste bud in my mouth. Heavenly."

Tom laughed quietly. "I love experiencing new things with you, Cassie." He leaned toward her for a kiss. "Delightful," he murmured.

Cassie moved beside him on his chaise lounge. "You've exceeded all my dreams. I love that we are here, together, gazing at this perfect sky, Tom…It makes me think of that song…you know, 'starry, starry night,'" she sang, her voice a near whisper.

"Another golden oldie," he said. "I'd say our parents had good taste…Shall we tour our accommodations?"

Every room in the villa provided breath-taking water views. The modern kitchen included every convenience—plus a stocked refrigerator and pantry.

"When did you have time to plan this?" Cassie asked.

"My secret. We can sit at the counter and see the beach." They walked through the living area to the enormous master suite.

Cassie stood in the middle of the room and slowly looked around. "Do you think people live here?" Her voice reflected awe she could not contain.

"I could," Tom said.

"Something new for my dream list…as long as you're with me." Cassie looped her arms around his neck. "Thank you for bringing me here." She reached to brush her lips against his.

"No one else I'd wish to share this with, babe. Let's check out the bathroom. You can relax in the jetted tub while I throw together something to eat…Unless you'd rather go out?"

Cassie shook her head. "I'd rather help you in the kitchen, then both of us can bliss out in the jetted tub."

58

The next few days flowed together. Each morning they walked on the beach, collecting exquisite shells and then discussing plans for the day over breakfast. Beach time included their private cabana surrounded by billowing gauze drapes with tiebacks and lunch at the poolside restaurant. Cassie loved their afternoon "naps," which included leisurely kissing, cuddling, and sweet lovemaking. Some evenings they dined at a recommended restaurant; other nights, they cooked in the suite, turning each meal into a romantic celebration.

Cassie felt the days slipping away and wished that she could click the "pause" button. She mentioned that dream to Tom one afternoon as they relaxed in the large jetted tub.

"Yeah, a pause button would definitely come in handy," Tom said. "Put that on your wish list—along with sunny days, turquoise water, and the most unique shells ever seen. You've already filled two buckets."

"I'll go through them and pick out our favorites before we leave. The rest I'll return to the beach for someone else to discover." Cassie loved sharing the jetted tub with Tom—especially when she leaned back against his chest. She turned to look at him, caressing his cheek with her palm, then urging his lips toward hers. *Heaven...paradise...*

nirvana. Wish we could stay and not return to Tampa...real life. My feelings for Tom grow deeper every day, but I worry about him and Andrew. What if Andrew never forgives me? What's the only choice Tom could make? Family first. Always.

While Cassie called Lauren one morning, Tom gave her a quick kiss and slipped from the villa. He wanted to find something that would remind Cassie of this week. He wandered toward a group of shops. *Does she realize how much I cherish our time together? We've connected in a way I've never experienced...* He wandered from shop to shop, finding so many trinkets that reminded him of Cassie. When he entered a small jewelry store, he knew he'd find the perfect gift among the selection of hand-crafted items. He examined several necklaces, rings, and bracelets. Nothing felt right…not as unique as he wished for his rainbow girl.

"I'm about to put some new pieces in the display case," the clerk told him. "Would you like to see them?"

"Please." Tom watched as she placed a black velvet cloth on the glass counter, then carefully added about a dozen new designs.

"These are unique. The jeweler only creates one of each item in a collection. You'd truly have an original piece of jewelry."

"Exquisite," Tom said as he carefully examined a necklace and bracelet. The stones reminded him of the colors of the sand and the sea.

"Then, we have a ring that matches this style." The clerk opened a small box and placed the ring on the velvet. Tom knew as soon as he saw it, he wanted to give Cassie this sign of his commitment to her. The translucent stone reflected the colors of the rainbow and changed continuously each time he moved the ring. *Perfect. As unique and beautiful as my girl.*

Cassie looked at her phone and took a deep breath. *Lauren said I really need to call Mom. Ignoring her puts Lauren in the middle...Lauren said I can decide if I tell her what happened...I'm not sure I want her to know...Ever. Maybe I could recap my plans to switch to full-time status next semester? Do I mention Tom?*

She pulled a bottle of water from the mini-fridge and took her phone to the balcony to place the call.

"Cassie? My long-lost daughter?"

"I'm sorry, Mom. I should have called you back earlier," Cassie began. "I've been preoccupied with classes. How's everything in Vancouver?"

Cassie exhaled a soft sigh of relief that her mom seemed in a good mood. She shared her plan to transfer to full-time status as of the summer semester.

"Good decision, Cassandra. When do you have to declare a major?"

"Not until I complete the core courses, so I'll have plenty of time to decide…still debating early childhood education or communications." Cassie opened her water bottle and took a quick drink. *Yesss! She sounds pleased about my plans. Relief that I'm going ahead with a degree? Maybe it's a good time to tell her about Tom? Daniel's accident?*

"Mom, I have some other news."

"More good news?"

"Some good; some not so good."

"Why don't you start with the 'not so good' news?"

Cassie stared at the ocean as she told her mother everything. It felt like a dam had burst, and words poured from her mouth. By the time Cassie assured her that Daniel had recovered with no after-effects, Cassie felt tears splashing against her cheeks.

Her mother didn't respond for a long moment. Cassie heard her sigh and braced herself for the lecture that would begin.

"Cassie, I can tell that this is still fresh and you're heartbroken. But, like Caryn told you, it was an accident. I had trouble keeping up with *you.* I can't imagine trying to entertain two toddlers…Should you have trusted your friend? Maybe not, but you just ran to the bathroom and grabbed a new shirt. See how fast toddlers can travel? Have you forgiven yourself?"

She thought about the question. Forgive herself? "I never even thought about that, Mom."

"It sounds like just about everyone has accepted it was an accident. Perhaps preventable, but still an accident. You saved the child's life. That's the important takeaway—not wallowing in guilt. Forgive yourself and move on with your life."

"Thanks, Mom. I need to think things through with that mindset." Cassie moved to a chaise and sipped some water.

"Please do that, Cassandra. I think you also had some good news to share?"

Cassie surprised herself by laughing quietly. "It's good news for me. I've been spending time with Andrew's brother. You'll like him… He's perfect—at least I think so."

"Is he taking classes at the university as well?"

So far, so good. "No, Tom's a physician—a neurologist. We have so much in common and started going out after American Thanksgiving…Tom's…"

"Cassie," Amanda interrupted. "A neurologist? What could you possibly have in common with someone who's settled in a career? How old is he?"

Cassie hedged. "He's not much older than me. He took extra classes year-round."

Her mother didn't speak for a moment, and Cassie bit her lip nervously.

"Well, you'll do what you want, but please don't start planning your wedding. He sounds like a brilliant young man. He may lose interest once you're enrolled in school full-time. Keep that in mind." Her mother paused. "Guard your heart—I don't want you disappointed when he meets someone who's more of a peer. Have you considered the dangers of getting involved with your employer's brother? Do they approve?"

"There's nothing to approve. I'm an adult, and so is he. Caryn said she's happy we got together. I really think you'll like Tom."

"If that time comes, I'll look forward to meeting your young neurologist."

Cassie set her phone aside and leaned back against the chaise, emotionally exhausted. She glanced at her watch. *We had a forty-five-minute phone call. And mostly positive—much better than expected. She didn't call me a failure or immature for allowing Daniel to fall into the pool. She comforted me and didn't ask me to return home. And she took the news about Tom reasonably well. Not too critical. She didn't go into her usual tirade about men. Just the comments about the age difference and warning about things not working out... Maybe I'm due for some good luck?*

When he returned to the suite, Tom found Cassie on the balcony, her hair loose and blowing in the wind as she stood near the edge gazing at the sea. The cut-off denim shorts and hot pink bikini top allowed him to appreciate her golden-tanned skin. His mind flashed through the many activities they could enjoy without leaving the suite.

Tom walked up behind her and closed his arms around her. "The Gulf's siren," he teased as he kissed her neck. "How many boats have you shipwrecked today?"

"Lost count," Cassie replied as she leaned back against him. "Missed you."

"Any news from Tampa?"

"Besides Lauren and Dave's house turning into a three-ring circus? Lauren says she's having a blast—absolutely loves his parents and siblings."

"I'm sure they love Lauren, too," Tom said.

"Have you heard anything from the Virgin Islands?" Cassie ventured, entwining her fingers with his.

"Not much...which means Caryn and Andrew don't want to return to reality. Especially not with the team heading to the Northeast in two weeks."

"And do you have to work straight through to make up for the shifts you traded?" Cassie turned to face him.

"I spread it out. I need my time with this beautiful girl who sometimes paints rainbows in her hair." He lifted her chin and sealed his words with a kiss. "What's on your bucket list for today?"

"You decide. We only have a couple days left." Cassie roped her arms around his neck. "Whatever you wish, doctor."

"Picked up a brochure for a dolphin and manatee boat tour. Do you get seasick?"

"No idea—but that sounds wonderful! Do we need to make reservations?" Tom saw the sparkle in her hazel eyes. "Can I swim with the dolphins?"

"I just need to book the tour," he answered her first question. "As for the dolphins, I didn't get a firm answer from any of the companies I contacted. Though, you could just jump in the water when you spot a pod of dolphins."

"So awesome even thinking about that!" Cassie showed no reluctance at all. "Do you have any bucket list items while we're here?"

"Maybe. Debating whether you'd enjoy it."

"I'll follow you anywhere and everywhere, you know."

Tom bit back a smirk as he leaned his forehead against hers. "That's a risky move, you know."

"Why? You planning to lead me astray?"

"Not exactly 'astray'... but I'd like to try parasailing before we leave." He watched Cassie's reaction and saw her momentary hesitation before her eyes flashed with excitement.

"Count me in. Can we go together?"

"That's the plan. I'm not letting my girl sail off into the sky without me."

Tom arranged a private dinner on the beach after sunset on the last night. Cassie commandeered the ensuite bathroom, and Tom showered and changed in the extra bath. Cassie wore the beautiful dress that Lauren gave her. She loved the feel of the silk fabric against her skin, and the vibrant colors enhanced her sun-kissed skin. She just applied eyeliner, mascara, and lipstick. Cassie's attempt to style her hair proved futile—instead of pulling it up into a way-too-messy bun, she opted to let it flow past her shoulders. *Wish I had some of my highlight colors. I'd work on an actual rainbow array around my face for my guy...*

Her legs felt wobbly in the espadrilles after spending the week in sandals. *Hope I don't trip or do a face plant. But these go perfectly with the dress...sandals just too casual.* With a final glance in the mirror, she opened the door and walked across the suite to look for Tom.

Her breath caught in her throat when she found him on the balcony, phone pressed against his ear and gazing at the beach. The white linen shirt and khaki slacks hugged his body in all the right places. With the darkened tan and two days' scruff, Tom caused her heart to skip a beat, and Cassie sank to the side of the sofa to enjoy watching—*gawking at?* —him. *Wish we could stay here forever. Hope it's not his work phone and a crisis with one of his patients. That could cast a shadow over our final evening in paradise.* Cassie noticed that his hair had picked up sun streaks that she liked very much. She fought the urge to interrupt the phone call and run her palm against his cheek and through the sun-lightened hair. *Tomorrow I'll have to share him with his family, friends, and work...but tonight, we can savor our alternate reality, and I can dream that nothing changes when we return to Tampa.*

59

Tom concluded the call with the resident, relieved that she'd just wanted to check if he agreed with the treatment plan she'd outlined for a new patient. *Can't escape reality, but we still have tonight and tomorrow morning...*He opened the French doors, stopping short when he saw Cassie.

He slowly ran his eyes over her as he moved toward her. "You're beautiful, Cassie. Exquisite." He gently cupped her chin in his hand and kissed her softly. "You intend to cause me to skip dinner?"

He watched her eyes dance in merriment. "Now, what makes you think that?" She ran her hand lightly against his cheek. "A romantic private dinner for two? On the beach? How could we *not* enjoy that?"

Tom chuckled. "We're having dessert in our room, babe. No discussion."

Cassie looped her arms around his neck. "Can't wait." She rose on tiptoes to kiss him.

Hand in hand, they followed the path toward the beach. Lanterns provided just enough light to reveal a single table beneath a cabana. A gentleman dressed in a tux awaited them. Tom offered his arm as Cassie stepped up on the platform, the delight reflected in her eyes.

He held a chair while she slid into it. Cassie's eyes widened as she took in the elegant surroundings. "It's magical," she whispered when he sat across from her.

Tom accepted the drink menu from the server and looked at Cassie. "What would you like to drink, sweetheart?"

"You choose," Cassie said, deferring. "Anything you pick will be perfect."

"Frozen margaritas?" Tom watched the frown forming, and then Cassie laughed.

"I think not, doctor. Maybe white wine?"

Tom looked at the menu and showed his selection to the waiter.

"Excellent choice, sir." He nodded and stepped away from the platform, loosening the tiebacks on the white curtains. Only the side facing the Gulf remained open.

"Tom, I feel like a princess."

Tom reached across the table for her hand. "You should know by now that you *are* my Princess Cassie. Thank you for sharing this week with me."

Cassie smiled tremulously and shook her head when she tried to speak. She flicked a tear from her cheek and took a deep breath. "I'll never...forget this week and how perfect you made it. I really, really don't want to go back to real life."

"Hey, we create our own reality, babe. I don't intend to change anything just because we return to Tampa. What we have right here is *our* reality, and we will take it with us when we leave."

They stopped as the waiter approached the table. Once Tom had tasted and approved the wine, he held his glass toward Cassie. "To many more weeks like this."

Cassie touched her glass against his, her smile wistful. "To too many weeks to count."

They sipped the wine, and Tom's eyes stayed fused to Cassie's. He reached across the table to take her hand. "After our week together, Cassie, I cannot imagine a future without you."

"I feel the same way." Her voice was just above a whisper.

Tom squeezed her hand as he continued, “So, you still want to continue our journey?”

“Very much.”

“I looked for something I could give you that would capture our week. Something to remind you how much you’re loved and that my commitment is forever with you.” He set the small box on the table in front of her. “When I saw this, I just knew it was created for you.”

He watched as Cassie opened the box, her fingers trembling as she held the ring he’d chosen. “Tom, this is so beautiful…the way it reflects different colors. I’ve never seen anything like this.”

“As unique as you.” Tom took the ring from her hand and slipped it on her finger. “So, will you wear this and remember our promise of a future together every time you look at it?”

Cassie looked up, her eyes blurred with tears. “I promise, Tom. And when you think about me, know that I love you in a way I never believed possible. Each day, my love grows…I’m yours for as long as you’ll have me.”

“That would be forever, babe.” Tom stood and walked around the table, then leaned to kiss her. “Forever—never forget or doubt that.” He held her hand and touched the ring. “When the time’s right, I plan to replace this with a diamond.”

He watched Cassie’s eyes widen. “You can’t replace this ring!”

Tom shook his head, not sure how to respond. *Too soon? Too much?*

A teasing smile crossed her face as she wiggled her other hand toward his face. “But this finger would love a diamond ring.”

Cassie woke before dawn, and she had no desire to move. Content cuddling with Tom, Cassie hoped to postpone her return to the real world as long as possible. She loved sleeping with Tom’s arms wrapped around her, their legs intertwined, and her head pressed against his chest. *If only we could awaken like this every day…Not likely to happen anytime soon in Tampa. I’ll never feel comfortable in Andrew and Caryn’s house. Would Tom feel any more comfortable at*

Lauren and Dave's home where we'd have less privacy? Or will we wait for getaways like this for "time alone?"

She touched the ring he'd placed on her finger, and her heart filled with love. *He said forever. I want forever...why do I feel I don't deserve this? Why am I certain "forever" will disappear when we return to Tampa? Am I over-reacting to what Mom said yesterday?*

Tom's hand played with the thin strap of the camisole she wore. "You're overthinking things," he commented.

"Did I wake you up? I tried to stay still."

"No, you didn't wake me. But I could feel your heartbeat suddenly quickening. What gives, Johnson?"

"Just wishing that this week never ended. I could stay here indefinitely."

"That's a wish I share, babe." He tightened his arms around her. "Promise, we can return; it's not that far from Tampa—a long weekend's always a possibility. Just need to coordinate our schedules."

Cassie laughed quietly. "My schedule's wide-open right now."

"Not for long. You'll jump head-first into whatever you decide is next for you."

Cassie shrugged. "Maybe."

Tom flipped her on her back, and she saw his eyes flicker in anticipation. "Move in with me."

Cassie shook her head. "Don't tease me, doctor."

"Not teasing, babe. Don't you think this week proves we're compatible…in *every* way?"

"I can't move in with you, Tom—even though I'd like to. I wouldn't feel comfortable in your apartment. Not with everything that happened."

"I will not touch that subject right now. I was thinking about an apartment downtown, close to school, and the hospital?"

"You never mentioned moving before. How can you leave your niece and nephew? Caryn and Andrew would protest. You have a perfect set up there."

"Not without you. After this week, I don't wish to go back to hoping our paths cross occasionally. I love you and want to spend as much time as possible with you." He lightly brushed his hand against her cheek. “We don’t need to decide anything now, Cass. I do know it’s time to quit freeloading off Andrew and Caryn. Andrew and I have had this discussion many times since I completed my residency. The thought of you moving in with me jump-starts the desire for my own place.”

Cassie blinked to contain the sudden onrush of tears. “You’re a major part of the family. What would Danny and Jenna do without Uncle Tommy? Or Caryn or Andrew?” She pressed her fingers against his lips. “I’ve seen how much everyone depends on you. Don’t take that away in the middle of the season. Caryn has enough stress with the twins.”

He shook his head as he leaned to kiss her forehead. “We won’t desert Caryn during the season. We can help as a couple…whatever makes you feel most comfortable. Let’s discuss this later, okay? But please think about choosing a place to live with me. Okay?”

Cassie nodded, then Tom continued.

“Let’s make the most of the time we do have in Sanibel. I’ll order breakfast, and why don’t you think if there’s anything you’d like to see or *do* this morning.” Cassie caught the emphasis on “do,” and his wink with a smirk sent warm tingly sensations rippling through her body.

60

The closer they drove toward Tampa, the deeper the anxiety crept into Cassie's brain. She'd spoken with Lauren earlier. The last of Dave's family had departed that morning. *So, I don't have to meet a bunch of new people and make nice. I'm sure Dave's family's just as wonderful as he is…just too much right now…brain's stuffed with emotions I need to sort through.*

What about college? Maybe there's a university in Fort Myers? Does Tom really want to move out of the house—or is he doing that just for me? How will "forever" feel to him once we're back in the regular routine? At least, his normal routine. My only schedule—going to class part-time. Maybe she could find a job to save more money before switching to full-time student status? Surely, she had the skill set to work in a boutique. Maybe where Amelie's working? *If she hasn't talked her way into becoming the twins' nanny…Why can't I just push all this negativity to the recesses of my brain? Overthinking much, Johnson?*

She closed her eyes, pretending to fall asleep. Will Tom experience a reality check when he spends time at home with Andrew and Caryn? Cassie absently twirled her new ring around her finger. Is it fair to hold Tom to a promise if it causes a rift between him and his brother's family? Especially a commitment made during a magical escape from reality?

Tom gently touched Cassie's shoulder after he'd pulled into the Martin's driveway. She'd slept most of the way back, and he hated to wake her. When she didn't respond, he walked around to the passenger side and leaned to brush his lips against her temple.

"Wake up, Sleeping Beauty." He saw the smile spread across her face as she murmured his name. When she didn't open her eyes, Tom reached across her to unfasten her seat belt. "Shall I carry my princess home?"

Cassie's eyes popped open, and she looked around her. "Tell me I didn't sleep the entire way home? I'm so sorry, Tom."

"For what? You make these adorable sounds when you're asleep."

Cassie cut her eyes toward him. "I was snoring?"

"Just a hushed little sound every so often." Tom stood and offered his hand to assist Cassie.

"I can't believe I failed as your navigator." Cassie slipped her arms around his neck. "Thank you for an unforgettable week. I felt like I was dreaming the entire time…I don't want to go back to the real world."

"Remember—reality is a state of mind. We can make every day amazing—just seeing you smile, whatever colors you use on your hair—that's as good as any dream. I'll call foul if you don't add those touches of color again."

"Your preference, my brave knight?"

Tom laughed and pulled her closer for a kiss. "Any and all colors." He popped the trunk open. "I'm jumping back into reality in a couple hours when I walk inside the hospital."

"Anyone home?" Cassie called when they opened the front door. When no one replied, she walked Tom toward her bedroom/Lauren's office. "Home, sweet…"

"I'd help you unpack if I didn't need to head into town." Tom set her suitcase on the bed. "I should be home tomorrow night."

He saw the smile that could brighten even the cloudiest day. "Can't wait." Cassie took his hand as they retraced their steps. "How can I ever thank you enough? Everything was just perfect."

"Start planning our next road trip, babe. I'd enjoy even just a couple days with you, Cassie." He brushed hair away from her face and his hand trailed against her cheek, before he kissed her. "Don't forget, I love you."

A devilish grin spread across her face. "Love you more."

Tom showered and changed into clothes suitable for work before walking to the main house. The happy sounds of toddler chatter greeted him, and he found his brother in the kitchen, preparing a meal for Jenna and Daniel.

"Discovering hidden talents?" Tom teased as he kissed Daniel, then Jenna.

"Hey, welcome back. Caryn's fighting a headache, so I suggested she take a nap and leave the dinner to me."

"Need some help?"

Andrew picked up the plates for Tom to view. "These two eat everything."

"Except peas." Tom tried to hold back a smug expression.

"That's on Caryn. Says she hated peas, so it looks like it's genetic." Andrew set the plates on the trays, then prepared their sippy cups.

"Caryn fighting a migraine?"

"I hope not. She's had so few since these rug rats joined the family, I almost forgot about them." Tom saw Andrew look at him, but his brother didn't bother to hide his smirk. "You look like you've spent a week on a beach."

"Sanibel's perfect. Highly recommend it for a get-away. How'd you like St. John's?"

"Very different from our other tropical trips, that's for sure. The island and beach—beyond my expectations. Trying to work in activities during the twins' schedule? Not so easy. But we enjoyed family togetherness—much needed since our schedule's crazy the rest of this season."

"Yeah, the league makes you pay for that bye-week." Tom caught Daniel's cup when he dropped it with excited chatter. "Before I go, could you check on Caryn—just in case she has a migraine brewing?"

"Sure, just watch where you stand if you don't want to change your clothes." Andrew took the sippy cup and placed it on the counter. "Not now," he said to Daniel's indignant protest.

Tom chuckled as father and son adopted the same facial expression. "You have your hands full with my boy."

Lauren spotted Cassie's new ring immediately after her "welcome home" hug. She held Cassie's arm and her other hand grasped her ring finger. Cassie saw the knowing smile cross Lauren's lips.

"So, you came home with a ring? That's stunning."

"I love it. Wait until you see all the colors it reflects."

"Am I correct in assuming that's a gift from Tom?" Lauren raised her eyebrows expectantly.

"Correct. I guess you'd call it a commitment ring."

"A commitment, as in love?"

Cassie tried to keep her neck and face from turning a splotchy rose. "Yes, I mean we love each other—and we…eh…said we want a forever love. But Lauren, you know I worry something will change 'forever' to heartbreak."

Lauren laughed. "Don't overthink it like I did with Marty. Just let the feelings wash over you. I'm happy for you, Cassie. I told you Tom's a keeper."

"He asked me to move in with him." When Cassie saw Lauren's momentary frown, she added. "He mentioned looking for something close to the hospital and the campus."

"He's moving out of the guest apartment?"

"Maybe. I don't know the time frame." Cassie shrugged. "I can't stay at Andrew and Caryn's home, and Tom wants us to spend more time together."

"I can understand that." Lauren's eyes gleamed mischievously. "You'll hear no objections from me." She paused a moment, then changed the subject. "Just so you know, Caryn misses you…a lot. I got the impression that she's apprehensive about the next road trip. Kelly, Terri, and I will rotate helping her, but it's not like having you right there."

"I wish I could help her, but you heard Andrew, Lauren. I can't go over there knowing Andrew doesn't trust me or want me near Jenna and Daniel." Cassie pinched the bridge of her nose. "Is she looking for someone new? Or thinking about Amelie?"

"Not that I know of." Lauren shrugged. "They're hardly back in town, and the road trip's not until next week. They'll work things out."

"It's not like Tom and I talked about moving tomorrow. We haven't even looked for a place." Cassie glanced out the window and watched a few birds perch on a feeder. "Besides, he may change his mind now that he's home. Especially if Caryn needs his help."

From the corner of her eye, Cassie caught Lauren's frown.

"Remember, no overthinking, Cass."

Don't overthink…easy to say, just tell my brain that. The conversation with Lauren replayed in Cassie's mind as she sorted through her clothes. An idea that sounded practical while walking on a beach looked different in actuality. She didn't expect Tom to immediately begin looking for an apartment. *Especially not if Caryn's feeling nervous about that road trip. He won't put any additional stress on her. I'd help her if I could. Tom may decide not to mention any plans to move. He may realize that's impractical—I'd understand.* She tossed the dirty clothes in her laundry basket and wished they were still in Sanibel…*Paradise. Fantasyland. Escape from real life. Should I research universities in Fort Myers?*

Her math textbook caught her attention. *Catching up on classwork —the perfect antidote to overthinking. Especially when trying to solve for x, y, or z…if it doesn't put me to sleep.* She opened the book to the chapters covered while she played in paradise. *Instant reality check.*

61

Her mother's ringtone jolted Cassie from deep concentration on her math assignment. *Another call so soon? Good excuse for a break.* She pushed the hair away from her face and swallowed a yawn before accepting the call.

"Mom, hi. How's everything in Vancouver?"

"Same as yesterday and the day before. You know how it is." Hearing her mother chuckle indicated a good mood. "A package from the university in Toronto arrived for you. I hope you don't mind, but I opened it."

"What kind of package?" Cassie's stomach churned as she waited for her mom's response.

"You're accepted—again—for summer or fall semester. They've offered a work-study program and a substantial scholarship. I thought I'd sign on your behalf and return the document right away."

"Sign what?"

"The acceptance form for the work-study and the scholarship."

"No! Mom, please send everything to me. I'll look it over—I haven't decided what or where I'll study." Cassie steeled herself for her mother's reaction.

"I would say this is an offer you can't refuse, Cassandra, and an extraordinary opportunity."

Cassie hated when her mother used that tone. *Like she's talking to a preschooler.* "Mom, my decision. Please, just forward the package to me—and any other mail you receive. I'll take care of it."

Cassie heard the light knock on the door and waved Lauren into the room. She mouthed "mother" as she listened to her response.

"Have you discussed your future with your father?"

"Yes, I've told him the same thing I told you." She cringed at her mother's loud sigh. "Could you just overnight everything? I'll go over it and let Lauren look at it, too."

"Do you promise not to ignore this until it's too late?"

"Yes, I promise. But I am not saying that I'll decide right away." She rolled her eyes when she met Lauren's gaze. "Yes, Lauren's right here." Lauren held her hand out for the phone. "I think she wants to talk with you."

"Yes, I'm interested in hearing how she enjoyed the house overflowing with Dave's family."

"Before I let you go, thanks for calling, and please hug my grandmother. I miss you."

Lauren took the phone and winked at Cassie as she greeted her sister. With hand gestures, Lauren indicated she'd return the phone after they chatted.

Taking a deep breath, Cassie fell back on the bed. She shoved her textbook and notes aside, then stared at the ceiling.

Not too bad, two "good" calls in a row. I know Mom expects me to accept the offer and move to Toronto—just like Lauren...last time we talked, she sounded positive about the courses I'm taking here.

Does she think if it's not a Canadian university, the credits don't count? A year ago, I would have been over the moon, receiving a ticket to leave Vancouver. Now, I don't want to leave Tampa or not explore possibilities in Fort Myers. If I accept the scholarship in Toronto, the countdown begins until the day I leave Tom. He says he'll wait for me. But do I want to live so far away until I get my degree? Now that I know how he feels about me, it's so much harder to consider leaving.

By the time Tom's shift ended, Sanibel Island felt like a distant memory, a mirage in the desert. He tapped a message to Cassie before he started his car. He knew she'd probably fallen asleep, but this would greet her in the morning. He wished he could come home to her every night. *We spent a week in paradise—can we make our own paradise here? About time I'd manned up and told Cassie how I felt...then, her response—yeah, a moment I won't forget. But, does she believe it's a forever kind of love, not just words? The last thing I want—make her feel pressured or overwhelmed—especially with her options for next year. Or worse, decline an opportunity that takes her away from Tampa. I can wait, she can have all the time she needs. We can visit each other frequently, no matter where she lives. But, will Cassie believe in us?*

He felt Cassie's absence the minute he entered his apartment—the sight of her head peeking over the back of the chair or sofa to greet him with a sheepish smile. She always insisted she hadn't fallen asleep, and he always pretended to believe her. He looked forward to their conversations when she joined him in the kitchen for a snack or meal. He knew he'd miss the times she studied in his apartment, especially the "distractions."

Tom usually prepared breakfast for the family any weekend day he didn't work. Surprised to find the kitchen empty, he looked in the refrigerator and pulled out eggs, bacon, milk, cheese, and fresh fruit. Andrew's voice startled him.

"Our personal chef back at work?"

Tom chuckled. "If you wish. Any requests?"

"Just the usual game-day menu."

"Gotcha...I'll make a double batch of eggs and bacon. You want pancakes, too?" Tom looked at his brother.

"I won't refuse it if you make them." Andrew poured a glass of orange juice before leaning against the counter.

Tom pulled ingredients from the pantry as he asked, "Caryn feeling better? No migraine?"

"Hopefully, no migraine, and she slept well last night. I told her to sleep in—I'll handle peanut-duty."

"They still like scrambled eggs?" Tom set two eggs aside for the twins.

"As of yesterday. We never know with Jenna, but Danny will eat everything."

"That's my boy." Tom glanced at his brother. "Cassie and I talked about getting an apartment together."

Andrew nodded and showed no surprise. "So, things going very well for you two?"

"Better than very well." Tom watched the smirk cross Andrew's face.

"Congratulations. You know you don't have to find something new. There's plenty of room here."

"Yeah, about that—I don't think Cassie would feel comfortable living here. We talked about looking for a place near the hospital and campus."

"Before you make a decision, I owe her a huge apology."

Tom didn't respond—he just raised his eyebrows.

"You probably know I went off on her the day of Danny's accident."

"I know the gist of it." Tom's gaze locked on his brother's eyes. "And you're apologizing for…"

"…blaming her for an accident. Accusing her of getting distracted when she should have been watching the twins." Andrew held Tom's gaze. "Telling her she's not welcome in this house."

"And you've changed your mind? Why?"

"Time and perspective, Tom." Andrew paused and drained his orange juice. "Instead of thanking her for saving Daniel's life, I blew up at her. She deserved nothing I said."

"No, she didn't. Though, she may let go of her guilt if you talk with her."

Andrew nodded. He placed his cup in the dishwasher as they heard the twins fuss. "I plan to apologize and thank her for saving his life. I hope I can talk to her today."

"Good. You need some help with your children?"

"I'll get them. If you can have their breakfast ready, they'll begin the day happy."

"On it."

62

Dave patiently explained solving Cassie's favorite quadratic equations again. "Let's try one more time."

"Why can I solve the equations with you, but when I'm alone, I make mistakes?"

Dave chuckled. "Lack of self-confidence. You can do this, Cass Maybe you can jot down the order in which you solve the components of an equation before you begin?"

The doorbell rang, and Dave excused himself. "Try it, kiddo."

"Okay." *Still don't know the benefit of this in real life—Dave's told me the order repeatedly.* Cassie took a sheet of paper and began listing the steps to solve equations. She'd barely started when Dave returned to the room. "Andrew wants to speak with you."

"About what?" Cassie felt her heart pound.

Dave offered his hand as she stood. "Relax, Cassie. It's nothing to worry about."

"How do you know?" Cassie looked at him and saw the smug expression on his face.

"Because he knows I'll beat his ass if he upsets you."

Cassie's laugh sounded only a little forced. "Thanks…I think."

Cassie fought to control her emotions before she met Andrew's eyes.

"Can I get either of you something to drink?" Dave offered. Both shook their heads, and he nodded toward the porch. "Why don't you guys talk out there? Give you some privacy."

"Thanks for seeing me, Cassie," Andrew said. Cassie studied his expression. *No anger, and he almost appears nervous…?*

"No problem. How are Danny and Jenna? And Caryn?"

"All well." After they both sat, he continued, "We've had absolutely no issues with Daniel. No cough, no fever, and guess who wanted to jump in the pool in St. John's? No fear."

Cassie nodded as Andrew looked at her. "I want to apologize, Cassie." His blue eyes locked with hers. "I'm sorry I blamed you for Daniel's accident."

"He was my responsibility."

"Yes, but accidents happen despite people's best intentions or efforts. It's not your fault Daniel fell into the pool. I should have thanked you for saving his life—for knowing what to do and not panicking. Instead, I accused you, told you it was your fault, and probably more that I don't care to remember." Andrew paused and Cassie watched as he took a deep breath, his eyes reflecting his emotions. "I'm sorry for putting you through that, Cassie. I know you love the twins and would never act carelessly with them. They ask for you every day—you've had such an impact on their lives. I'm not expecting you to accept my apology, but I do want you to know that no one blames you. You're welcome in our home any time, any day. I sincerely hope you'll visit the twins soon—and Caryn, who's miserable without you."

Cassie nodded as she tried to contain her emotions. She pinched the bridge of her nose to stop the tears that threatened. "There's nothing to forgive, Andrew. You had every right to be furious with me. I don't blame you for anything you said." She paused for a deep breath. "Thank you for telling me you realize it was an accident and no longer blame me. I do appreciate that, but I'll never forget Danny almost drowned on my watch. That's the truth; I can't forget that or forgive myself." She swiped her hand across her face.

Andrew reached to grasp her hand. "Please, Cassie, accidents happen. If I can admit that, so should you. If you think you can't forgive yourself, please remember no one—not even me and my inexcusable temper—believes it's your fault. We're incredibly grateful you knew what to do…that you took those courses on your own time just in case such a situation occurred. We didn't ask you to give up your free time to take them. Like Caryn said, if you or Tom hadn't been there, we would have had to wait for the paramedics."

"So…are you signed up for the courses?"

"Caryn has registered. I'll take mine after the season ends." He squeezed her hand. "I meant what I said about everyone missing their 'Ca Ca.' Please, consider visiting us soon."

Cassie laughed even as she choked on her tears. "Thank you, that means a lot."

He stood and shook his head when she started to follow him. "I'll let myself out. Before I go, know also that we could not be happier that you and Tom found each other. No pressure, but Caryn really hopes to have a sister in the family soon."

When Cassie had the chance to relay her conversation with Andrew via phone, Tom didn't express surprise.

"I told him 'it's about time' when he said he needed to apologize to you. I know he's sincere," Tom said. "Both he and Caryn worry you'll avoid them and not visit the twins."

"It's just hard, Tom. I'm not comfortable walking into their house. I miss Daniel and Jenna terribly, but I'm not sure I can look at the pool without it haunting me."

Tom paused for a long moment. "Just a head's up—Caryn's going to invite you, Lauren, and Dave for dinner. Small get together, just the six of us. Maybe that can ease some of your anxiety. But don't tell her I said anything. You're my date, just don't leave me hanging."

"I won't. Maybe with that group—and if I don't look at the pool—I can relax. Maybe help break the ice?"

"Yes, I hope so. I miss you in my apartment. I want you to come and go whenever you want. Use my office to study. Surprise me when I come home. Wake up with you next to me. I told Andrew he's not off the hook until that happens."

"Is this an invitation?"

"Whenever you're ready, baby. You have the key."

Cassie shared the acceptance package from the university in Toronto with Lauren as soon as it arrived from Vancouver.

"I promised Mom I'd ask your opinion. Do you mind?"

"Of course not. Could you leave it with me? I have a client conference call in thirty minutes—I don't want to rush through this, Cassie." Lauren placed the package on the counter.

"That's perfect. Thanks—I have a couple assignments to turn in this afternoon. Take your time—I'll work in the screen porch. Sunshine's calling." Cassie collected her laptop and textbooks, then organized her workspace.

Amelie's ringtone sounded before she opened her laptop. They hadn't seen each other or communicated by text since *"that day."*

"Hey, Amelie. How are you?"

"I've missed you. Stuck in classes while you and your hot doc enjoyed a mysterious vacation."

"Eh…how did you know? I didn't get the chance to call before we left. Last-minute decision."

"When I couldn't reach you, I tried to contact Lauren, then Caryn. I know things were crazy getting ready to go to the All-Star weekend. Caryn returned my call and mentioned that you and Tom had plans."

"Hmm, yes, the best surprise. I'm sorry I didn't get your call. What did you need?" Cassie's kept her voice friendly, yet neutral.

"I didn't need anything. I wanted to ask you if I should give details about how Danny got to the pool…Now it's probably not important."

"You didn't need my permission to tell Caryn and Andrew what happened. I still don't know how Danny even got near the pool," Cassie said. "Did you tell them?"

"Not until I could speak with you. I wanted to be sure our stories matched."

Cassie took a deep breath. "Stories match? That doesn't matter. I told them everything I could. Caryn and Andrew deserve as many details as we can provide. I think Lauren has your phone…she said the screen showed numerous texts received."

"I wish I'd known before I got a new phone. Oh well, no big deal."

"Were you texting when Daniel disappeared? Is that why you didn't notice?" Cassie tried to tamp her anger.

Amelie took a moment before replying. "The truth is that I don't know. Yes, I had a couple texts, but he was beside me making car sounds as he lined up those little cars. Jenna started acting silly, climbing on me—we were laughing. Next thing I know, you're asking me about Daniel." Her voice hitched a bit. "I feel so guilty, I have trouble sleeping."

"Tell me about it. I think you should talk to Caryn and just tell her what you just said," Cassie said. "It's not about blame, Amie. Caryn and Andrew need to make sure Danny or Jenna never get to the pool unsupervised again."

"Will you tell them?"

"No, you should answer their questions, Amelie. The twins were my responsibility, and I made a poor decision by allowing anything to interfere with keeping them safe. All you're going to do is fill in some blanks for them." Cassie paused a long moment. "Everyone knows that what happened to Danny was an accident. They're not pointing fingers. Maybe you'll feel better if you talk to them."

63

Lauren joined her niece on the porch later that afternoon. "Working on math?" Cassie made a face while she dug in her bag for a folder. She pulled out a sheet of paper and handed it to Lauren. "Your latest test? Seventy-three's passing, right?"

"It is when I'm testing out of remedial algebra." Cassie couldn't hold back her smile. "I decided this morning to just try that test one more time. I was going to wait until Dave's here to tell you both."

Lauren hugged her. "Congratulations! I won't say anything to Dave—I'm so proud of you."

"I feel like this huge boulder just fell off my shoulders. Now I can complete the core courses, then decide on my major." Cassie rolled her eyes. "Maybe double major if I can't decide."

"You can do anything you put your mind to, Cass. And it looks like my alma mater believes in you, too. That's an impressive acceptance package."

"You sound like Mom." Cassie looked at her nails. "I really need a manicure." She shrugged and met Lauren's eyes. "I'm supposed to discuss Toronto with you. I told her I had enrolled here and already started classes…she just waved that aside as if Tampa doesn't count."

"What if this had come last year?"

"I'd have been on the next plane to Toronto. Across the country from Mom…but things have changed in a year. I don't want to leave Tampa."

"You don't want to leave Tom," Lauren corrected gently.

"Is that wrong?"

"Have you mentioned this to him?"

"Since I don't plan to accept, what's the point of telling Tom?" Cassie stared at the lake behind the porch.

"Full disclosure…if he finds out later, he may assume you hid the information because…"

"He might encourage me to accept the offer," Cassie completed the thought. "Okay, I get it. I need to tell him, but I don't want to go to school that far away. How often would we see each other? His schedule already limits our time together. If I go to Toronto, we might see each other two or three times a year. Plus, I'd have that work-study."

"True. Remember, Tom and Andrew grew up in Toronto. Their parents live there, also."

"Lauren, do *you* think I should accept this offer? Leave Tampa and freeze my butt off in the 'cold, white north?'"

She watched Lauren's eyes they revealed nothing. "Cassie, I'm playing devil's advocate. Tell me this—if Andrew and Caryn ask you to continue as the twins' nanny, would you accept?"

Cassie stood and walked toward the side of the porch closest to the water. "Thought I saw an alligator, but I guess it's a turtle." She turned to look at her aunt. "They haven't asked me to come back, so don't you think it's irrelevant?"

"Not necessarily. I'd be surprised if Caryn doesn't, so you really should consider that possibility."

Cassie shrugged. "Give me some reasons why I might want to accept the university in Toronto?"

She watched as Lauren thought for several moments. "I'm just speaking from my experience. I didn't have someone like Tom in my life to consider. I learned how to function independently for the first time in my life. I enjoyed the freedom of deciding what and when I wanted to take classes, go out with friends, enjoy a party or two. I met my best friend, whose boyfriend introduced me to Dave…I'd go back and do it all over again in an instant. Those four years were the best therapy for me after all that crap at home."

Cassie walked back to the table and hugged Lauren before she sat next to her. "I'm beyond happy you got away from home and had those experiences. I'm in awe of everything you've accomplished. Maybe I'd have a similar experience there…or maybe I'm already experiencing it in Tampa—or even at those colleges I'm researching in Fort Myers. I'm just not ready to commit to accepting that scholarship."

"You have time—isn't the due date in April?"

"I think so." Cassie picked up the packet and looked through it again. "I guess you're right, though. I'll tell Tom. He said that no matter what I want to do, he'll wait for me…even if I just wanted to travel, have new experiences…"

"Told you he's a keeper."

"The thought of leaving him for three years—at least—scares me, Lauren. I love him. I want to be with him, not over a thousand miles away…"

"I do understand that, honey, and I am *not* pushing you to go to college in Toronto. Just some suggestions to consider, okay? Then, you make the right decision for yourself."

Tom knew Cassie had something on her mind. Not exactly distracted, his rainbow girl's personality felt muted, like a beautiful bird whose wings had been clipped. *Still not at peace with what happened with Daniel? Feeling pressure from her parents? Undecided about her future?* He resolved to give her space and wait for her to share.

With the Suns out of town and Lauren joining Caryn, Kelly, and Terri for a "girls' evening" at Caryn's home, Cassie invited Tom for dinner, Chez Martin.

"I'll come directly from work, babe. But don't worry about dinner. My turn to cook."

Cassie laughed. "You count picking up takeout as cooking, doctor? I haven't prepared a home-cooked meal in weeks."

"Studying for mid-terms gives you extra latitude. You're done, right?"

"Thank heavens. I had a nightmare last night about the math exam, woke up in a panic, and *then* remembered I'd tested out of the course. I think I really do have a math phobia."

"Sounds like it, but don't obsess about it. With any luck, you're done with college math." Tom paused a beat. "If you haven't already shopped and begun preparing dinner, let me bring it tonight. The end of mid-terms calls for a celebratory meal."

"In that case, the kitchen's all yours. I'll provide the drinks and...*dessert.*"

Tom loved the seductive tone, promising a sweet after-dinner treat.

He shopped at Whole Foods on the way home. He took his time selecting a variety of seasonal vegetables—all locally grown. He looked forward to the community garden at the hospital reopening for planting. He hoped to bring Cassie with him also. She'd asked many questions about the produce he brought home last summer and said she had wished to live on a farm when she was young. Of course, her vision of a farm included chickens, cattle, pigs, and other animals raised purely as pets. She told him she wouldn't care if rabbits shared some of the produce—she'd just plant more if necessary. With those thoughts in mind, he planned a vegetarian meal of roasted vegetables and air-fried sweet potatoes, and then picked up a bottle of wine and fresh flowers.

As if she'd been waiting at the window, Cassie opened the front door and rushed to the car seconds after he parked in the driveway. She opened his door, grabbing his hand as if to pull him up and out of the car. He caught the spark in her eyes and quickly released the seatbelt.

"I missed you so much!" Cassie said, jumping into his arms as soon as he exited the car.

"Perfect welcome after a double shift." Tom lifted her off her feet, so they were eye-to-eye. "I missed you, too, Princess Cassie." Their kiss may have continued indefinitely had not another car slowly passed the house. "Later," Tom said, brushing his fingers across her cheek.

He reached into the car and gave her the large bouquet of spring blooms, followed by the bottle of wine. "To celebrate successful midterms."

"And an entire weekend off for my hot doc." Cassie looked up at him as she smelled the blooms. "No changes in your schedule?"

"None." He kissed her cheek. "Get the flowers in water—I'll meet you inside, babe."

Cassie's conversation with Lauren had replayed in her mind all week. She needed to talk with Tom but feared he'd encourage her to move to Toronto. *I don't want to totally rule out Toronto, but do I want to live so far away from family and Tom? Truly on my own? How did Lauren do it? She had no support growing up, but she thrived once she moved so far away. Between growing up as a "Daddy's Girl" and Mom smothering me and never wanting me to grow up, the only time I did something in my own—"disappearing" for twenty-four hours at a four-star hotel—colossal fail. Then, as soon as I graduated, I moved to Tampa knowing I'd have Lauren and Dave nearby. That rapidly expanded to the Chadwicks...especially Tom.*

Cassie arranged the flowers in one of Lauren's vases, then carried it to the table she'd set overlooking the screen porch. Maybe she needed to admit that it frightened her to think of putting herself thousands of miles from her support system. She'd checked—Toronto was over thirteen-hundred miles from Tampa; about twice that to Vancouver. *Pretty scary if anything happened.*

Couldn't she learn independence living on campus in Tampa or moving three hours away to Fort Myers...or even the University of Florida or Florida State? *Adulting's so much more complicated than I imagined. I loved my job, Tampa, and beginning classes downtown. Then everything changed.*

She felt Tom's hands grip her shoulders and pulled her back against him. "Where'd you go, Cassie? You look like you're a million miles away."

She leaned her head back against his shoulder and angled her face to smile at him. "No, I'm right here with you. Need help with dinner?"

"Under control. Join me for a glass of wine?"

"Of course."

64

Cassie continued her internal debate through dinner. Tom deserved to know her options for school, but what if he agreed with her mother that the Toronto offer overshadowed all other school choices and made them insignificant?

After they'd cleared the meal and each carried a glass of wine to the porch, Tom broke the ice. "Babe, what's weighing on your mind?"

She leaned to kiss his cheek before sitting on the wicker loveseat beside him. "That obvious? I'm sorry if I've seemed distant…I do need to get your opinion on something. I've been putting it off. Nothing serious; I'm just confused."

He took her hand. "Maybe I can help, sweetheart. Or just listen."

"You know my plans to take classes full-time next semester and hopefully live on campus…"

"Or we get an apartment," he added.

"Mm, yes, that." Cassie's smile felt genuine. "Complication. My mom forwarded an acceptance package from the University in Toronto—scholarship and work-study."

"Congratulations, Cass. That's impressive. Are you excited?"

Cassie shrugged and made a face. "Honestly, not at all. I guess I'm flattered, but now all I feel is pressure to accept it."

"How so?" Tom pulled her to his side, and Cassie snuggled against him.

"I thought I had everything figured out. Complete my core courses in Tampa, then decide on my major…I started looking at the universities in Fort Myers, too. Then this offer comes out of nowhere…My mom's over the moon about it. She's finally proud of me, and for once, I exceeded her expectations."

"And you don't want to disappoint her?"

"Not that so much. Lauren said leaving Vancouver for Toronto allowed her to live independently, make her own decisions, gain self-confidence, make new friends." Cassie grasped Tom's arm that held her securely against his side. "Moving to Tampa helped me to feel independent, but with security, knowing Lauren and Dave live so close. And now I have you." She pulled away long enough to kiss him. "Just thinking about attending school in Fort Myers makes me anxious, but you're only a couple of hours away. Moving all the way to Toronto terrifies me." She turned to meet his eyes and read the empathy and concern.

"Do you want to visit the campus? I'll fly up there with you—I need to see my parents soon. Would that help at all?"

"My parents will know I seriously considered it. You'd do that for me?"

"In a heartbeat." Tom kissed her forehead. "I'd enjoy having the chance to introduce you to my parents, show you my old stomping grounds, see a few of my professors. You could tour the communication and education buildings, check out the dorms. Then compare it with your other options—it might help you make your choice."

"I could do that. Can you get away for a few days?"

"We just need to coordinate our schedules. It may be in the middle of the week, but we can make anything work."

Cassie reached for their wine and handed a glass to Tom. "Cheers to an upcoming Toronto adventure." She took a sip, then smiled at him with a wink. "I think I'm ready for your dessert. What do you think?"

"More than ready." He tapped his watch. "Lauren say when she's due home?"

"She promised to call first." She tapped his chest. "We can take All. The. Time. We. Want."

Two weeks later, Cassie's enthusiasm for the trip increased when Tom mentioned that Caryn had arranged for her father's corporate jet to take them to and from Toronto. He'd kept that a secret until they were driving to the airport.

"How long have you known this?"

"Confirmed yesterday. Caryn's father has it on standby in case somebody needed to fly for business purposes. Caryn offered as soon as I told her about our plans—her parents enjoy helping with stuff like this. I'm sure you'll meet them at some point."

"They live in…Ottawa?"

"Yes, and I have another surprise—Caryn invited us to stay at her townhouse. It's very close to campus. I check on things whenever I visit Mom and Dad, and Caryn practically shoved the key into my pocket. I hope you don't mind?"

"Mind? My excitement level just rose ten times."

Tom laughed quietly. "Wow, should I take offense?"

Cassie playfully swatted his arm. "Having you with me is so beyond any excitement level—I didn't include that. It's just the whole campus tour thing."

"Good save, kiddo. So, no phobias about small jets?"

"If Caryn and Andrew use it to fly with the twins, I'm good. And I can't wait to see their townhouse—I've heard it's fabulous!"

"It will give us close access to the campus, plus the area's very vibrant with shops, restaurants, sports bars. We may luck out on the weather—Mom said it's not too cold right now."

Cassie rested her hand on Tom's leg. "Hope so—don't want to have to buy a coat!"

Tom covered her hand for a moment. "I'm sure Caryn has several you can borrow. No need to invest in a coat."

"Besides, you'll keep me warm, doctor, won't you?"

"Count on that, babe."

Cassie had scheduled her campus tour and meeting with the admissions office first thing the following morning. As soon she got through *that*, she could begin to enjoy the impromptu vacation with Tom. The day was mild for early March—in Toronto. Cassie took a step outside, then added a sweater under her jacket.

"Your blood's already 'thinned.'" Tom teased her as he walked with her to the admissions office. Cassie placed her free hand against his cheek. Tom pulled away reflexively, and she laughed when she caught the surprise in his expression.

"I love the way you understate the obvious." Cassie turned and slipped her hands under his coat. "Notice all the students not even wearing a jacket?"

"You know how it is. After months of snow and below freezing temps, this feels like summer."

"Snow." Cassie shuddered. "I didn't even think to pack gloves. Smart move."

"We're almost to the admissions office. We'll find gloves after your meeting and tour."

Cassie reluctantly pulled her hands away from the warmth of his body and shoved them in her pockets. "Where do I find you afterward?"

"Just text me. I won't be that far. I'm meeting a friend from med school at the Hortons down the street." He walked Cassie up the stairs and opened the door. He hugged her and then nodded toward the admissions office. "Relax and remember that you're interviewing *them*." He kissed her briefly. "No question's off-limits."

Cassie swallowed a giggle. "My first is whether they have a heated underground tunnel connecting the buildings."

Cassie had prepared herself for a boring meeting and did not expect to hear anything that would attract her to the university. After meeting the admissions director and reviewing her acceptance package, she introduced Cassie to the student who'd conduct the tour.

"Marc's work-study assigned him to our office. You do a bit of everything around here, don't you?"

Marc looked at Cassie with a warm smile. "You're work-study, too?" When she nodded, he spoke positively about the experience. "Shall we come back to you after the tour?"

"Just to wrap up. Cassie, speak up if there's anything special you want to see."

"The dorms and student union are just across from here. Let's start there."

"What year are you? What's your area of study?" Cassie shoved her hands back inside her pockets, but when the wind didn't blow, the sun felt warm. *Not too bad.*

"I'm a senior biology major. I'm waiting to hear if I'm accepted to med school," Marc said.

"Here?"

"Or McGill. Whichever will have me." His self-deprecating smile made Cassie feel more comfortable with him.

"My boyfriend graduated from med school here. He's planning to visit some of his professors while we're in town." Cassie looked around as they entered one of the dorms. She liked the option of a two- or four-bedroom suite that shared a kitchen and a large living room. "Do you need to find roommates, or do you just get assigned to an apartment?"

"Both. You can request specific people, or you can complete a survey that will match you with people with similar preferences. Early riser or night owl? Share groceries or maintain your own supply? Need to study in quiet surroundings, or does music help you concentrate? Are you okay with guys visiting? Stuff like that. The computer does a pretty good job matching people, but you have a month to request a change if the roommates don't work out. For any reason. You can also request a private room, but it's more expensive and not as easy to meet new people."

Marc showed a typical four-bedroom apartment, and Cassie was surprised by the large size of all the rooms, plus the private bathrooms. *Really is like an apartment except for the shared common areas. Good that it's a co-ed dorm—but no co-ed apartments.*

By the time they toured the food court's meal opportunities and both the education and communication buildings, Cassie thought she had a good sense of the campus. *Wonderful environment, friendly students. Maybe I could see myself here. Perhaps...*

When they returned to the admissions office, Cassie asked Marc if he'd like to talk with Tom about medical school. She sent Tom a quick text before her wrap-up meeting with the admissions director.

"Any questions unanswered, Cassie?"

"Marc did a super job as the tour guide. I think I saw everything. If I were to enroll summer semester, when would I need to make a decision?"

"April first, for summer and fall. Summer's less crowded, so it would allow you to get settled on the campus, make friends, and decide which of the dorms you'd like to choose. Summer has its own atmosphere...more relaxed, outdoor student activities, weekend excursions to places like Montréal, Ottawa."

"Thanks so much," Cassie said. "So much to consider, but I will contact you before the deadline. The scholarship and work-study are very generous and definitely will play a huge role in my consideration." They shook hands, and Cassie walked outside to find Tom chatting with Marc.

"So, you didn't need me for introductions." She sent a teasing smile Tom's way.

"I have class across campus, so I asked all the questions I could," Marc said. "Thanks, both of you."

"And thank you for the tour."

Tom pulled his wallet from his pocket and handed Marc a business card. "That's my direct line—the cell phone on the back. Give me a call if you think of any more questions or if I can help you."

65

After a quick lunch and ducking into a shop to buy a pair of gloves, Cassie readily agreed to visit Tom's parents.

"I'm looking forward to meeting them. Your mom and dad must be exceptional to raise two such amazing and successful sons." Cassie caught the smirk that hinted at the corners of Tom's mouth.

"Suck up," he lobbed back at her.

"Would you rather I use 'two such smug and scorching hot sons?'"

Tom grabbed her by the waist and held her face-to-face. "How 'bout we not comment on either?"

Cassie shrugged, then slipped her arms around his neck. "You could persuade me."

"I could, but we'd never make it to my parents. Trust me for a rain-check?"

"I suppose." Cassie tried to contain a giggle. Tom's mouth caught hers, and the kiss threatened to delay their departure.

"Consider this a small down payment."

Cassie followed Tom across the courtyard to the garage, where Andrew kept a car for use when either visited Toronto. "This is the *spare* car?"

Tom chuckled as he unlocked the Range Rover. "Much more practical for Toronto winters. He decided it would be overkill for Tampa." He helped Cassie climb into the car.

"I can't imagine driving this in Tampa traffic. Too big!"

"But it conquers snow like a tank. And it's built like one too." Tom opened the garage door and allowed the car to warm up. "You know the car I drive?"

"The Beemer?"

"Yeah, that was Andrew's first purchase when he signed with the Leafs. Not practical in Toronto, but awesome in Tampa." He shook his head. "Caryn drove it until she became pregnant, then only a Volvo would satisfy Andrew."

"So, you inherited the BMW?"

"Yeah, tough, right?"

Cassie watched a smattering of snow as they drove outside the downtown area. "I hope we don't see more snowflakes."

"Not in the forecast—at least last time I checked. Hopefully, no surprise arctic freezes."

Cassie knew that Tom and Andrew's father suffered an injury many years ago as an electrician. A live wire threw him off the equipment he used, and he landed on concrete, many meters below. Although he'd survived thanks to the quick response of paramedics, his back had broken, and the spinal cord damaged below his chest.

Although needing a wheelchair, his dad and mom attended every hockey game—peewee to the NHL. They made an effort to continue to enjoy the city's many cultural activities, but as the years passed, his strength sapped, and now he required live-in help. Tom mentioned how he and Andrew had played the guilt card before his mother accepted the help.

"He told her that since we both were in Tampa, she needed to allow us to provide live-in help—or one of us would move back to Toronto, no matter what it took. Dad finally took our side, so the guys outnumbered her. Now she says she doesn't know how she'd coped without the help."

"Both your parents sound remarkable. Your father has problems with pneumonia?" Cassie asked. "Caryn mentioned it one day."

"Yes, his ability to breathe deeply has deteriorated over the past several years, so he's prone to infections, especially during the winter months. Vicious cycle—get rid of the pneumonia, then back under treatment in a couple weeks. We've had a few scares."

Cassie touched his arm and reached to kiss his cheek. "That's very hard for you, isn't it?"

"Watching him deteriorate and knowing there's nothing I can do to stop it? Yeah, that pretty much describes hell."

"You're a good son, Tom. Your parents must be so proud of you and Andrew."

Cassie's nerves over meeting Tom's parents disappeared the moment Jean Chadwick enveloped her in a hug.

"We're so happy to meet you! I feel like I know you—Tom's told us so much about you."

"Thank you. I've wanted to meet you for a long time—you have two incredibly amazing sons."

Tom's father, Jim, had Andrew's blue eyes and Tom's knowing smirk when he grasped Cassie's hand. "We almost lost hope he'd bring a girl to meet us." His voice sounded raspy and it took a moment before he could continue. "Instead, suddenly, he's introducing us to a beautiful young woman."

Cassie's throat suddenly constricted, and she had to flick away a couple tears. "Thank you."

Tom slipped his arm around her waist, and Cassie pressed against his side. "Don't start using that blue-eyed charm on my girl, Dad." That same smirk hinted on Tom's face.

"Guilty as charged," Jim Chadwick replied.

Cassie helped Tom's mother prepare a tray of snacks and drinks. The afternoon passed quickly—his father delighted in reminding Tom of the antics he and Andrew had attempted. Tom shook his head when Jim started to tell the tale of *The Day They Skipped School.*

"Let's just call that a major fail, Dad. I think you figured out what we were up to even before the school called." He looked at Cassie. "We were maybe nine and ten. He made sure we were assigned to the after-school maintenance crew for at least a month. Only the beginning of hockey practice lifted that sentence."

"And you never skipped school again?"

Tom raised his eyebrows but kept his expression neutral.

"So, you never got caught?" Cassie guessed. She looked at Jean. "They must have kept you on your toes."

"You have no idea, Cassie. But we have to agree they left childhood as responsible and respectful adults."

When Tom noticed his father beginning to tire, he exchanged a glance with his mother and then reached for Cassie's hand. "Shall we head back to the townhome? Maybe sneak in a nap?" When she nodded, he stood and offered his hand to assist. "We've had a long couple of days."

"I don't know how Tom manages those long shifts," Cassie said. "Thank you for spending the afternoon with us. I'm so happy to meet you—and I loved the stories of the not-so-angelic childhood."

"You cannot repeat them, Cassie." Tom pretended to adopt a stern tone.

"Ruin your image as the perfect doctor?"

"Well, yeah, besides not setting a good example for the twins." He winked at his father. "Payback's hell, don't you agree?"

"Hush, don't speak about our grandchildren like that," Jean said. "They were perfect angels at Christmas."

"That's before Demo Danny emerged. Fearless and a force to be reckoned with. Andrew's going to have his hands full down the road." He squeezed Cassie's shoulders, and then both said their goodbyes.

Jean hugged Cassie one last time before they walked out the door. "I do hope you'll visit again soon. With or without your doctor."

"So once again, I'm yesterday's news—or whatever you call it." Tom teased Cassie as they walked to the car. "Feel colder to you?"

"I'm freezing. It smells like snow." Cassie looked at the sky as she climbed up into the passenger seat. "Much cloudier now."

Tom started the car and switched on the heated seats. "We'll check the forecast when we get to the townhome. As much as I'd love to get snowed in with you, I can't afford to get stranded in Toronto due to the weather."

"Très romantic," Cassie said. "Fireplace, hot chocolate, and major cuddling."

"We could always pretend at home—turn the AC way down, close the shutters, and light candles in lieu of a fireplace."

"Cuddling with you anywhere works for me."

By the time they returned to the townhome, and Tom adjusted the heat setting in the garage, the wind shifted, blowing briskly from the Northwest and bringing pellets of sleet.

"Your prediction of snow looks more likely now. Let's check the forecast, then I'll call Caryn to see if we should book a commercial flight home." Tom kissed Cassie's cheek as he helped remove her coat. "I wanted to take you to a couple of our favorite restaurants and clubs, so hopefully, it's a passing sleet shower."

Cassie watched as Tom pulled his phone from his jacket and opened a weather app. He frowned and shook his head, then selected a second app.

"Bad news?"

"More like no news or updates to the forecast. Would you mind checking the TV while I call Caryn?"

By the time Cassie located the remote and navigated to the weather station, Tom stood beside her in the cozy living room. "Well, at least they're predicting the same forecast as Caryn had received from our pilot. She gave him my number. He'll call once he contacts the crew, and the forecast looks more definite." He kissed her temple. "I hate that our weekend may wind up a twenty-four-hour turnaround."

"Maybe a snow-check?" Cassie smiled and put her arms around Tom's chest. "I'm glad I met your parents. You and Andrew don't know what a blessing you had growing up. They're wonderful."

"We may not have realized it at the time, but looking back, we did have it pretty good—tough love and all." Cassie watched his smile spread to his eyes. "We did test the limits."

"I can't imagine." Cassie rolled her eyes, then grew serious. "How do you handle living so far away...your father's condition must worry you constantly?"

"Both Andrew and I worry." Tom looked in the cupboards until he found some instant hot chocolate. "Sorry, no marshmallows." Cassie watched as he set the tea kettle of water on the stove. "One of us speaks with them every week, and I check in with his caregiver. Though, I didn't expect to find him that much weaker...Andrew didn't mention it at Christmas, so I need to compare his observations with mine."

Cassie saw the shadow cross his face. "That must be hard to watch...Do you think moving them to Tampa could help—even sitting on the pool deck in the middle of winter?"

"Definitely. Andrew and Caryn chose their home specifically because of the apartment. Everything's accessible, no stairs, and close to family."

"While maintaining their privacy and some independence," Cassie added. She pulled back and looked at him. "Have they resisted moving?"

Tom's wry smile didn't reach his eyes. "Let's say that 'stubbornness' is genetic in the Chadwick DNA. But this time we may need to play bad cop. Even with a fantastic caregiver, they're too far away. And you're right—getting fresh air year-round could do wonders for both of them. Maybe stop the cycle of pneumonia all winter—really nine months out of twelve." He pressed his lips against the top of her head as the teapot began to whistle. "Andrew and I will come up with a plan and double-team them."

Cassie took her hot chocolate upstairs to the loft and relaxed on the love seat. Small snowflakes swirled above the skylight. The forecast on her iPhone showed the changing weather conditions, and she set it aside with a sigh. *Could so imagine Tom and me living in a place like this. Very cozy. Maybe even here in Toronto with him to keep me warm. I can see why Caryn loves this home so much. It's their refuge away from the crazy schedules. Caryn said they hoped to add an addition in the back for bedrooms for Danny and Jenna.*

She sipped the last of her hot chocolate as she heard Tom walk up the stairs. "See the snow?" Cassie asked, pointing up to the skylight.

"And much more to come. The pilot says we have a sixty-to-ninety-minute window to leave. Now they're predicting almost a foot of snow tonight."

Cassie set her mug on the table and began to strip the sheets from the bed. "Do your parents have everything they need?"

"I checked. My mom informed me that as lifelong Toronto natives, their emergency basket is well-stocked…and to worry about getting ourselves to the airport instead of them."

Cassie giggled. "Your mom totally has everything under control. What should I do with the sheets? I don't have time to wash them."

Tom pointed at the laundry basket. "They have an arrangement with a cleaning service. They'll come by this week. No perishables, so no rush." He glanced toward their suitcases. "Just a few things to pack and we're good to go." Tom grabbed Cassie and pulled her with him onto the bed. "Guess I owe you a couple of romantic nights in Toronto?"

"As long as it's in July," Cassie whispered as she drew his mouth toward hers.

66

Tom listened as Cassie described her campus visit during the flight back to Tampa. "Great campus, good programs, student housing better than expected…I met a communications professor who taught both Lauren and Caryn. That was pretty cool…"

"And?" Tom prompted.

"It's a new city where I don't know anyone. That's the first time I've visited Toronto. I'm not like Lauren; she'll talk to anyone and makes friends easily. Look how long it took for me and Amelie to truly click."

"So, you worry that you'll feel isolated?"

"Exactly—and the larger the crowd, the more anxious I get. If Lauren hadn't graduated from Toronto, I wouldn't have even applied. Now I wish I hadn't." *Tom understands…I hope my parents realize that a large university isn't a good match.*

"No one's forcing you to go. That's your decision, babe. Large universities aren't for everyone. You're comfortable at the Tampa college?"

"Well, I do have a huge security net all around me." Cassie laughed quietly. "I also want to explore the universities in Fort Myers. Does that make me immature?"

Tom pulled her close to his side. "Immature? Not to me. Self-aware is a better description." He tucked her under his arm, and she lay her head against his chest. "Now, if Mom and Dad dig in their heels and absolutely refuse to move, I'll probably apply for a job in Toronto."

"That's a giant game-changer. If we're together, nothing else matters."

Tom hooked a finger under her chin and lifted her face. "You're my forever…We're together until you kick me to the curb."

"Not happening," she whispered as his mouth claimed hers. The kiss chased away all thoughts except her love for the incredibly thoughtful, sensitive, romantic—and all hers—hot hockey doc.

Cassie asked Tom if they could stop by Caryn and Andrew's before he took her home. She wanted to thank Caryn for arranging their travel on her father's private jet and the use of her townhome. When he pulled into the driveway, Cassie felt a sudden panic—she had not set foot in the house since the day Daniel almost drowned. Tom grasped her hand as soon as he turned off the car.

"Cassie, I promise you'll make Caryn very happy."

She trailed a half step behind him when he entered the front door. "Back from wonderful, snowy Toronto."

"Hi, Tom, I hate that the snowstorm ruined your weekend." Caryn greeted him, then noticed Cassie behind him. "Oh my God, Cassie! Come here…I need to hug you."

"Hi, Caryn." Even though she was petite like Lauren, Caryn's fierce hug nearly knocked the breath out of Cassie. "Please thank your parents for making the trip so luxurious. And your townhome—Now I know why you call it your summer retreat."

"I'm sorry you had to cut your visit short—come in, let's get something to drink and tell me all about your visit."

She grabbed Cassie's hand and pulled her into the kitchen.

"It's too quiet," Tom commented. "Where are my brother, niece, and nephew?"

"On a short walk up the street." Caryn laughed as she pulled glasses from the cupboards. "Beer? Wine? Iced tea? Water?"

Tom glanced at Cassie as she scooted up on a counter chair. "I'd love a beer," he said. "Cass, you've had a busy day. Ready to relax with a beer or wine?"

"Whatever is easiest, Caryn. Whatever you're drinking."

Cassie felt odd sitting at the island with Caryn serving her. She should be on the other side helping, not sitting like a guest. She sipped the beer Tom handed her and glanced around the rooms she thought of as home. Cassie felt the pull of the pool and chanced a brief look. Her heart pounded, even as she saw the black fencing enclosing the pool. She quickly shifted her eyes to the play area.

"Where are the toys?"

Caryn laughed. "I'll show you their playroom. I tripped over one too many blocks and cars. Everything's contained in the bedroom across from your room. I don't know why we didn't think of that sooner."

"Your room." Does Caryn still think of it as my bedroom? I wish I could turn the clock back. Make everything like it was before I made the worst mistake of my life. She picked at the label on her bottle as Tom relayed his parents' greetings to the family.

"They may have this 'thought' about you and Andrew leaving the twins with them this summer—maybe for a week or so."

Cassie swallowed a laugh when she caught the distressed look that crossed Caryn's face. Andrew and the twins burst through the front door, capturing everyone's full attention. Each gripped one of Andrew's hands, calling excitedly to "Momma."

"Show Momma what you found."

As the twins hurried toward the kitchen, Andrew greeted Cassie and Tom with hugs and an empathetic smile. "Weather ruins another trip. Forties yesterday, snow warning tonight? Another extreme winter."

"How did you all manage?" Cassie asked.

"We didn't know any better," Tom said. "We thought it was the same everywhere. Who knew?" He nodded to his brother. "Then, when Andrew and Caryn moved to Tampa…"

"Caryn said, 'You mean people actually *live* here?'" Andrew finished the thought. "Hope we never need to move elsewhere." Andrew turned his attention to Tom. "You had a good visit with Mom and Dad?"

"Yes. We need to talk, though."

Before Andrew could respond, excited voices echoed with little footsteps leaving the kitchen. "Ca! Ca! CaCa!"

Cassie slipped from the chair, her throat constricting. "My munchkins," she said, kneeling and holding her arms out as they walked and crawled toward her.

Andrew motioned to the sunroom. "You have time to talk now, Tom?"

He nodded, then squeezed Cassie's shoulders as she gathered the children into a wobbly hug. When their eyes met, she nodded when he indicated the sunroom.

The twins had Cassie flat on the floor within a few short minutes. She laughed with them, pretending to understand their twin-speak and looked at Caryn when Daniel began to pull on her hand. "CaCa, now."

"I think he wants to show you the new toys."

"I can't believe all the new words. Do you mind if they show me the playroom?"

"A few moments peace and quiet? Please, please, Cassie! If you and Tom don't have plans, I thought I could invite Lauren and Dave for dinner."

Cassie read the hope in Caryn's expression. "That's a wonderful plan—all my favorite people and munchkins together." She laughed as Daniel insistently continued to pull on her hand.

"Go before he sprains your wrist, Cassie. I'll call the Martins. I hope you enjoy the playroom!"

Andrew and Tom compared their impressions about their father's health. "We didn't notice anything at Christmas that was different from our last visit, Tom. Do you think it's the pneumonia or that he's that much weaker?"

"Maybe a combination of the two. Mom told me that his pulmonologist said his function has definitely deteriorated, which aids in this never-ending cycle of fluid in his lungs. The only times he goes outside —when he has a doctor appointment."

"You think it's time to force the issue?" Andrew asked.

"If they won't agree to move here, he really needs to move to an acute care facility."

"Will he need that level of care here?"

Tom shrugged. "Hard to say. The healing power of warmth and sunshine may give him more good days than bad. You know he'd hate an acute care facility."

"Yeah, he would. We can offer privacy, a completely accessible apartment and house, and all the grandchildren they can tolerate." Andrew smiled wryly. "You realize you'll be moving to smaller quarters with less privacy."

"I'll get my own space. I've always known you intended that apartment for Mom and Dad. Don't even put that in your consideration. The one thing I do know—if they flat refuse to move, I'll find a job in Toronto."

"Thanks, Tom. If necessary, I'll use that as a threat to get them here. Between that and their grandchildren, how could they *not* move?"

Cassie waited until Tom and Andrew confirmed a definite timeline for their parents to move to Tampa before declining the Toronto opportunity. She hoped she'd left the door open should circumstances change. Her father supported her decision. He told her that he took pride, knowing that Cassie had considered the opportunity seriously, visited the campus, and made an educated choice.

She asked Lauren to please join her on the more difficult call to her mother. Amanda's voice indicated pleasure that Cassie had visited the campus—and had even met one of her aunt's professors. Cassie could hear the disappointment in her tone after she explained why she declined the opportunity. She also speculated that Cassie had allowed her "relationship" with the "older physician" to influence her decision.

"I hope you're not sacrificing your future for a man." That familiar anti-male tone grated on Cassie's nerves like the sound of nails on a chalkboard. "I hope you don't regret it."

Cassie looked at Lauren, who spoke up. "Amanda, I've known Tom since I was a sophomore. He's an incredible person, a talented neurologist, and he treats Cassie like she's a princess." Both Cassie and Lauren heard Amanda's groan. "Not in a bad way, Amanda, the best possible manner. He respects her, makes her laugh, and understands her better than any of us. You couldn't hope for a better man in Cassie's life."

"Cassie, you're just about to celebrate your twenty-first birthday. Don't rush into a lifetime commitment."

"I'm not rushing. You'd like him if you met him. Just like Dave."

"Why don't you visit us this spring?" Lauren suggested. "We could celebrate Cassie's twenty-first birthday—a family celebration."

"Do you expect your father there, too?"

"Amanda, just plan a visit, if you can, around Cassie's birthday," Lauren interrupted.

"Nothing would make me happier than to celebrate with our entire family…you know, like when I was young." Cassie's voice was wistful.

Both heard Amanda's snort. "You're still a dreamer. Is your grandmother included?"

"Of course, I'd love to see her," Cassie replied.

Lauren said, "Then you can meet Dr. Tom Chadwick." After the call ended, Lauren collapsed next to Cassie. laughing. "I almost said she could meet your hot hockey doc."

"That would have gone over like a bucket of ice water."

"Cassie, it's your twenty-first birthday. I promise you'll enjoy a celebration that you'll never forget. Leave the planning to me."

67

Time moved at a rapid clip as if the brisk March winds sought to push life forward. When Cassie didn't have classes, she helped Tom look for an apartment or condo to rent. She knew he had no pressure to find another place. In fact, he had numerous offers of places to stay. Andrew and Caryn had said he could live there indefinitely; Dave mentioned to Tom that they had several guest rooms available. Kelly and John Peterson offered the apartment at their home, Kelly half-joking that he could reverse the CamKarma that remained in that space.

"Have any of these 'spoken' to you?" Tom asked after a Saturday looking at apartments.

"I don't know, Tom. I'm easy to please." Cassie flashed a smile at him. "Have you seen anything you like?"

"Not really. We can keep looking…maybe we should rethink our decision not to move into any of the condos, villas, or apartments where the younger players live." Tom looked at her, inviting a response.

"Maybe. But not on the same floor." Cassie clutched his arm. "Remember, you have an open invitation from Lauren and Dave."

"Let's go a little further away from the hospital and campus next time. We'll figure it out."

Andrew placed a file folder on the coffee table when he joined Tom in the living area. "Good news—the team arranged for the company that handles player relocation to work with us on Mom and Dad's move."

"That's a relief. They're not planning to bring that much, right?"

Andrew shrugged with a wry smile. "You may find yourself with an apartment full of furniture."

"Don't think we've seen anything large enough. Wait until we get the manifest from the moving company—then we can figure out what to do with any extra furniture."

Andrew nodded, then handed the file folder to his brother. "Take a look at these. Some options you may not have considered."

Tom flipped through the contents and shook his head. "This is way out of our price range, Andrew. Not sure I could afford it even if I switched to private practice."

"Do me a favor?"

Tom raised his eyebrows in a silent question.

"Please go with Cassie and look at these properties. Pick out your top choices, then let's talk."

"Andrew, we can…" Tom stopped when his brother held up his hand.

"Okay, we'll talk first. Once Mom and Dad move here, it puts a huge responsibility on Caryn with the twins and our parents—especially during the season. We'll arrange the live-in help, but I know Caryn will stress about something happening when she's here alone."

Tom nodded but didn't speak.

"If you're at work or living in town, you're thirty-to-forty-five minutes away—on a good day. We've had you as our personal physician for years. I can never repay you for everything you did from the night I was injured to the day I was cleared to get back on the ice."

"Andrew, you don't need to repay anything. We're family," Tom said.

"Correct. And we accepted your help. All we're asking is to allow us to help you find a home in our neighborhood. We'll continue relying on your help—soon more than ever. Will you please take Cassie and look at homes in this neighborhood?" Andrew locked gazes with Tom. "We can work something out about the finances if that helps you consider this. Just remember, we've got more money than we, our children, their children, yadda yadda yadda can ever hope to spend."

"You drive a hard bargain," Tom said.

Tom saw the smirk forming on his brother's face. "I'd prefer not to put the money in some irrevocable trust for you—let's keep this simple." Andrew slapped Tom's knee as he stood. "You want to ride to the game with us?"

"Sounds good. Maybe once Mom and Dad are settled, Caryn can enjoy attending your games again." Tom paused a beat. "You guys *could* always ask Cassie to babysit."

"I'm pretty sure I torpedoed any chance of her agreeing to babysit again." Andrew turned to walk away.

"Hey, Andrew?" Tom waited until his brother met his gaze. "You ever consider that by not asking her, Cassie may think you don't trust her with the twins? Just saying."

Cassie felt awkward, expressing an opinion on a prospective home that Andrew and Caryn wished to buy for Tom. *Even though he says it's for both of us, I can't assume that we'll get married and raise a family in the home. We've talked about forever, but nothing about marriage. It's too soon to expect that kind of commitment, right? I can dream about the house, picket fence, three or four children, and a dog and a cat... but that's all it is right now—a dream. Tom might run if he knew about my fantasy. Couldn't blame him—and he hasn't met my parents yet. My mom as Tom's mother-in-law? Nightmare in Tampa.*

Cassie told Tom she'd enjoy living in any of the homes—*who wouldn't?* however, he wanted specific feedback on each house or condo they visited. She tried to give pros and cons on each property until they all began to look alike.

"I'm not sure about a condo—when the twins visit, I don't want to worry about them stomping on the floor or thin walls."

Tom looked at her with a wink. "The twins won't be the only ones generating noise complaints."

Cassie swatted his chest and pretended to look through the properties for sale. She handed one to Tom. "Did we see this one? I don't remember."

"I don't think so. Looks like a smaller footprint, but larger front and back yards." She saw the teasing glint in his cinnamon brown eyes. "Nice size pool; perfect for laps…and skinny dipping."

"If there's a privacy fence."

"Understood. Let's take a look." He looked at the community map and located the lot—it was about a block away from Dave and Lauren's home. Tom texted the agent as they walked in that direction. He slipped the phone into his pocket and pulled Cassie against his side. "Last house today—promise."

Tom glanced at Cassie's expression and knew this house checked all the right boxes. Not small by any sense of the word—*except in this community*—the home featured an open concept floor plan. Cassie commented on the two large islands in the kitchen. One contained a cooktop and plenty of counter space while the second island comfortably accommodated eight people.

"I like this better than a breakfast nook," she mentioned. "Look, you can see the entire living area from the kitchen."

"Makes it easier to keep track of rug rats."

"You're calling my love bugs 'rug rats' now?" Cassie accused.

"No, I'm saying 'rug rats' in general. I might like three or four running around." Tom waited for Caryn's reaction.

"You 'might?' Is that a decision you plan to make on your own?" Cassie cut her hazel eyes toward him.

"Of course not. But if my wife wants six kids, we're looking at the wrong house." Tom watched as Cassie took her time before replying.

"Your wife, you say? Shouldn't *she* be the one looking at these homes with you?"

"Hypothetical wife." Tom suppressed a chuckle. "I told you that you're my forever…and to me that means the entire package: life partner, children, maybe a dog or two. Or even a couple cats. Fair warning. If your vision of forever is different, let's talk."

He watched Cassie think about his statements. *Too much too soon? She may not want that or want to consider it right now. Maybe walk it back?*

Cassie met his eyes. "I'm not ready to commit to…" She held up her hand to keep Tom from interrupting. "Two dogs? Two cats? Seriously, doctor? Jump in the deep end without checking if there's water in the pool. Maybe consider starting with *one* pet?" She giggled as Tom laughed in relief.

"Definitely negotiable. Now tell me which of the houses you liked best, Princess Cassie."

"First, you pick your favorite." Cassie's hazel eyes challenged him.

"I liked all the homes. Definitely not the condos—the noise factor you pointed out. So, four or five bedrooms? Pool, screen porch, or both? Do we need a formal dining room? Media room…"

"You mean Man Cave," Cassie corrected with a smug expression. "I like the backyard here—if we fence it in, we could plant our own garden. You definitely need a lap pool—would this one be large enough? I may never leave some of the master suites we've seen. Four bedrooms? Five? I wished I'd had a sister to share my bedroom. So, any 'rug rats' in our future may share space."

"Can you see yourself in this house?"

"Can I? Holy guacamole, Tom, look around—it's more than I could have ever envisioned. Who wouldn't want to live here?"

"Suitable castle for my princess?"

Cassie swatted his chest. "If you promise we can create a cozy space just for us?"

"Easy promise to keep."

68

April felt like a sprint toward an unknown destination. With finals approaching, Cassie didn't even think about her upcoming birthday. Lauren had not mentioned whether either of her parents had scheduled a trip to celebrate as a family. *Disappointed? Not really. Family celebrations were just memories of a happy childhood cut short.* Cassie resolved to give her future children positive family memories. She'd try her best to avoid the helicopter mom syndrome. She definitely would not create a cocoon of bubble wrap to prevent children from experiencing life—the positives as well as the negatives.

She thought Tom would share the same philosophy. Their children would experience both success and falling short of expectations; they would learn that victory comes with defeat—and how to deal with disappointment. Most of all, she longed to give their children the extended family she never had. She hoped their children would grow up with cousins, aunts and uncles, and of course, doting grandparents.

Cassie laughed to herself, thinking how Lauren would react if she only knew how many Martin cousins she wanted–*expected!* Caryn and Andrew, too.

Tom stood at the door to her room, watching the pensive expressions cross her face, along with a winsome smile. He didn't want to disrupt her daydream, but curiosity won. She didn't notice him, so he tapped lightly on the door. He saw Cassie shake her head, then she looked at him with a guilty smile.

"Doesn't look like there's much studying here." He leaned to kiss her, then flipped pages in her textbook. "You have your Florida History nailed?"

"Kinda. I was just daydreaming."

"Care to share?"

"Just thinking about my childhood—after the divorce—I promised myself I'd never repeat my parents' actions and reactions post-divorce." Cassie looked up at him, her cheeks turning slightly pink. "No one will accuse me of acting like either a Tiger Mom or a Helicopter Parent."

"Sounds more like a life plan, not a daydream. We'll compare notes on raising children." He brushed his hand against her cheek. "Do you have time to take a break?"

"With you? Of course."

Tom offered his hand. "Let's get some fresh air. It's not too hot."

Cassie looped her arm through his and intertwined their fingers. "You have a game tonight, don't you?"

"Yep—opening round of the playoffs. Do you want to ride with me?"

Cassie shook her head and bit back a grin. "I'm not going tonight." Tom raised his eyebrows in question. "Caryn and Andrew asked if I would babysit the twins. How could I say no to a few hours with my love bugs?"

"That's great—Jen and Danny will be bouncing off the walls with excitement."

"I may join them."

Tom saw genuine happiness reflected by her eyes. "Shall I bring dinner when I come back?"

"Like I'd ever refuse a meal with you."

Cassie suddenly realized they were headed toward their future home. "Do we have a closing date yet?"

Tom shook his head. "Waiting on the inspection report, appraisal, and survey. Usual hoops to jump through, so I hear."

"I can't wait to start decorating. Okay, if I work with Lauren and Caryn's interior designer? I have an idea, but probably need help to execute it."

"Whatever you need, princess. I wanted to give you a head's up. Dan asked me to attend a conference in Seattle at the end of April—rehab after TBIs—he wants me to present Andrew's case."

"Congratulations! That's quite an honor. Is Andrew okay with that?" Cassie asked. They stopped across the street from their future home.

"Yes, but I don't plan to identify him as the patient. Another physician will present long-term effects of childhood concussions." Tom glanced at Cassie. "The end of April is your exam week, isn't it?"

Cassie nodded, disappointment flooding her face. "I could see if I can take them early?"

"Highly unlikely any professor would agree to that—hopefully, you'll be supervising our home makeover."

"Not so much a makeover, but a new color palette. No knocking down walls, relocating the kitchen, or any of that fun stuff you see on HGTV. The biggest expense's likely replacing the carpet with wood and tile." She met his eyes with a bright smile. "Maybe I'll have samples to choose among when you get back."

"My goal—in the house by your birthday."

"Best. Gift. Ever."

With the semester winding down, Cassie rechecked the courses she'd selected for the summer session. None appeared difficult, as she'd decided to knock out required core courses—music appreciation, PE, art history, beginning French. *Nothing scary; maybe I can practice my French with Amelie. Then I can decide next steps...Early childhood education? Or earn a childcare certification much more quickly than a bachelor's degree? I'd love to work with children from infants through pre-school. Maybe I could specialize in educating at-risk infants and toddlers? I could always go back for the bachelor's degree.*

She flashed on the disappointment Cassie knew she'd hear in her mother's voice when she shared her decision. For once, she shrugged it off. As an adult paying for her own education, this decision was hers to make.

Cassie missed Tom and checked off each day he attended the conference. She didn't know how Lauren, Caryn, and the other hockey wives coped with the constant travel. Even when Tom pulled a double shift, Cassie knew he was just minutes away.

The conference wrapped up with an optional breakfast on the final day. Tom stopped in briefly to say goodbye to a few friends, then drove up to Vancouver. Cassie had no idea that he had arranged to meet her father and mother—separately. Tom wanted to make face-to-face contact and answer any questions either may have. *Like my intentions toward their daughter?* He also hoped they'd see him as a responsible, mature person and understand that his plans were the result of a friendship that grew into love. Cassie didn't know about these meetings, but Tom thought she'd appreciate his reasoning later.

Lunch with Cassie's father began with Trevor greeting Tom like an old friend. "Thanks for driving up to meet with me. I feel like I already know you from talking with Cassie. You're a frequent topic."

The next hour passed quickly. Tom answered every question Trevor posed—his profession, whether he planned to remain in Tampa, and how was he attracted to a younger woman, unsure of her goals?

The conversation flowed naturally bonded by their mutual love for Cassie. Tom looked at Trevor. "I want to tell you my intentions regarding your daughter."

Trevor nodded, a smile crossing his face. "Yes, *the* question. What *are* your intentions?"

"I love Cassie and everything about her. I realize there's an age difference and that I'm settled in my profession while she's deciding what she wants to do. I will never discourage her from chasing a dream, even if she decides to study in Paris for the next three years. She knows I will wait for her."

"Cassie's seriously considering Paris?"

Tom shook his head with a chuckle. "She hasn't mentioned it. Her friend studied there for two years and may return. But, even if her dreams take her away from Tampa, we'll see each other as often as possible. She knows I'll work to make a long-distance relationship flourish."

"From what she tells me, she has no desire to leave Tampa. She's enrolled in what they call a community college?" After Tom nodded, Trevor continued, "When we talk, she's happier than I've ever seen her—even more than when she received my blessing for this gap year."

"She's an incredibly responsible and mature woman. It's like she has blossomed in the past eleven months," Tom said. "I love her, and I hope to spend my life with her. She fills a void I never realized existed. I want to propose on her birthday, and I'm asking for your blessing."

Trevor locked eyes with Tom. "You're not concerned that proposing could be a risky move considering everything we've discussed?"

"When Cassie says she loves me, I believe her. I know what makes her happy, sad, or frightened. Other than with my brother, I have not experienced that depth in a relationship. She knows me better than lifelong friends. Cassie tells me that I know her deepest secrets—which I'll never divulge."

"Do you plan to marry soon?"

"Not in the immediate future. I think we'll both know when it's time." Tom paused a moment. "Full disclosure—I'm buying a home and Cassie's planning to move in."

"You'll propose before she moves in?"

"Yes, sir, and I pray she says, 'Yes.'"

Trevor stood, a smile on his face. "I'll let you sweat that out, doctor."

As they walked outside, Trevor met Tom's gaze. "Are you meeting with Amanda?"

"Next stop."

"Final piece of advice. Make crystal clear to Amanda and her mother that this is a surprise for Cassie." He clapped a hand on Tom's shoulder. "Thank you. I will be proud to have you join our family."

69

Amanda did not answer the door when Tom knocked. He double-checked the address before trying again. He knew he had arrived on time, but maybe something had come up. Tom waited in his car for a half-hour before deciding to drive back to Seattle. *No way I'm missing that flight. My girl's waiting for me.*

He opened a notepad he'd received at the conference and penned a short note to Cassie's mother, putting the mix-up on his shoulders. He wrote in all caps—"CASSIE DOESN'T KNOW I'M HERE—Planning a surprise for her birthday. Please don't mention anything. I hope we can meet soon."

He folded it and slipped it through the letter slot on the door. He also sent Trevor a quick text explaining he had not spoken to Amanda. As he drove south toward the border, Tom felt that all things considered, he'd had a productive trip.

Tom asked Andrew to come with him to choose an engagement ring.

"Did you get her ring size from Lauren? Any idea what you're looking for?"

"Yes, to the first," Tom answered. "Definitely not a cookie-cutter diamond ring. It needs to reflect Cassie's spirit—an original."

"There's a family-owned jeweler who's a huge Suns fan. I've seen some of his designs—they're all custom created. I saw an anniversary bracelet for one of the guy's wife. I'm thinking of doing something for our fifth anniversary." Andrew shook his head. "Jenna and Daniel also need to give her jewelry for Mother's Day."

"Hope you left your credit card at home," Tom said. "Helping me look for a ring could turn into an expensive trip for you."

Tom flipped through a binder featuring custom engagement rings. *So many choices...gold, white gold, yellow gold, rose gold, platinum. I'm supposed to pick one?* He remembered the first time they met at the airport—Cassie's hair featured pink highlights. He also thought of the many times she used a rose-gold tint.

Andrew introduced him to the owner/craftsman, Marcus Vallejo, who chatted with Tom while Andrew wandered around to look at displays.

"Describe your Cassie's personality. Does she prefer classic styles? Or does she embrace the contemporary look or something totally original?"

"A little of each, but leaning toward something original. She paints different color subtle highlights in her hair—I never know which color she'll select. She reminds me of a butterfly—pastels and brilliant colors." He shrugged as Marcus took notes, then began sketching ideas for a ring.

"Was there anything that caught your eye in our portfolio?"

"One ring had a diamond in the middle, then somehow looked like a butterfly. Another was the heart-shaped diamond with smaller stones outlining the diamond and continuing around the band."

"Yes, I know both rings. Very beautiful, and we can custom choose the size of the diamond, the color or colors of the smaller stones. I think platinum will make the colors pop." He quickly sketched the rings. "Or you could go with a braided band and focus attention on the heart-shaped diamond and surrounding stones. Do you know her birthstone?"

"Emerald."

"And yours?"

"Sapphire."

"Lovely combination. I can create several designs—similar to costume jewelry? I could have them ready in a few days—if you don't like any of them, we'll keep talking. Figure two weeks once you decide on a design."

Tom pulled a card from his wallet and circled his email address and personal phone number. "Just let me know when you have the designs. I may need to make an after-hours appointment, depending on my schedule."

Marcus stapled the card to the design sheet. "That will not pose a problem, Dr. Chadwick."

Between finals, supervising the few renovations in the new home, and choosing furniture, Cassie lost track of time. She only remembered her birthday when Tom mentioned taking her out for dinner.

"What an airhead—I completely forgot! Of course, I'd love to go *anywhere* with you."

Tom stifled a laugh by kissing her forehead. "Since you only turn twenty-one once, I'm taking you to an elegant restaurant."

"So…I need to dress up?"

"Yes, my princess. But remember, so do I. No takeout or late dinner on the couch this time, babe." Tom closed his arms around her. "I promise an evening you will not forget."

She nestled against his chest, tucking her head against his shoulder. If she were a kitten, she'd purr contentedly. "I can't wait."

"Before we get side-tracked, I'll pick you up at seven. This Saturday," he emphasized.

"I won't forget." She put her hands on his cheeks and pulled his face toward her for a kiss. "And the house should be move-in ready next week."

"Guess we need to start looking at furniture. You have time this weekend?"

"Always. The master bedroom set came today—I hope you like where everything's placed."

"The bed has a mattress?" Tom couldn't resist the smirk.

"Yes. Sheets, too."

"Perfect." Tom teased his fingers across her cheek.

"And I've ordered linens and towels online. Some kitchen items. I'm storing everything in the garage until the work's complete. I'll show you the order confirmation—I probably forgot something essential."

"That's why Walmart's open twenty-four-seven. Or we know several neighbors who can loan us anything we *can't live without.* Don't sweat it." Cassie caught the self-satisfied smile. "Any work underway on the pool deck?"

"It's finished. I hope you like the flooring—we can test our pool if you have time," Cassie offered.

"What time does the contractor close shop for the day?"

Cassie couldn't resist Tom's tone and wink. She glanced at her watch. "About thirty minutes ago. Shall we check it out?"

"Grab your bikini of the day and a towel," He paused for a moment. "Damn, I forgot about the privacy fence. I'll have it installed next week. PG-only swimming until then."

Caryn proposed that she and Andrew host the birthday celebration along with Lauren and Dave. Tom gratefully accepted the offer.

"Only if you hire an event coordinator and caterer. I want you both to enjoy the party, not worry about anything." Tom looked at each of them until they nodded. "And use the debit card I gave you, Caryn."

"You still want Jenna and Daniel there? We can manipulate their naps, so they crash early," Caryn said.

"Cassie would insist they join us if she knew. Don't disappoint my girl." His smile softened the warning. "Speaking of disappointment, I haven't spoken with Cassie's mother. I don't know what else I can say to get a call back."

"I'll call her," Lauren said. "If she knows Trevor's committed to coming, she may do a one-eighty. One will stay with Kelly, the other with Terri." She rolled her eyes. "Whoever gets stuck with Amanda and Allyssa gets a case of wine." She squeezed Tom's arm. "Don't worry about her—she's disappointed Cassie so many times that it won't faze her if only Trevor attends."

Lauren offered her wardrobe to Cassie. "No need to buy a dress. Some of these should actually live in *your* closet. Pick some and try them on—there's a turquoise sequin sheath that suits your personality more than mine. Only worn once."

Lauren pulled the dress from the garment bag and handed it to Cassie.

"How could you only wear this once? It's beautiful!" Cassie held the dress in front of her and looked in the full-length mirror.

"Really not my style—but you, my dear, could definitely pull off this look. I have a pair of Jimmy Choo's I bought for this dress—also only worn once."

Cassie shook her head. "This dress is beautiful—elegant, but fun."

"And it will showcase those long legs. Très chic—and sexy,"

Lauren offered several other dresses, but Cassie tried on the first and waved off the others. "I love this, Lauren."

"Let's see the shoes," Lauren said.

Cassie slipped on the four-inch stilettos and tried to walk without wobbling. "How do you stay upright?"

"Look at the mirror. There's your incentive. Keep them on and practice—be careful not to get a blister."

Cassie hugged Lauren. "You're the best. If I get wobbly, I'll just walk very, very close to Tom."

70

Lauren rapped on the bedroom door and pushed it open. "Rise and shine, birthday girl!"

Cassie shook her head as she sat up and brushed the hair away from her face. She smiled when she noticed the bed tray Lauren held. "What did you do? I forgot it's my birthday."

"Your twenty-first birthday, Cassie! Today, you do nothing but relax. Everything can wait for another day…except your dinner date with my favorite doctor tonight." She set the tray on the bedside table. "Blueberry pancakes, chocolate chip muffins, a mimosa."

"Yum, my stomach's rumbling." Cassie pushed the covers back and got to her feet. She hugged Lauren before going into the bathroom. "Thank you, Lauren, all my favorites."

"Don't take too long—those chocolate chip muffins are calling my name."

Cassie returned, refreshed by splashing cold water on her face, brushing her teeth, and running a brush through her hair.

"Yay, I'm twenty-one," she laughed as she passed a chocolate chip muffin to Lauren. She set the tray on the bed and indicated for Lauren to sit opposite her. Cassie plucked a fresh blueberry from the top of her pancakes and popped it into her mouth. "You're the best, Lauren." She sipped the mimosa and offered it to her aunt. “I thought I’d feel different today—like a ‘grown-up.’ I can legally order a drink in Tampa, and I think renting a car’s possible.”

Lauren chuckled as Cassie enthusiastically tackled her pancakes. “I have more if you’re still hungry.”

“We’ll see after I lick the syrup off this plate. I’ll save the muffin for later so I can appreciate it properly. This was a great surprise!”

“I wanted to be the first to welcome you to official adulthood.” Lauren passed a card to Cassie. “Just a little celebratory cash from Dave and me.”

Cassie first read the card and the comments written by each. “You guys always give me leaky eyes.” When she looked at the check, Cassie started to shake her head. “It’s too much.”

“No, you deserve every penny. Buy something extravagant, pay for books and tuition, pick out something special for your new home. Guilt-free money, Cass. Just spend it on something that makes you happy.”

Cassie reached for her aunt and enveloped her in a hug. “I love you, Lauren. You’re my aunt, my sister, and on occasion, my mother. You helped me shed that protective bubble where Mom tried to stash me.”

“You know, she loves you very much and did everything she could to ensure you stayed innocent and safe. But you grew up and became your own person. You’ve matured so much since you moved to Tampa.” Lauren chuckled as Cassie’s phone rang. “You can let Tom think he wished you a happy birthday first.”

Cassie scrunched her nose at Lauren as she reached for the phone. “Is this my favorite physician?”

“Hope so. Happy birthday, Princess Cassie. I’d have preferred to awaken you with a kiss. Owe you one later.”

“Just one?” Cassie couldn’t contain her giggle. “Maybe one for each birthday I’ve had?”

“And then one to grow on, I suppose.”

“Complaining?”

“Not a bit.”

Tom’s voice sounded so seductive that Cassie wished she could drive to the hospital to collect a few of his kisses. "Do you think you'll get to leave at four this afternoon?"

"I have back-ups for the back-ups. We'll have our special dinner."

"No hint where we're going?"

"Nope, a surprise for my rainbow girl."

Lauren had booked a spa day for both, complete with mani-pedi, facial, massage, hair styling, and make-up.

"I've never felt so pampered," Cassie said.

"Once a month, Cassie. It always lifts my spirits, and I get that guilty pleasure when Dave realizes where I've been. Lights his fire every time."

"Uh-oh, poor Tom!" Cassie closed her eyes, enjoying the foot massage. "Have you brought Dave for a couple's massage?"

"Oh, Cassie, we had one in our suite on the cruise. Absolutely incredible. We didn't leave the room for the rest of the day."

"I do like the sound of that."

Cassie laughed nervously as Lauren helped her dress. "I feel like an imposter. The makeup, the hair, this dress—I can't believe it's me."

"A beautiful 'imposter,' then. Adding the turquoise highlights was brilliant. It's like your hair reflects your dress."

When the doorbell rang, Cassie steadied herself with the headboard to slip into the stilettos. "Say a prayer I don't face-plant."

"You won't." Lauren handed her the small white beaded bag. "Enjoy tonight."

Dave knocked on the bedroom door, and Lauren quickly opened it. "Almost ready. Did you offer Tom something to drink?"

Cassie saw him give Lauren a "Give me a break" look and giggled. "Just a few minutes," she said. "I need to find my balance with these shoes on."

"You look beautiful, Cass. Absolutely breathtaking."

"Thanks, Dave. Please tell Tom I'll be out in a few minutes."

Cassie walked back and forth across the room until she felt steady on her feet. "The downside to wearing flip-flops, sandals, and sneakers every day."

"Just like a runway model," Lauren said. "Ready to make your debut?" When Cassie nodded, Lauren kissed her cheek. "Enjoy, birthday girl."

Tom might have ended up on his rear if he weren't seated at the counter. Cassie caught the periphery of his vision before she completely turned the corner. She always stirred his heart with her beauty, but at that moment, she morphed into an angel, a true princess. He allowed his eyes to rove up and down as she walked toward him. Cassie's eyes glistened, and she clutched the tiny white purse.

He met her halfway. "Happy birthday, Princess. You won't break if I hug you?"

Cassie shook her head. "Please…I need a hug."

Tom quickly complied, kissing her temple as her fresh citrus scent intoxicated him. "You're stunning, babe," he spoke softly into her ear. "I'll enjoy undressing you later." She pressed against him with a soft sigh, cut short by Tom's sweet birthday kiss. "Ready?"

Cassie stepped back and took her time admiring her doctor in a perfectly tailored suit. "You clean up very nicely. My handsome prince."

"At your command, milady. Ready for a twenty-first birthday celebration?"

Tom drove half-way downtown before he suddenly felt the pocket inside his coat. "Damn it."

Cassie watched as he began to check his other pockets. "You're looking for…"

"Wallet."

Cassie heard the aggravation in his voice. "You keep your hand on the wheel, sir. I'll check." She flashed a smile as she patted the other pockets on the jacket, then unsnapped her seatbelt so she could reach both of the pants' pockets.

Tom gently guided her back to her seat. "Buckle up. Don't look out your window. The guy in the car beside us enjoyed your…eh…display a bit too much."

Cassie felt her cheeks flaming. "I forgot about my dress. Did I really give a show?"

Tom maneuvered into a left turn lane, then stopped at a red light. "No comment."

Cassie saw the smirk on his face as he glanced beyond her. "Just keep looking at me, babe."

Cassie patted his arm. "I'm calling BS, Tom."

"For what?"

"You'd let some random guy look at me and do nothing?"

"I did push you back into your seat. You want me to go road rage on the guy?" Tom struggled to keep a straight face.

"Well…you could have at least flipped him off."

"Honey, I guarantee he thought this woman with a gorgeous ass in the air was doing more than checking my pockets."

Cassie covered her face, the mortification suddenly a million times worse. "Just tell me when that car is gone."

Tom did a U-turn with the left turn signal and headed back home. "And now you're in the clear."

Cassie peeked at him through her fingers. "Please say you were teasing me."

Tom's tone sounded robotic. "I was teasing you."

"Tom…"

"Don't worry about it, babe. Our secret, okay?"

Cassie saw the mischievous smile and shrugged. "Whatever you say, doctor."

71

"Shall I wait for you in the car?" Cassie looked at Tom when he stopped his car in the driveway.

"Nope. You stick with me—don't want you reaching for something in the backseat or if you drop your purse on the floor by my seat. I think I left the wallet on the counter—talked with Andrew and Caryn before I left."

He offered both hands to help her stand. "Okay?" he asked as she grabbed his arm until she stopped wobbling in the stilettos. Cassie nodded, and Tom slipped his arm around her waist as they approached the front door. The house looked unusually dark.

"Did they go somewhere?" Cassie asked, blinking her eyes against the dark. "Looks like blackout shades in there."

Tom shrugged. "Maybe they want extra privacy—or everyone crashed early." He slipped the key into the lock and opened the door. Cassie hung back, waiting for Tom to flip the light switch. He kept his hand against her lower back and guided her forward.

Tom held her hand in his as he reached for the switch. Cassie blinked her eyes against the bright light then staggered against Tom when the room exploded with shouts of "Surprise!" and "Happy Birthday!"

"Oh my..." Cassie gazed around the room with wonder. Lauren, Dave, Andrew, Caryn, Terri, Steve, Kelly, John, Amelie, Trevor... Amanda, and her grandmother. She blinked back tears as she looked at Tom. "How?" she croaked.

Tom kissed her quickly before the crowd overwhelmed them. Caryn hugged her and took her other hand. "Welcome, birthday girl."

Caryn led the way to the great room, transformed into an exclusive restaurant. Cassie tried to look everywhere at once. Flowers and candles on each table, glittering white lights overhead, countless greetings with hugs...Cassie's head began to spin. She clutched Tom's arm, and then attempted to contain the tears when her father hugged her.

"I can't believe you're here."

"And in the same room as your mother," Trevor spoke softly into her ear. "Nothing could keep either one of us away from our daughter's twenty-first birthday party." He kissed her cheek. "We'll talk later. Go share some love with your mom."

Tom guided her the few feet to where her mother and grandmother waited.

"Happy birthday, Cassie. You've grown into a beautiful young woman." Her mother whispered in her ear. "And your young man's absolutely delightful."

Cassie suppressed her tears until she hugged her grandmother. Her family had come—all the way to Tampa—for her birthday celebration. Something she had believed existed only in her memories. Lauren handed her tissues.

"You didn't suspect?"

"Never. My heart's beating so fast, my head's spinning."

"Breathe," Tom said quietly. "Let's get you seated." They looked at Caryn, who grinned and pointed to a table set for two in the center of four round tables. Cassie laughed through her tears.

"You surprised me, doctor. I still can't catch my breath. Everyone I love is here..." She looked around. "My love bugs. Where are they?"

"Coming out in a few minutes," Caryn said. "They took a late nap, but they just woke up."

Tom pulled a chair back. "Sit and catch your breath." He accepted two glasses of champagne and handed one to Cassie.

"How did you manage this?"

"Lots of help—everyone in this room loves you." He swiped his finger under her eyes. "My parents send their love—said they will see you soon."

"I…I'm overwhelmed…never dreamed…" She leaned toward him while grasping his hand and tried to pull him closer. Tom stood and moved to her side of the table to claim his kiss. "Thank you is not enough…where did you leave your white horse?"

"At your castle." He kissed her forehead, then returned to his seat as servers went from table-to-table distributing flutes of champagne. "Enjoy every moment tonight. Your turn to shine."

Tom glanced about the room and caught Andrew's eye. His brother nodded, confirming that all the guests had received champagne. He lightly tapped a spoon against the crystal and stood. He caught Cassie's eye and winked before he spoke.

"Thank you for joining us tonight to celebrate an exceptional woman who has captured the love of many new friends. Cassie knew Lauren and Dave before moving to Tampa, but almost a year later she's managed to wiggle her way into the hearts of everyone here. First, let's raise a toast to Cassie on her twenty-first birthday—she's brought sunshine and joy into our lives. Happy birthday, Cass!" He clicked his glass against hers, their eyes locked as they each took a sip. Tom waited until the room quieted and stepped closer to Cassie, guiding her to stand beside him.

"The day we met, you had beautiful pink highlights in your hair. I can see you now, navigating the crowded terminal at the airport looking for Lauren. Remember, I had to convince you I wasn't a serial killer before you'd leave with me?" He heard Cassie's laugh, and the warmth of love filled his body.

"I'm pretty sure I fell in love with you that day, Cassie. I stayed in denial because I didn't want to explain to your aunt, my brother and sister, and ultimately your parents how I fell for my best friend's younger niece, my brother's nanny, and a beautiful girl just beginning her journey as an adult. That's the stuff you read in romance novels—and that's a general 'you' because I haven't read any of those books. But many of you have taken the time to remind me of those facts."

He stopped a moment for a sip of champagne. If her eyes strayed anywhere but his face, she'd see the anticipation on many expressions. "Once I explained that I'm not 'really old'—actually Andrew's *younger brother*—we first became friends. Sometime during the past year, we realized that our friendship had grown into something much more profound. Cassie, you're my best friend, my confidant, my sunshine when it rains, and the woman I want to hold when I come home after a double shift. You've changed my life in the best possible way." Tom touched her cheek when Cassie closed her eyes against the tears that gathered.

When she opened them, he'd taken one knee and grasped both her hands. "Cassie Johnson, I love everything about you. You've claimed a huge chunk of my soul—and you are my future."

Cassie covered her mouth and choked back a sob when Tom reached in his pocket and pulled out a tiny box. "Will you join me on a lifetime of adventures? Will you marry me?"

Tom may have been the only person to hear her response, but there was no mistaking her intent when Cassie launched herself into Tom's arms, crying and laughing at the same time.

Tom gathered her close. "She said, 'Yes.'" Cassie bobbed her head in the affirmative, then Tom slipped the ring on her finger. Cassie placed her hands on his face and pulled him into a kiss that erased any doubts.

Neither appeared aware of the applause, whistles—or anything except the kiss, the love they shared, and the promise of a lifetime of adventures they'd explore together.

EPILOGUE

Cassie gazed at the Gulf as it brightened in the predawn glow. Her wedding day. The two-year engagement sometimes felt like an eternity. Still, the images of her twenty-first birthday celebration and Tom's proposal flowed through her mind as clearly as that night.

Earning her certification in early childhood education opened a vast array of opportunities. But when Tom mentioned he noticed that the hospital's on-site Child Learning Center for employees had several job opportunities, Cassie applied. She'd begun training in May, but after the wedding and honeymoon would accept a managerial position. She loved the prospect of traveling to work with Tom, when their schedules meshed—added opportunities for lunch or break time together.

First, she would cherish every minute of this beautiful dawn. She yearned to share the moment with Tom, but after deciding to include a few customs, they agreed not to see each other after the rehearsal dinner until the sunset wedding ceremony. *Tom even has a suite in a distant section of the resort—shared with Caryn, Andrew, and the twins. Dave and Lauren share my suite...I know Lauren will steady my nerves...but if I could see Tom for one minute.* She needed another of the kisses that snatched her heart. When they parted late last night—early morning—she had to blink away tears.

Lauren scheduled an active day…beginning with a bridesmaid brunch. As Cassie's Matron of Honor, Lauren hosted the meal at a shady outside terrace overlooking the Gulf. Caryn, plus both mothers, Tanya, and Cassie's grandmother comprised the rest of the guests. Then an afternoon at the spa for "the works," as Lauren called it. Mani-pedi, facial, massage, makeup, and hair. Then back to the resort for dressing and finally the ceremony.

Lauren also vowed to run interference with Cassie's parents. Cassie cringed at the thought of her mom and grandmother seated in the first row, and her dad sitting directly behind them with his wife and son. *A disaster waiting to materialize. Though Lauren and Dave monopolized my mom and grandmother at the rehearsal dinner by seating them at their dinner table. Trevor, Tanya, and Tyler joined Tom's parents, along with Andrew and Caryn and the twins. Now, if we can make it through the day with no drama.*

Cassie knew that as Tom's Best Man, Andrew had organized activities for the guys in the wedding party. Those arrangements were *Top Secret*—no doubt to ensure that Tom's and Cassie's paths never crossed.

She glanced up with a grin as Dave stepped on the veranda, carrying a Coke for her and a cappuccino for himself. "May I?"

"Yes! Thank you—exactly what I need." She sipped her cola. "Where are you headed this morning?"

Her honorary brother shrugged. "Heck if I know. Just that we're to meet in about an hour."

Cassie feigned indifference. "Where are you guys meeting?"

She caught the smile that turned into a smirk as Dave chuckled. "That's on a Need-to-Know basis."

Cassie pretended to sulk. "You're no fun, Dave."

"He won't even tell me," Lauren added as she joined them. "Just like he wouldn't say anything about the Bachelor Party. Ignorance is bliss, right, Cass?"

"Um…I guess so?" She cut her eyes toward Dave. "Just so my doctor's not hung over today."

"Are you?" he challenged.

"Didn't drink last night. Alcohol doesn't mix properly with my nerves."

"No need to fret about Dr. Tom," Dave said.

Tom had trouble inserting the cufflinks on his dress shirt. After bouncing them off the dresser twice, swallowing an expletive, he was ready to toss them off the terrace. Andrew walked into his room just in time to avoid any further annoyance.

"Let me give you a hand. Caryn always attaches mine—you're not alone." Andrew clapped Tom's shoulder when he finished. "Anything else? Help with your tie?"

"I've got that. Do you notice the silence?"

"Caryn took Jenna and Daniel down to the bride's dressing area," Andrew said. "Caryn's questioning her decision to include them in the procession."

Tom chuckled. "No matter what happens, they're so adorable no one will mind."

"Just hope neither throws a tantrum. Jenna may keep all the blossoms, and Daniel could decline to give up the rings."

"Andrew, just go with the flow. Mom's on standby just in case something goes sideways." Tom glanced at his watch. "About time to head down?"

Andrew nodded and handed Tom the tuxedo jacket. "The wedding planner has the boutonnières."

"You have the rings?"

Andrew patted his pocket. "I tried to talk Caryn into letting Danny carry some fake rings, but no go. The wedding planner assumes responsibility for them until the ceremony."

Tom fixed his jacket as he glanced in the mirror. "Dave and Lauren's wedding at sea sounds better and better."

"At least you're not having two ceremonies like Caryn and I did."

"Correct. My favorite's the one on campus. The full production at the Cathedral of Notre Dame in Montréal? Over the top," Tom said.

"You know Caryn's parents." Andrew stopped short of rolling his eyes. "But nothing like two precocious grandchildren to capture their attention. Ready to head down? Martin's meeting us in the lobby."

Cassie smoothed the satin sheath over her hips and shifted to peer at herself from all angles. She loved the simplicity of the dress, from the semi-modest v-neck to the crisscrossed thin strips of material on her back—a row of bows to her waist. No veil, but she'd requested the hairstylist to weave thin pastel-hued ribbons in her hair—a surprise for Tom. Her heart always skipped a beat when he called her "His Rainbow Girl." *Tonight he'll find rainbows in my hair.*

She wore an antique pendant necklace from her mom as her "something old." The something new came from Lauren—a pair of beautiful glass beaded flip-flops. She borrowed the exquisite diamond tennis bracelet from Caryn, and the single blue ribbon in her hair added the something blue.

"You look stunning, Cassie," Lauren said.

Cassie held out her trembling hands. "Taking deep breaths…"

Laurent hugged her. "You'll relax the instant you see Tom. Fair warning—don't let your mouth hang open—he looks absolutely smoking in that tux!"

The door opened, and the wedding coordinator brought the bouquet to Cassie. She showed Cassie where to put her hands and how to carry it. "Lovely, dear. Your father's outside. The mothers have taken their seats. And those adorable twins can't wait to do their job."

Lauren and Caryn slipped out the door, and Cassie's father took their place. "My beautiful daughter," he sighed, brushing her cheek. "Ready to greet your prince?"

Cassie nodded, then squeezed the bridge of her nose to quell any tears.

"Just hold on to me," Trevor said, passing a white handkerchief to her. "Thought this might come in handy. You can hide it under your bouquet."

Cassie laughed and took a deep breath. They heard music, and the coordinator opened the door.

"Wait for my cue, then go to the back of the aisle, just like we rehearsed. You'll know to proceed when you hear the opening chords."

The next few moments blended into a blur, Cassie so grateful her father took charge and ushered her on cue. She focused on not stumbling on the turf and only glanced up when they reached the center aisle. There, not a hundred feet away, awaited her doctor, so elegant in his tux, a smile that melted her soul and beckoned her forward. Their eyes locked and Cassie looked only at her groom until the moment came for her father to leave her with Tom.

"Be happy, Cassie. I'm so proud of you." He shifted to Tom. "I wish for you and Cassie a lifetime of happiness and love." He hugged his daughter, then settled her hand in Tom's. "Take care of each other."

Tom stole a kiss before escorting his rainbow girl to the flowered trellis. "Perfect timing," he whispered in her ear. "Almost sunset."

Cassie handed the bouquet to Lauren and clutched both of his hands. "I'm beyond excited." Again, Cassie lost herself in his darkened cinnamon eyes, scarcely hearing the minister's comments. When they exchanged their vows, Cassie felt a cloak of overwhelming love surround them. Tom winked when she guided the ring toward the wrong hand and moved his hands, so the correct finger received the ring.

When the minister declared them husband and wife, Tom didn't wait for permission to kiss his bride. He cupped her face in his hands, murmured his love, and their mouths met in a kiss that began soft and demure…Cassie looped her arms around his neck. Tom lifted her and continued the kiss, deaf to the cheers and ovations from their friends. "I love you, Mrs. Chadwick."

"Love you more, Doctor Chadwick," Cassie said with the hint of a smirk. Tom nodded to the Gulf behind them. The sun slipped past the horizon with a slight burst of fire. Their eyes met, and neither could resist another kiss. Tom shortened it and sighed in her ear.

"Let's get this party underway, Mrs. Chadwick."

Cassie gripped his arm and drew him toward the aisle. "Maybe a hint about our plans after the reception?"

"A night you'll never forget."

She turned to gaze into his eyes. "Sounds perfect to me."

Thank you for taking the time to read Risky Move. If you enjoyed it, please consider telling your friends or posting a review where you purchased the book. Word of mouth is an author's best friend and much appreciated.

Sign up for our newsletter for exclusive pre-release sneak peeks and the upcoming release dates for future books. You can find more information on the following pages. New subscribers have the opportunity to receive a copy of one of my books.

Special thanks to those who have followed this saga from the very beginning. You keep the muse flowing. If you're a first-time reader, I hope you'll read all the interconnected books in these two series. All books are available at Amazon, Apple Books, Barnes & Noble, GooglePlay and Kobo.

Many thanks,

Robyn

Please keep reading for an exclusive excerpt from the next book in the Tampa Suns Hockey Series, ***Timely Assist.***

PREVIEW: TIMELY ASSIST

This is an unedited sample from Timely Assist. It may or may not appear in the published book.

Brilliant silver eyes flashed in irritation as the man's gaze swept over her body. Instead of flashing the million-watt smile that had swept her away, his lips curved in mockery. "I don't know you, sweetheart—believe me, I'd remember if we'd hooked up. Mistaken identity." He turned to walk away, but Shannon Mackenna grabbed his arm.

"Two months ago, just before Christmas. You came into the club—Maloney's—with your teammates to celebrate a win." She lowered her voice. "Y'all invited us to join you. Does that ring a bell?"

"Not even a ping. Everyone knows where the team hangs out after games. Lots of chicks join us...never met you, sweetheart." His eyes slowly raked over her again. "We didn't hook up. You've confused me with someone else."

"You made sure I got home safely," she persisted. "We both were a bit buzzed. I invited you in, we had a snack, then things progressed..."

His expression softened for a moment, then he shook his head. "Sorry, no clue. Can't help you."

"Do you want the pregnancy test results?"

"I don't need to see anything, sweetheart. We didn't meet, never hooked up. You need to look somewhere else for the father."

He lifted her hand off his sleeve and turned as a dark-haired man, leaning against an obviously new sports car, called out to him.

"You coming with us, man—or do you have other plans?" He nodded toward Shannon.

"Give me a sec." He shifted his glance back to Shannon. "If you need money, drive over to the Benz and hook up with one of the football stars. We don't make much playing AHL hockey out here in the burbs."

"I want nothing from you!" Shannon's temper flared. "I'm not asking for money or your name. Absolutely nothing. For some insane reason, I thought you should know you're going to be a father."

"Sorry, you've confused me with someone else." The darkened silver eyes searched her face. "If you don't believe me, call my lawyer." He reached inside his jacket and removed his wallet. He wrote something on a card and held it toward her. "He'll take care of you."

His flippant tone slapped her face like an icy hand. She grabbed the card he offered. "Like I said, I don't want your help. Just know, this child will never know you as his or her father." Shannon spun away before her rage bubbled over. *Not worth it.* She squared her shoulders and held her head high as she walked toward her car. *How dare he... stand there and lie—not even flinch when I told him about the baby. Thinks I'm looking for money? Call his lawyer to "take care of me?" What an ass.* She crumpled the card in her fist, then flicked it aside.

Atlanta's wet January winds whipped through her, but she refused to run to her car. She heard an engine roar and watched a silver SUV race toward the exit. Shannon blasted the heat and leaned back in her seat. Slowly, warmth seeped through her. *How did I think he'd react? One night... maybe magical for me, obviously not for him. No names. No phone numbers. Nothing but... mutual lust? Gone before dawn, no note, nothing.*

She'd pushed the experience to the back of her mind, chalking it up to an alcohol-influenced mistake. She knew what she'd wanted that night. No promises, no strings. Out of sight, out of mind… well, until she missed her second period. Now, with confirmation from the on-campus clinic, reality shoved the memories of that night back in her face.

Not knowing how to contact him, Shannon had waited in the arena's parking lot, hoping she'd recognize her one-night stand. As soon as she saw the golden hunk with the cocky smile, she knew. He even turned on the charm until she pulled him aside to confide her reality.

What did you expect? The Hallelujah Chorus and "Thank you,

Jesus?" Not exactly, but she never imagined he'd dismiss her outright. She had expected skepticism and researched DNA testing, knowing he deserved proof—but to deny the possibility outright and mock her...worse, pity her? What a fool to think he'd want to know—just another jock collecting notches on his hockey stick. Shannon sat up straight and shook the fog from her mind as she shifted her car into drive. *Fine. He will never know the child he just rejected.*

Order from Amazon Apple Books, Barnes & Noble Nook, Google Play, and Kobo

ORDER OF BOOKS

Please note, for your enjoyment* ***This Piece of My Heart, This Piece of My Soul**, and* ***This Piece of Our Being*** *should be read in order.*

All other books are *standalone romances in the* ***Tampa Suns Hockey series.*** *These sweet and sensual full-length novels can be read on their own—no cliffhangers, no cheating and a guaranteed Happily Ever After.*

This Piece of My Heart
Andrew Chadwick and Caryn Stevens' story Part 1

This Piece of My Soul
Andrew and Caryn's story Part 2

This Piece of Our Being
Andrew and Caryn's story Part 3

Clearing the Ice Box Set
Includes: This Piece of My Heart, This Piece of My Soul, This Piece of Our Being)

Healthy Scratch
Lauren Gentry and Dave Martin's story

Risky Move
Tom Chadwick and Cassie Johnson's story

Timely Assist
Cliff Camden and Shannon Mackenna's story

Secret Plays, a Tampa Suns Christmas
(TBD)

THIS PIECE OF MY HEART

CLEARING THE ICE, BOOK ONE

A Hockey Romance

She had her future all planned...until she met him.

Struggling to live up to the high expectations of overprotective parents and a hefty family name, Caryn Stevens only wants one summer of fun before she focuses on finishing her college degree. She knows her destiny—to lead her dad's multi-million dollar business. But that plan changes forever the day she runs into—literally—sexy and single professional hockey player, Andrew Chadwick.

Sparks instantly fly between the two, and Caryn can't resist his charms as she discovers that Andrew has a reputation of winning—both on and off the ice. One of the most eligible singles in Toronto, Andrew could have any woman he wants, and he's got Caryn in sights. But when Caryn's parents disapprove of the match and threaten to disinherit her, and his hockey team trades him to a new city, it may take more than love for the couple to survive this penalty play.

****This Piece of My Heart*** *is the first book in the Clearing the Ice trilogy. ***

THIS PIECE OF MY SOUL

CLEARING THE ICE, BOOK TWO

A Tampa Suns Hockey Romance

Love may not conquer all...

One of pro-hockey's golden couples, Andrew and Caryn Chadwick live in the limelight reserved for elite professional athletes. On their second anniversary, Andrew receives an unexpected contract offer to join the Tampa Suns. As they look forward to a new adventure, neither foresees an event that challenges their love and threatens their marriage.

A sudden and senseless accident threatens Andrew's life and inexplicably drives a wedge between the couple. Shattered by the incident, paralyzed by fear that it could happen again, Caryn finds herself at odds with her husband and unable to provide the support he needs—at the time he is most vulnerable.

****___*This Piece of My Soul*___ *is the second book in the* ___*Clearing the Ice trilogy*___*. For your enjoyment, please read This Piece of My Heart,* ___*free*___ *on major ebook online stores.*

THIS PIECE OF OUR BEING

CLEARING THE ICE, BOOK THREE

A Tampa Suns Hockey Romance

She no longer believes that love conquers all.
He questions his convictions.
Alone, each faces an uncertain future.
However, Fate has other ideas.
Now, they are about to find out if they're stronger together or if this is their last skate.

***This Piece of Our Being is the third and final book in the Clearing the Ice trilogy. It is strongly recommended that you read This Piece of My Heart and This Piece of My Soul, both out now!**

HEALTHY SCRATCH

TAMPA SUNS HOCKEY

A Tampa Suns Hockey Romance

He wants out of the friend zone...she doesn't believe in happily ever after.

Relationships are not in Lauren Gentry's playbook. The only kind she's willing to consider are friends-with-benefits, and even a red-hot and sexy hockey player like Dave Martin isn't going to change that. Right?

When those chocolate brown eyes threaten to melt her defenses, she has to remind herself that demons from her past could rise up at any moment. Which is going to be pretty hard to do, since she loses herself every time they touch.

Dave used to love the benefits that came easily to professional athletes; especially when they were in the form of puck bunnies who only wanted one night. But when he meets the pint-sized girl with bewitching green eyes and sun-streaked auburn hair his outlook suddenly changes.

He wants forever with Lauren. Now he just has to convince her.

Can Lauren risk everything for the man she's secretly been falling for? Or will her past stop her from taking a chance on love?

Healthy Scratch—book one of the ***Tampa Suns Hockey Series****—is a standalone romance whose main characters' lives are intertwined with those introduced in* ***The Clearing the Ice Trilogy.*** *You do not need to read the trilogy to enjoy* ***Healthy Scratch.*** *The book stands on its own,* *promises HEA, and no cliffhangers! To heighten your enjoyment of the Tampa Suns Hockey Series, you may wish to read* ***The Clearing the Ice Trilogy.***

TIMELY ASSIST

TAMPA SUNS HOCKEY

A Tampa Suns Hockey Romance

She has no time for romance.
He's not looking for love.
Neither sees the slap shot life sends their way.

Shannon Mackenna's life revolves around her family, with her four-year-old daughter at the center. She knows firsthand how life can change in an instant. Her parents' unexpected death taught her never to take things for granted.

She lives with no regrets—not even the one-night-stand with a minor league hockey player that resulted in a surprise pregnancy. When she tried to contact him, he denied even recognizing her, and Shannon vowed to raise her daughter on her own.

Cliff "Cam" Camden embraced the bad-boy-athlete persona the moment he was drafted. He enjoyed all the perks and has long stopped counting notches on his hockey stick.

Now, Cam wants more than off-ice conquests. It's time to put his career first. He's not looking for distractions—until he meets the beautiful, sassy owner of Shamrock Fitness. Intrigued by the elusive, private woman, Cam hopes for the chance of something more.

Shannon fears her past has collided with her carefully scripted life. Still, she finds it difficult to resist Cam's devilish smile and brilliant blue eyes. His thoughtfulness outshines his obvious sex appeal, and every time she sees him, her heart skips a beat—and not just because of the way his touch lights up her whole body.

Neither denies the mutual attraction, but Shannon must protect her secret at all costs—even if it means walking away from her happily ever after.

******Timely Assist*** *is a standalone book in the* ***Tampa Suns Hockey*** *series. This sweet and spicy full-length novel can be read on its own—no cliffhanger, no cheating, and a guaranteed Happily Ever After.*

ABOUT THE AUTHOR

Chicago born, honorary Atlanta native, Parisienne at heart. Proud 60's Flower Child. "Fearless" barrier-breaker for female sports journalists and minor league "batpersons." While at UGA, she scored a PR internship with an NHL team during its first season. Interviewed future MLB and NHL Hall of Fame members, published in a variety of print media. Wife, mom, PR professional, and finally, 35 years later, published author. Two Westie grand-dogs pretty much run the household.

As do many writers, Robyn chooses to write using a pseudonym—hers is a combination of her sons' names, a contribution from her youngest nephew.

Robyn loves to hear from fellow sports fans and readers who enjoy sports romances. Get the latest news from her newsletter. Connect on Facebook, Twitter, BookBub, or her website. Join Robyn's Readers in the Center Ice Lounge Facebook Group, where you can grab a drink and chat for a while—books, hockey, sports, binge-worthy shows, hot guys, favorite athletes...did we say "hot guys?" Members receive exclusive contests, giveaways, and sneak peeks about future books.

All books are available at Amazon, Apple Books, Barnes & Noble, GooglePlay and Kobo.

Made in the USA
Monee, IL
04 November 2026

67380842R00223